MR Spectroscopy of the Brain

Editor

LARA A. BRANDÃO

NEUROIMAGING CLINICS OF NORTH AMERICA

www.neuroimaging.theclinics.com

Consulting Editor
SURESH K. MUKHERJI

August 2013 • Volume 23 • Number 3

ELSEVIER

1600 John F. Kennedy Boulevard • Suite 1800 • Philadelphia, Pennsylvania, 19103-2899

http://www.theclinics.com

NEUROIMAGING CLINICS OF NORTH AMERICA Volume 23, Number 3
August 2013 ISSN 1052-5149, ISBN 13: 978-0-323-18610-0

Editor: Pamela M. Hetherington
Developmental Editor: Teia Stone

Neuroimaging Clinics of North America (ISSN 1052-5149) is published quarterly by Elsevier Inc., 360 Park Avenue South, New York, NY 10010-1710. Months of issue are February, May, August, and November. Business and editorial offices: 1600 John F. Kennedy Blvd., Suite 1800, Philadelphia, PA 19103-2899. Business and editorial offices: 6277 Sea Harbor Drive, Orlando, FL 32887-4800. Periodicals postage paid at New York, NY, and additional mailing offices. Subscription prices are USD 342 per year for US individuals, USD 489 per year for US institutions, USD 172 per year for US students and residents, USD 396 per year for Canadian individuals, USD 612 per year for Canadian institutions, USD 502 per year for international individuals, USD 612 per year for international institutions and USD 246 per year for Canadian and foreign students and residents. To receive student/resident rate, orders must be accompanied by name of affiliated institution, date of term, and the *signature* of program/residency coordinator on institution letterhead. Orders will be billed at individual rate until proof of status is received. Foreign air speed delivery is included in all *Clinics* subscription prices. All prices are subject to change without notice. POSTMASTER: Send address changes to *Neuroimaging Clinics of North America*, Elsevier Health Sciences Division, Subscription Customer Service, 3251 Riverport Lane, Maryland Heights, MO 63043. Telephone: 1-800-654-2452 (U.S. and Canada); 314-447-8871 (outside U.S. and Canada). Fax: 314-447-8029. E-mail: journalscustomerservice-usa@elsevier.com (for print support); journalsonlinesupport-usa@elsevier.com (for online support).

Reprints. For copies of 100 or more of articles in this publication, please contact the Commercial Reprints Department, Elsevier Inc., 360 Park Avenue South, New York, NY 10010-1710. Tel.: 212-633-3812; Fax: 212-462-1935; E-mail: reprints@elsevier.com.

Neuroimaging Clinics of North America is covered by *Excerpta Medical/EMBASE*, the RSNA Index of Imaging Literature, *MEDLINE/PubMed (Index Medicus)*, MEDLINE/MEDLARS, SciSearch, Research Alert, and Neuroscience Citation Index.

Printed and bound by CPI Group (UK) Ltd, Croydon, CR0 4YY

Transferred to digital print 2013

PROGRAM OBJECTIVE

The goal of Neuroimaging Clinics of North America is to keep practicing radiologists and radiology residents up to date with current clinical practice in radiology by providing timely articles reviewing the state of the art in patient care.

TARGET AUDIENCE

Practicing radiologists, radiology residents, and other healthcare professionals who utilize neuroimaging findings to provide patient care.

LEARNING OBJECTIVES

Upon completion of this activity, participants will be able to:
1. Review the use of magnetic resonance spectroscopy in multiple sclerosis and related disorders.
2. Discuss techniques for the neuroradiologist in the use of proton magnetic resonance spectroscopy.
3. Recognize the use of magnetic resonance spectroscopy in the evaluation of epilepsy.

ACCREDITATION

The Elsevier Office of Continuing Medical Education (EOCME) is accredited by the Accreditation Council for Continuing Medical Education (ACCME) to provide continuing medical education for physicians.

The EOCME designates this enduring material for a maximum of 15 *AMA PRA Category 1 Credit*(s) ™. Physicians should claim only the credit commensurate with the extent of their participation in the activity.

All other health care professionals requesting continuing education credit for this enduring material will be issued a certificate of participation.

DISCLOSURE OF CONFLICTS OF INTEREST

The EOCME assesses conflict of interest with its instructors, faculty, planners, and other individuals who are in a position to control the content of CME activities. All relevant conflicts of interest that are identified are thoroughly vetted by EOCME for fair balance, scientific objectivity, and patient care recommendations. EOCME is committed to providing its learners with CME activities that promote improvements or quality in healthcare and not a specific proprietary business or a commercial interest.

The planning committee, staff, authors and editors listed below have identified no financial relationships or relationships to products or devices they or their spouse/life partner have with commercial interest related to the content of this CME activity:
Julio Alonso, PhD; Debora Bertholdo, MD; Roberta Biancheri, MD, PhD; Lara A. Brandão, MD; Cristiana Caires, MD; Mauricio Castillo, MD, FACR; Kim Cecil, PhD; Rakesh Gupta, MD; Pamela Hetherington; Brynne Hunter; Kamlesh J. Jobanputra, MD; Jason Johnson, MD; Kejal Kantarci, MD; Sandy Lavery; Jill McNair; Suresh K. Mukherji, MD; Lindsay Parnell; Otto Rapalino, MD; Eva-Maria Ratai, PhD; Sandra Rincon, MD; Andrea Rossi, MD; Alex Rovira Cannelas, MD; Mariasavina Severino, MD; Karthikeyan Subramaniam; Ron Thibert, DO; Arvemas Watcharakorn, MD; Abhishek Yadav, PhD; Tina Young Poussaint, MD.

The planning committee, staff, authors and editors listed below have identified financial relationships or relationships to products or devices they or their spouse/life partner have with commercial interest related to the content of this CME activity:
Meng Law, MD is on speaker's bureau for Toshiba America Medical, iCAD, Inc., and Bracco; is a consultant/advisor for Bayer Healthcare Pharmaceuticals; has stock ownership in Prism Clinical Imaging; and has research grants with National Institutes of Health and Bayer Healthcare Pharmaceuticals.

UNAPPROVED/OFF-LABEL USE DISCLOSURE

The EOCME requires CME faculty to disclose to the participants:
1. When products or procedures being discussed are off-label, unlabelled, experimental, and/or investigational (not US Food and Drug Administration (FDA) approved); and
2. Any limitations on the information presented, such as data that are preliminary or that represent ongoing research, interim analyses, and/or unsupported opinions. Faculty may discuss information about pharmaceutical agents that is outside of FDA-approved labelling. This information is intended solely for CME and is not intended to promote off-label use of these medications. If you have any questions, contact the medical affairs department of the manufacturer for the most recent prescribing information.

TO ENROLL

To enroll in the *Neuroimaging Clinics of North America* Continuing Medical Education program, call customer service at 1-800-654-2452 or sign up online at http://www.theclinics.com/home/cme. The CME program is available to subscribers for an additional annual fee of $212 USD.

METHOD OF PARTICIPATION

In order to claim credit, participants must complete the following:
1. Complete enrolment as indicated above.
2. Read the activity.
3. Complete the CME Test and Evaluation. Participants must achieve a score of 70% on the test. All CME Tests and Evaluations must be completed online.

CME INQUIRIES/SPECIAL NEEDS

For all CME inquiries or special needs, please contact elsevierCME@elsevier.com.

NEUROIMAGING CLINICS OF NORTH AMERICA

DOWNLOAD Free App!

Review Articles
THE CLINICS

NOW AVAILABLE FOR YOUR iPhone and iPad

Contributors

CONSULTING EDITOR

SURESH K. MUKHERJI, MD, FACR
Department of Radiology, University of
Michigan Health System, Ann Arbor, Michigan

EDITOR

LARA A. BRANDÃO, MD
Neurorradiologist, Clínica IRM - Ressonância
Magnética; Chief of Neuroradiology, Clínica
Felippe Mattoso, Barra da Tijuca,
Rio de Janeiro, Brazil

AUTHORS

JULI ALONSO, PhD
Department of Radiology, Magnetic
Resonance Unit (IDI), Vall d'Hebron Research
Institute, Vall d'Hebron University Hospital,
Barcelona, Spain

DÉBORA BERTHOLDO, MD
Research Fellow, University of North Carolina
at Chapel Hill, Chapel Hill, North Carolina

ROBERTA BIANCHERI, MD, PhD
Infantile Neuropsychiatry Unit, Istituto Giannina
Gaslini, Genoa, Italy

LARA A. BRANDÃO, MD
Neurorradiologist, Clínica IRM - Ressonância
Magnética; Chief of Neuroradiology, Clínica
Felippe Mattoso, Barra da Tijuca,
Rio de Janeiro, Brazil

CRISTIANA CAIRES, MD
Neuroradiologist, Clínica Felippe Mattoso,
Barra da Tijuca, Rio de Janeiro, Brazil

PAUL A. CARUSO, MD
Director of Pediatric Neuroimaging, Division of
Neuroradiology, Department of Radiology,
Massachusetts General Hospital, Harvard
Medical School, Boston, Massachusetts

MAURICIO CASTILLO, MD
Professor of Radiology; Chief of
Neuroradiology, Division of Neuroradiology,
Department of Radiology, University of North
Carolina School of Medicine, Chapel Hill,
North Carolina

KIM M. CECIL, PhD
Department of Radiology, Pediatrics,
Neuroscience and Environmental Health,
Cincinnati Children's Hospital Medical Center,
Cincinnati, Ohio

RAKESH K. GUPTA, MD
Professor, MR Section, Department of
Radiodiagnosis, Sanjay Gandhi Post Graduate
Institute of Medical Sciences, Lucknow,
Uttar Pradesh, India

KAMLESH J. JOBANPUTRA, MD
Resident, MR Section, Department of
Radiodiagnosis, Sanjay Gandhi Postgraduate
Institute of Medical Sciences, Lucknow,
Uttar Pradesh, India

JASON JOHNSON, MD
Division of Neuroradiology, Department of
Radiology, Massachusetts General Hospital,
Harvard Medical School, Boston,
Massachusetts

KEJAL KANTARCI, MD, MS
Associate Professor of Radiology, Division of Neuroradiology, Department of Radiology, Mayo Clinic, Rochester, Minnesota

TINA YOUNG POUSSAINT, MD
Professor of Radiology; Attending Neuroradiologist, Division of Neuroradiology, Department of Radiology, Boston Children's Hospital, Harvard Medical School, Boston, Massachusetts

OTTO RAPALINO
Division of Neuroradiology, Department of Radiology, Massachusetts General Hospital, Harvard Medical School, Boston, Massachusetts

EVA-MARIA RATAI, PhD
Division of Neuroradiology, Department of Radiology; Athinoula A. Martinos Center for Biomedical Imaging, Harvard Medical School, Massachusetts General Hospital, Boston, Massachusetts

SANDRA RINCON
Division of Neuroradiology, Department of Radiology, Massachusetts General Hospital, Harvard Medical School, Boston, Massachusetts

ANDREA ROSSI, MD
Pediatric Neuroradiology Unit, Istituto Giannina Gaslini, Genoa, Italy

ÀLEX ROVIRA, MD
Department of Radiology, Magnetic Resonance Unit (IDI), Vall d'Hebron Research Institute, Vall d'Hebron University Hospital, Barcelona, Spain

RON THIBERT, MD
Epilepsy Service, Department of Neurology, Massachusetts General Hospital, Harvard Medical School, Boston, Massachusetts

ARVEMAS WATCHARAKORN, MD
Research Fellow, University of North Carolina at Chapel Hill, Chapel Hill, North Carolina

ABHISHEK YADAV, PhD
Postdoctoral Fellow, MR Section, Department of Radiodiagnosis, Sanjay Gandhi Postgraduate Institute of Medical Sciences, Lucknow, Uttar Pradesh, India

Contents

Brain Proton Magnetic Resonance Spectroscopy: Introduction and Overview

Débora Bertholdo, Arvemas Watcharakorn, and Mauricio Castillo

> Magnetic resonance (MR) spectroscopy offers a noninvasive means of assessing in-vivo brain metabolites that shed light on cellular concentrations, cell function and dysfunction, cellular energetics, presence of ischemia, and presence of necrosis, among others. Studies obtained at higher field strengths are evolving toward sampling of smaller tissue volumes, greater signal-to-noise ratio, and higher metabolic spatial resolution. This article discusses the usefulness, from the clinical standpoint, of MR spectroscopy in various disorders. However, to be valid and significant the results of MR spectroscopy should always be correlated with their imaging counterparts.

Proton Magnetic Resonance Spectroscopy: Technique for the Neuroradiologist

Kim M. Cecil

> Magnetic resonance spectroscopy (MRS) provides information on neuronal and axonal viability, energetics of cellular structures, and status of cellular membranes. Proton MRS appeals to clinicians and scientists because its application in the clinical setting can increase the specificity of MR imaging. The objective of this article is to provide descriptive concepts of the technique and its application in vivo for a variety of patient populations. When appropriately incorporating MRS into the neuroradiologic evaluation, this technique produces relevant information to radiologists and clinicians for their understanding of adult and pediatric neurologically based disease processes.

Magnetic Resonance Spectroscopy in Common Dementias

Kejal Kantarci

> Neurodegenerative dementias are characterized by elevated myoinositol and decreased N-acetylaspartate (NAA) levels. The increase in myoinositol seems to precede decreasing NAA levels in Alzheimer's diseases. NAA/myo-inositol ratio in the posterior cingulate gyri decreases with increasing burden of Alzheimer's disease pathologic conditions. Proton magnetic resonance spectroscopy (^{1}H MRS) is sensitive to the pathophysiologic processes associated with the risk of dementia in patients with mild cognitive impairment. Although significant progress has been made in improving the acquisition and analysis techniques in ^{1}H MRS, translation of these technical developments to clinical practice have not been effective because of the lack of standardization for multisite applications and normative data and an insufficient understanding of the pathologic basis of ^{1}H MRS metabolite changes.

Contents

Magnetic resonance spectroscopy (MRS) is indicated in the imaging protocol of the patient with epilepsy to screen for metabolic derangements such as inborn errors of metabolism and to characterize masses that may be equivocal on conventional magnetic resonance imaging for dysplasia versus neoplasia. Single-voxel MRS with echo time of 35 milliseconds may be used for this purpose as a quick screening tool in the epilepsy imaging protocol. MRS is useful in the evaluation of both focal and generalized epilepsy.

Magnetic resonance spectroscopy (MRS) is a powerful clinical tool for investigating the metabolic characteristics of neurologic diseases. Proton (^{1}H)-MRS is the most commonly used and widely available method. In this article, a brief introduction regarding technical issues of ^{1}H-MRS applied to the study of metabolic diseases is followed by a description of findings in some of the most common entities in this large, heterogeneous group of neurologic disorders. The aim was to provide a focused representation of the most common applications of ^{1}H-MRS to metabolic disorders in a routine clinical setting.

Hypoxic ischemic injuries are a very common clinical situation in the pediatric population. This article focuses on the metabolic signature of hypoxic ischemic injuries and metabolic indicators of prognosis.

Proton magnetic resonance spectroscopy (^{1}H-MRS) is an unconventional technique that allows noninvasive characterization of metabolic abnormalities in the central nervous system. ^{1}H-MRS provides important insights into the chemical-pathologic changes that occur in patients with multiple sclerosis (MS). In this review article we present the main brain and spinal cord ^{1}H-MRS features in MS, their diagnostic value in differentiating pseudotumoral demyelinating lesions from primary brain tumors, and their relationship with clinical variables. Last, some data related to the use of ^{1}H-MRS in therapeutic trials is presented.

Infection of the central nervous system can be life-threatening and hence requires early diagnostic support for its optimal management. Routine definitive laboratory diagnostic tests can be time-consuming and delay definitive therapy. Noninvasive imaging modalities have established themselves in the diagnosis of various neurologic diseases. In this article, a pragmatic review of the current role of magnetic resonance spectroscopy in the diagnosis and management of intracranial infections is addressed.

Pediatric brain tumors are the most common solid tumor of childhood. This article focuses on the metabolic signature of common pediatric brain tumors using MR spectroscopic analyses.

Proton magnetic resonance spectroscopy (H-MRS) may be helpful in suggesting tumor histology and tumor grade and may better define tumor extension and the ideal site for biopsy compared with conventional magnetic resonance (MR) imaging. A multifunctional approach with diffusion-weighted imaging, perfusion-weighted imaging, and permeability maps, along with H-MRS, may enhance the accuracy of the diagnosis and characterization of brain tumors and estimation of therapeutic response. Integration of advanced imaging techniques with conventional MR imaging and the clinical history help to improve the accuracy, sensitivity, and specificity in differentiating tumors and nonneoplastic lesions.

Foreword

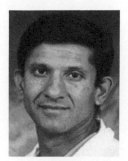

Suresh K. Mukherji, MD, FACR
Consulting Editor

It is my distinct pleasure to thank Lara Brandao for editing this edition of *Neuroimaging Clinics*. Dr Brandao had focused this edition on MR spectroscopy (MRS). One can argue that MRS was one of the first "molecular imaging" techniques that was introduced to clinical imaging. MRS has lost some "STEAM" (pun intended!) in the United States due to the payment challenges; however, it is still a very robust technique that is gaining greater worldwide acceptance.

This edition also highlights the tremendous talent of individuals outside the usual confines of the United States and Europe. With her expertise and vast experience, Dr Brandao is the perfect person to write this comprehensive and state-of-art edition. She has assembled an outstanding group of contributors from all corners of the world and I personally thank all of them for their efforts.

I also want to personally thank Lara. She is a bit of a "Superwoman"(!) to me. I am still not quite sure how she accomplishes everything she does with all of her other personal and professional obligations and completes her tasks with such quality. I guess my wife was right when she said, "if you want something done right, give it to a woman!" Thank you very much, Lara!!

Suresh K. Mukherji, MD, FACR
Department of Radiology
University of Michigan Health System
1500 East Medical Center
Ann Arbor, MI 48109-0030, USA

E-mail address:
mukherji@med.umich.edu

Preface

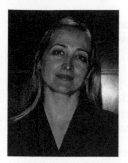

Lara A. Brandão, MD
Editor

This issue of *Neuroimaging Clinics* focuses on the main technical aspects as well as the main clinical applications of magnetic resonance spectroscopy (MRS) of the brain.

In the beginning of this issue the readers are provided with two articles describing the principles behind proton MRS in a practical fashion. Technical concerns, such as chemical shift, short TE versus long TE, single-voxel spectroscopy (SV-MRS) versus multivoxel spectroscopy (MV-MRS), benefits and challenges at fields 3T and higher, signal-to-noise ratio, spectral dispersion, shimming, water and lipid suppression, and localization methods are discussed. The main metabolites and their meaning are also described. In addition, postprocessing, interpretation, spectral changes related to normal development and normal aging, and protocols are addressed.

The remaining topics were selected to provide an overview of the current clinical applications of MRS in the brain, including hypoxic encephalopathy, epilepsy, metabolic disorders, infections, multiple sclerosis, dementia, and brain tumors in children and adults.

MRS is useful in estimating the prognosis of patients presenting with hypoxic encephalopathy, suggesting the etiology of chronic seizures in children, distinguishing among different metabolic disorders, and better characterizing brain infections and dementia disorders. Concerning MS, MRS may help characterize acute and chronic plaques as well as explain the clinical-radiologic discrepancy of the disease by demonstrating normal-appearing white matter compromise. MRS is also a very useful tool in neuro-oncology. In this setting it may help suggest tumor histology by demonstrating typical spectral patterns in some tumors. Differentiation between primary and secondary neoplasms may be possible by demonstrating tumor cell infiltration (high choline) into the peritumoral edema, consistent with the diagnosis of high-grade glioma. Significant elevation of the choline peak, along with reduction of the NAA, Cr, and mI peaks may help indicate high-grade versus low-grade glioma, which is crucial for therapeutic planning.

By demonstrating the area of highest tumor cell density (highest choline peak), multivoxel MRS may help indicate the ideal site for biopsy. Also, tumor extent may be better estimated by MV-MRS than by conventional MRI. Finally, after treatment, multivoxel MRS may help to distinguish tumor recurrence from radiation-induced changes.

Another important clinical application of MRS addressed in this issue is the differentiation between focal brain lesions that may simulate brain tumors, including infarcts, infection, and tumefactive demyelinating plaques. From the data presently available, one may conclude that MRS has numerous clinical applications.

In this issue we intend to share our experience with performing and interpreting MRS for more than 12 years, as well as to offer the readers an

Neuroimag Clin N Am 23 (2013) xiii–xiv
http://dx.doi.org/10.1016/j.nic.2013.03.006

extensive literature review. The articles were written by experienced radiologists and address relevant topics of daily practice.

I would like to sincerely thank all of the authors of this issue for their invaluable contributions. I wish to express my gratitude to the consulting editor, Dr Suresh Mukherjy, for the opportunity to lead this project. I would also like to thank the series editors, Pamela Hetherington and Nicole Congleton, for their guidance and support during the preparation of this work. Thanks also to my friend and partner, Alice Brandão, MD, for helping me with patient reports while I was involved in researching and writing. Thanks also to my friend, Anderson Sales, for his tremendous help with the literature searching.

I would like to dedicate this issue to my husband, Sergio, and my daughters, Carolina (8 years) and Camila (4 years), for their support, love, incentive, and understanding during the process of preparing this work.

To my parents, Adelmo and Maria Helena, for always instilling integrity and hard work in all aspects of my life!

Lara A. Brandão, MD
Clínica Felippe Mattoso
Av. Das Américas 700, Sala 320
Barra da Tijuca, Rio de Janeiro 22640-100, Brazil

Clínica IRM - Ressonância Magnética
Rua Capitão Salomão, 44-Humaitá
Rio de Janeiro 22271-040, Brazil

E-mail address:
larabrandao.rad@terra.com.br

Brain Proton Magnetic Resonance Spectroscopy
Introduction and Overview

Débora Bertholdo, MD, Arvemas Watcharakorn, MD,
Mauricio Castillo, MD*

KEYWORDS

- ^{1}H Magnetic resonance spectroscopy • Stimulated echo acquisition mode • Brain metabolites
- Brain tumors

KEY POINTS

- Magnetic resonance (MR) proton spectroscopy is a technique which mainly provides biological information regarding cellularity, energy, neuron viability, necrosis and ischemia.
- MR spectroscopy is ideal to assess the limits of brain tumors when planning surgery.
- MR spectroscopy allows identification of some metabolic disorders guiding further laboratory analysis.

INTRODUCTION

Magnetic resonance (MR) spectroscopy is an analytical method used in chemistry that enables the identification and quantification of metabolites in samples. It differs from conventional MR imaging in that spectra provide physiologic and chemical information instead of anatomy.

MR spectroscopy and MR imaging have their origin in nuclear magnetic resonance (NMR). NMR was first described in 1946 simultaneously by the Nobel Prize winners Edward Purcell, from Harvard University, and Felix Bloch, from Stanford University. At that time, NMR was used only by physicists for purposes of determining the nuclear magnetic moments of nuclei. It was only in the mid 1970s that NMR started to be used in vivo, after Lauterbur, Mansfield, and Grannell introduced gradient into the magnetic field, enabling them to determine the location of the emitted signal and to reproduce it on an image. In vivo NMR was renamed MR imaging because the term "nuclear" had been consistently (but erroneously) associated with nuclear medicine.

For the same reason, NMR spectroscopy used in vivo is now named MR spectroscopy. During the 1980s, the first MR imaging medical scanners became available for clinical use. Since then improvements have been made, especially in relation to higher field strengths.

MR spectra may be obtained from different nuclei. Protons (^{1}H) are the nuclei most used for clinical applications in the human brain, mainly because of their high sensitivity and abundance. The proton MR spectrum is altered in almost all neurologic disorders. In some diseases, proton MR spectroscopy (^{1}H-MRS) changes are very subtle and are not reliable without a statistical comparison between groups of patients. In these cases, ^{1}H-MRS is usually used for research. In clinical practice, ^{1}H-MRS is mostly used for more detailed analysis of primary and secondary brain tumors and metabolic diseases.

This article discusses the physical basis of ^{1}H-MRS, emphasizing the different techniques, the normal spectra in adults and children, its clinical applications, and the significance of brain

University of North Carolina at Chapel Hill, Room 3326 Old Infirmary Building, Manning Drive, Chapel Hill, NC 27599, USA
* Corresponding author.
E-mail address: castillo@med.unc.edu

Neuroimag Clin N Am 23 (2013) 359–380
http://dx.doi.org/10.1016/j.nic.2012.10.002
1052-5149/13/$ – see front matter © 2013 Elsevier Inc. All rights reserved.

metabolites under both normal and abnormal conditions, particularly in the evaluation of brain tumors.

PHYSICAL BASIS

Many nuclei may be used to obtain MR spectra, including phosphorus (^{31}P), fluorine (^{19}F), carbon (^{13}C), and sodium (^{23}Na). The ones mostly used for clinical MR spectroscopy are protons (^{1}H). The brain is ideally imaged with ^{1}H-MRS because of its near lack of motion (this prevents MR spectroscopy from being used in the abdomen and thorax without very sophisticated motion-reduction techniques). The hydrogen nucleus is abundant in human tissues. ^{1}H-MRS requires only standard radiofrequency (RF) coils and a dedicated software package. For nonproton MR spectroscopy, RF coils tuned to the Larmor frequency of other nuclei, matching preamplifiers, hybrids, and a broadband power amplifier are needed.

Different field strengths are used for conventional clinical MR imaging, ranging from 0.2 to 3 T. Because the main objective of ^{1}H-MRS is to detect weak signals from metabolites, a minimum of 1.5 T is advised. Units with higher field strength have the advantage of higher signal-to-noise ratio (SNR), better resolution, and shorter acquisition times, making the technique useful in sick patients and others who cannot hold still for long periods of time.

^{1}H-MRS is based on the chemical-shift properties of the atom. When a tissue is exposed to an external magnetic field, its nuclei will resonate at a frequency (f) that is given by the Larmor equation:

$$f = \gamma B_0$$

Because the gyromagnetic ratio (γ) is a constant of each nuclear species, the spin frequencies of certain nuclei (f) depend on the external magnetic field (B_0) and the local microenvironment. The electric shell interactions of these nuclei with the surrounding molecules cause a change in the local magnetic field, leading to a change on the spin frequency of the atom (a phenomenon called chemical shift). The value of this difference in resonance frequency gives information about the molecular group carrying ^{1}H and is expressed in parts per million (ppm). The chemical-shift position of a nucleus is ideally expressed in ppm because it is independent of the field strength (choline, for example, will be positioned at 3.22 ppm at 1.5 or 7 T). The MR spectrum is represented by the x axis that corresponds to the metabolite frequency in ppm according to the chemical shift, and the y axis that corresponds to the peak amplitude.

Some metabolites such as lactate have doublets, triplets, or multiplets instead of single peaks. These peaks are broken down into more complex peaks and are explained by J-coupling, also named spin-spin coupling. The J-coupling phenomenon occurs when the molecular structure of a metabolite is such that protons are found in different atomic groups (eg, CH_3- and CH_2-). These groups have slightly different local magnetic fields, thus each ^{1}H resonates at a frequency that is characteristic of its position in the molecule, resulting in a multiplet peak.

Techniques

The ^{1}H-MRS acquisition usually starts with anatomic images, which are used to select a volume of interest (VOI), where the spectrum will be acquired. For the spectrum acquisition, different techniques may be used, including single-voxel and multi-voxel imaging using both long and short echo times (TE). Each technique has advantages and disadvantages, and choosing the right one for a specific purpose is important in improving the quality of the results.

Single-voxel spectroscopy

In single-voxel spectroscopy (SVS) the signal is obtained from a voxel previously selected. This voxel is acquired from a combination of slice-selective excitations in 3 dimensions in space, achieved when an RF pulse is applied while a field gradient is switched on. It results in 3 orthogonal planes whose intersection corresponds to the VOI (Fig. 1).

One of two techniques is typically used for acquisition of SVS ^{1}H-MRS spectra: pointed-resolved spectroscopy (PRESS) and stimulated

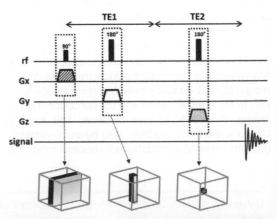

Fig. 1. Slice selection in single-voxel spectroscopy. The 3 radiofrequency pulses (rf) select 3 orthogonal planes (Gz, Gy, and Gx). Their intersection corresponds to the volume of interest (VOI). TE, echo time.

echo acquisition mode (STEAM). The most used SVS technique is PRESS. In the PRESS sequence, the spectrum is acquired using 1 90° pulse followed by 2 180° pulses, each of which is applied at the same time as a different field gradient. Thus, the signal emitted by the VOI is a spin echo. The first 180° pulse is applied after time TE1/2 from the first pulse (90° pulse), and the second 180° is applied after time TE1/2 + TE. The signal occurs after a time 2TE (Fig. 2). To restrict the acquired sign to the selected VOI, spoiler gradients are needed. Spoiler gradients dephase the nuclei outside the VOI and reduce their signal.

STEAM is the second most commonly used SVS technique. In this sequence all 3 pulses applied are 90° pulses. As in PRESS, they are all simultaneous with different field gradients. After time TE1/2 from the first pulse, a second 90° pulse is applied. The time elapsed between the second and the third pulse is conventionally called mixing time (MT), and is shorter than TE. The signal is finally achieved after time TE + MT from the first pulse (see Fig. 2). Thus, the total time for the STEAM technique is shorter than that for PRESS. Spoiler gradients are also needed to reduce signal from regions outside the VOI.

The STEAM sequence uses only 90° pulses, which results in 50% lower SNR than for PRESS. As described, the PRESS sequence is acquired using 2 pulses of 180°. The use of these 180° pulses results in a less optimal VOI profile and leads to a higher SNR. However, because the length of 180° pulses is longer than 90°, PRESS cannot be achieved with a very short TE. Another disadvantage of the PRESS sequence is the larger chemical-shift displacement artifact, which is described later in this article. Therefore, STEAM is usually the modality of choice when a short TE and precise volume selection is needed. Nevertheless, PRESS is the most used SVS technique because it doubles the SNR, which is an important factor that leads to better spectral quality.

Magnetic resonance spectroscopy imaging

MR spectroscopy imaging, also called spectroscopic imaging or chemical-shift imaging, is a multivoxel technique. The main objective of MR spectroscopy imaging is to simultaneously acquire many voxels and a spatial distribution of the metabolites within a single sequence. Thus, this ^{1}H-MRS technique uses phase-encoding gradients to encode spatial information after the RF pulses and the gradient of slice selection.

MR spectroscopy imaging is acquired using only slice selection and phase-encoding gradients, besides the spoiler gradients. A frequency encoding gradient is not applied. Thus, instead of the anatomic information given by the conventional MR imaging signal, the ^{1}H-MRS signal results in a spectrum of metabolites with different frequencies (information acquired from chemical-shift properties of each metabolite).

The same sequences used for SVS are used for the signal acquisition in MR spectroscopy imaging (STEAM or PRESS). The main difference between MR spectroscopy imaging and SVS is that, after the RF pulse, phase-encoding gradients are used in 1, 2, or 3 dimensions (1D, 2D, or 3D) to sample the k-space (Fig. 3). In a 1D sequence the phase encoding has a single direction, in 2D it has 2 orthogonal directions, and in 3D it has 3 orthogonal directions.

The result of a 2D MR spectroscopy imaging is a matrix, called a spectroscopy grid. The size of this grid corresponds to the field of view (FOV) previously determined. In the 3D sequence, many grids are acquired within one FOV. The number of partitions (or voxels) of the grids is directly proportional to the number of phase-encoding steps. The spatial resolution is also proportional to the number of voxels in

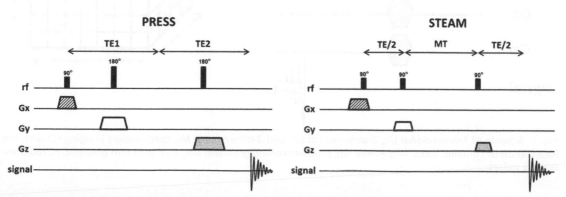

Fig. 2. Schemes of PRESS and STEAM sequences. To simplify, only slice selection gradients are shown. Gz, Gy, and Gx, orthogonal planes; MT, mixing time; rf, radiofrequency pulses; TE, echo time.

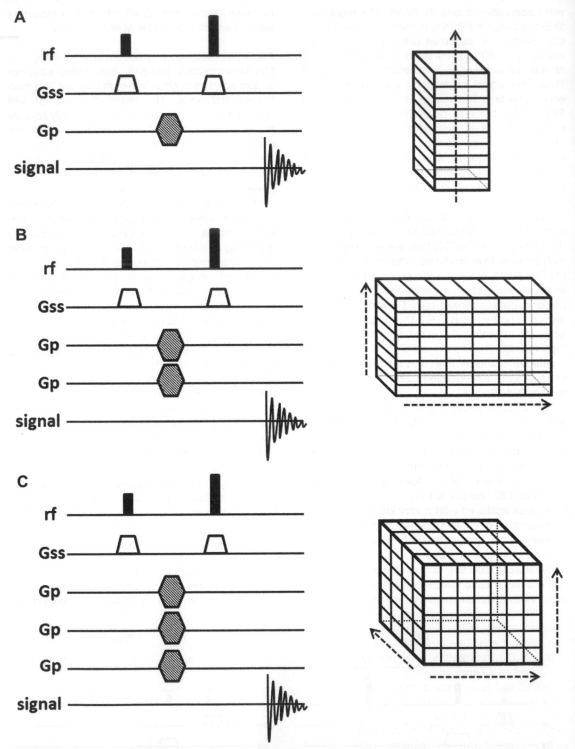

Fig. 3. Scheme of 1-dimensional (*A*), 2-dimensional (*B*), and 3-dimensional MR spectroscopy imaging (*C*) with the localization of columns, slices, and voxels. Gp, phase-encoding gradient; Gss, slice-selection gradient; rf, radiofrequency pulses.

a determined FOV (more voxels give a better spatial resolution). However, for a larger number of voxels, more phase-encoding steps are needed, and this implies a longer time for acquisition. Spatial resolution is also determined by the size of the FOV (a smaller FOV gives better spatial resolution) and by the point-of-spread function (PSF).

PSF on an optical system is defined as the distribution of light from a single point source. For MR spectroscopy imaging, the PSF is related to voxel contamination with signals from adjacent voxels, also called voxel "bleeding." This same effect corresponds to the Gibbs ringing artifact seen on conventional MR imaging. The shape of PSF is determined by the k-space sampling method and the number of phase-encoding steps. PSF can be avoided when more than 64 phase-encoding steps are applied, which leads to a scanning time not feasible in clinical practice. To reduce PSF, methods such as k-space filtering and reduction are used. For k-space reduction, the measured data are restricted to a circular (2D) or spherical (3D) region.

Another concern about MR spectroscopy imaging is the suppression of unwanted signals from outside the brain, particularly from the subcutaneous fat, because lipids have a much higher signal than brain metabolites. Because the FOV is always rectangular and does not conform to the shape of the brain, some techniques must be implemented to optimize the FOV. The use of outer-volume suppression (OVS) is the technique most used for this purpose.

All techniques that help optimize the MR spectroscopy imaging sequence by reducing voxel bleeding, and by increasing spatial resolution and the amount of phase encoding needed to acquire a 2D or 3D MR spectroscopy image, have a time cost. Therefore to minimize scan time without reducing quality, fast MR spectroscopy imaging techniques are used. A large FOV means a longer MR spectrum acquisition time. A simple way to reduce time is to use the smallest possible FOV consistent with the dimension of the object to be analyzed.

Reducing the k-space sampling by measuring the data inside a circular or spherical region instead of a rectangular one is another way to reduce scan time. Other techniques used for this purpose are turbo-MR spectroscopy imaging (using multiple spin echoes), multislice MR spectroscopy imaging, 3D echo-planar spectroscopic imaging, and parallel imaging methods. These techniques are beyond the scope of this article, and more details on these methods can be found elsewhere.[1-3]

SVS versus MR spectroscopy imaging

SVS and MR spectroscopy imaging have advantages and disadvantages, depending on the specific purpose (**Table 1**). The SVS technique results in a high-quality spectrum, short scan time, and good field homogeneity. Thus, SVS technique is usually obtained with short TE because longer TE has a decreased signal owing to T2 relaxation. SVS is used to obtain an accurate quantification of the metabolites.

The main advantage of MR spectroscopy imaging is spatial distribution, compared with SVS that only acquires the spectrum in a limited brain region. Moreover, the grid obtained with MR spectroscopy imaging allows voxels to be repositioned during postprocessing. On the other hand, the quantification of the metabolites is not as precise when using MR spectroscopy imaging because of voxel bleeding. Therefore, MR spectroscopy imaging can be used to determine spatial heterogeneity.

Short TE versus long TE

^{1}H-MRS can be obtained using different TEs that result in distinct spectra. Short-TE studies (typically 20–40 milliseconds) have a high SNR and less signal loss because of T2 and T1 weighting. These short-TE properties result in a spectrum with more metabolites peaks, such as myoinositol and glutamine-glutamate (**Fig. 4**), which are not detected with long TE. Nevertheless, because more peaks are shown on the spectrum, overlap is much more common, and care must be taken when quantifying the peaks of metabolites.

^{1}H-MRS spectra may also be obtained with long TEs, from 135 to 288 milliseconds. Long TEs have a poorer SNR; however, they have more simple spectra because of the suppression of some signals. Thus, the spectra are less noisy but have a limited number of sharp resonances. On 135- to 144-millisecond TEs, the peak of lactate is

---

Table 1
Differences between single-voxel spectroscopy (SVS) and MR spectroscopy imaging

SVS	MR Spectroscopy Imaging
Short TE	Long TE
One voxel	Multivoxel
Limited region	Many data collected
Fixed grid	Grid may be shifted after acquisition
More accurate	Voxel bleeding
Quantitative measurement	Spatial distribution

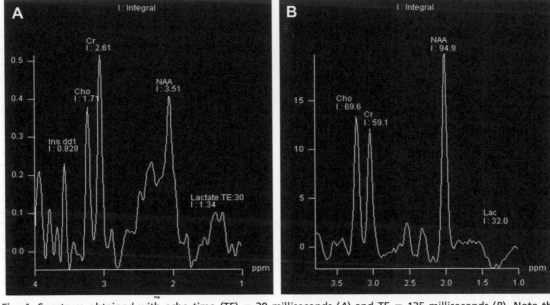

Fig. 4. Spectrum obtained with echo time (TE) = 30 milliseconds (*A*) and TE = 135 milliseconds (*B*). Note the inverted lactate peak (doublet) with long TE acquisition and the increased number of sharp resonances with short TE. Cho, choline; Cr, creatine; Ins dd1, myoinositol; NAA, *N*-acetylaspartate.

inverted below the baseline. This factor is important because the peaks of lactate and lipids overlap in this spectrum. Therefore, 135- to 144-millisecond TEs allow for easier recognition of the lactate peak (see **Fig. 4**) because lipids remain above the baseline. With a TE of 270 to 288 milliseconds there is a lower SNR and the lactate peak is not inverted.

Water Suppression

^{1}H-MRS–visible brain metabolites have a low concentration in brain tissues. Water is the most abundant, and thus its signal in the ^{1}H-MRS spectrum is much higher than that of other metabolites (the signal of water is 100,000 times greater than that of other metabolites). To avoid this high peak from water to be superimposed on the signal of other brain metabolites, water-suppression techniques are needed (**Fig. 5**). The most commonly used technique is chemical-shift selective water suppression (CHESS), which presaturates the water signal using frequency-selective 90° pulses before the localizing pulse sequence. Other techniques sometimes used are variable pulse power and optimized relaxation delays (VAPOR) and water suppression enhanced through T1 effects (WET).

Postprocessing

Quantification and analysis methods of collected data are as important as the acquisition

techniques used to obtain the spectra. Using an incorrect postprocessing method may lead to wrong interpretations. There are many postprocessing techniques that may be used before and after the Fourier transform (FT).

The properties of the spectrum can be manipulated using digital filters before the FT. Zero-filling, multiplication with a filter, eddy-current correction, and band-reject filters are some examples of postprocessing steps in the time domain. The use of zero-filling results in a higher digital resolution in the spectrum. Band-reject filters are used to remove residual water signal when the water-suppression technique used during signal acquisition does not completely eliminate it. Eddy-current correction is used to eliminate eddy-current artifacts (explained in the Artifacts section) using a reference signal such as unsuppressed water signal and applying a time-dependent phase correction. After the FT, in the frequency domain, phase and baseline correction are usually used. All these postprocessing methods may be used with SVS and MR spectroscopy imaging. However, because MR spectroscopy imaging uses phase-encoding gradients, other filters need to be applied before FT (eg, Hanning, Hamming, and Fermi filters).

Artifacts

^{1}H-MRS is prone to artifacts. Motion, poor water or lipid suppression, field inhomogeneity, eddy

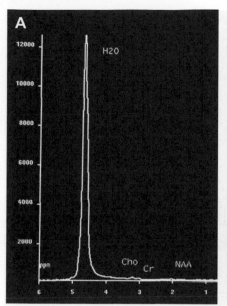
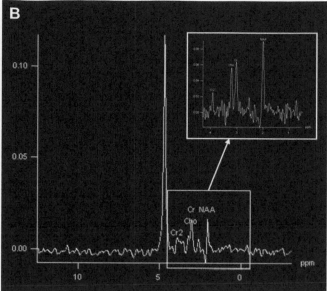

Fig. 5. Water-signal suppression with chemical shift selective water suppression (CHESS). Spectrum before CHESS (*A*) and after CHESS (*B*). CHESS reduces the signal from water by a factor of 1000, allowing brain metabolites to be depicted on the spectrum. Cho, choline; Cr and Cr2, creatine; NAA, *N*-acetylaspartate.

currents, and chemical-shift displacement are some examples of factors that introduce artifacts into spectra. One of the most important factors that predict the quality of a spectrum is the homogeneity of the magnetic field. Poor field homogeneity results in a lower SNR and broadening of the width of the peaks. For brain ¹H-MRS, some regions are more susceptible to this artifact, including those near bone structures and air-tissue interfaces. Therefore, placement of the VOI near areas such as inferior and anterior temporal cortices and orbitofrontal regions should be avoided. Paramagnetic devices also result in field inhomogeneity, leading to a poor-quality spectrum when the VOI is placed near them.

Eddy currents are caused by gradient switching. A transient current results in distortion of the peak shapes, making spectrum quantification difficult. This artifact is more commonly seen in older MR imaging units. However, even modern units produce smaller eddy-current artifacts, and eddy-current correction (used postprocessing) is needed.

Chemical-shift displacements correspond to chemical-shift artifacts on conventional MR imaging. The localization of the voxel is based on the precession frequency of the protons. Because this frequency is different for each metabolite, the exact position of each metabolite is slightly different. This artifact is larger with higher magnetic field strengths. To solve this problem, strong field gradients must be used for the slice selection.

Higher-Field ¹H-MRS

Higher-field MR imaging (3 T, 7 T, and above) is used in many centers mostly for research purposes. In the past decade 3-T MR imaging has started to be routinely used for clinical examinations, resulting in better SNR and faster acquisition time.

¹H-MRS at 3 T has a higher SNR and shorter acquisition time than when performed at 1.5 T. It had been assumed that SNR increases linearly with the strength of the magnetic field, but SNR does not double with 3-T ¹H-MRS because others factors are also responsible for the SNR, including metabolite relaxation time and magnetic-field homogeneity.

Spectral resolution is improved with a higher magnetic field. A better spatial resolution increases the distance between peaks, making it easier to distinguish between them. This aspect is important, particularly for resonances from coupled spins such as glutamate, glutamine, and myoinositol. However, the line-width of metabolites also increases at higher magnetic field because of a markedly increased T2 relaxation time. Thus, a short TE is more commonly used with 3 T. The difference in T1 relaxation time from 1.5 to 3 T depends on the brain region studied.[4]

3-T ¹H-MRS is more sensitive to magnetic-field inhomogeneity, and some artifacts are more pronounced (eg, susceptibility and eddy currents). Chemical-shift displacement is also greater at 3 T, and this artifact increases linearly with the magnetic field.

Receiver coils have also improved. The use of multiple RF receiver coils for ¹H-MRS provides higher local sensitivity and results in a higher SNR. These coils also allow a more extended coverage of the brain.

SPECTRA

¹H-MRS allows the detection of brain metabolites. The metabolite changes often precede structural abnormalities, and ¹H-MRS can demonstrate abnormalities before MR imaging does.[5] To detect these spectral alterations, it is fundamental to know the normal brain spectra and their variations according to the applied technique, patient's age, and brain region.

¹H spectra of metabolites are shown on x and y axes. The x (horizontal) axis displays the chemical shift of the metabolites in units of ppm. The ppm increases from right to left. The y (vertical) axis demonstrates arbitrary signal amplitude of the metabolites. The height of metabolic peak refers to a relative concentration, and the area under the curve to metabolite concentration.[5]

Long TE sequences result in less noise than short TE sequences, but several metabolites are better demonstrated with short TE. In 1.5-T MR scanners, long TE sequences (TE = 135–288 milliseconds) detect N-acetylaspartate (NAA), creatine (Cr), choline (Cho), lactate (Lac) and, possibly, alanine (Ala). Short TE sequences (TE = 20–40 milliseconds) demonstrate the metabolites seen with long-TE acquisitions and, in addition, lipids, myoinositol (Myo), glutamate-glutamine (Glx), glucose, and some macromolecular proteins (**Fig. 6**).

Brain Metabolites

N-acetylaspartate

The peak of NAA is the highest peak in normal brain, assigned at 2.02 ppm. NAA is synthesized in the mitochondria of neurons, then transported into neuronal cytoplasm and along axons. NAA is exclusively found in the nervous system (peripheral and central), and is detected in both gray and white matter. It is a marker of neuronal and axonal viability and density. NAA can additionally be found in immature oligodendrocytes and astrocyte progenitor cells. NAA also plays a role as a cerebral osmolyte.

Absence or decreased concentration of NAA is a sign of neuronal loss or degradation. Neuronal destruction from malignant neoplasms and many white-matter diseases results in decreased concentration of NAA. By contrast, increased NAA indicates Canavan disease, although it may also

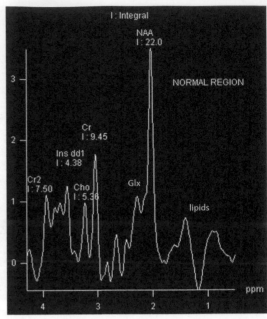

Fig. 6. Normal spectra obtained with short TE sequence. (TE = 30 milliseconds). Cho, choline; Cr, and Cr2, creatine; Glx, glutamate-glutamine; Ins dd1, myoinositol; NAA, N-acetylaspartate.

be demonstrated in Salla disease and Pelizaeus-Merzbacher disease. NAA is not demonstrated in extra-axial lesions such as meningiomas or intra-axial ones originating from outside of the brain such as metastases, unless there is a partial volume effect with normal parenchyma.

Creatine

The peak of the Cr spectrum is assigned at 3.02 ppm. This peak represents a combination of molecules containing creatine and phosphocreatine. Cr is a marker of energetic systems and intracellular metabolism. The concentration of Cr is relatively constant, and it is considered a stable metabolite. It is therefore used as an internal reference for calculating metabolite ratios. However, there is regional and individual variability in Cr concentrations.

In brain tumors, the Cr signal is relatively variable (see later discussion). Gliosis may cause minimally increased Cr, owing to increased density of glial cells (glial proliferation). Creatine and phosphocreatine are metabolized to creatinine, then the creatinine is excreted via the kidneys.[6] Systemic disease (eg, renal disease) may also affect Cr levels in the brain.[7]

Choline

The Cho spectrum peak is assigned at 3.22 ppm and represents the sum of choline and choline-containing compounds (eg, phosphocholine). Cho is a marker of cellular membrane turnover (phospholipids synthesis and degradation) reflecting cellular proliferation. In tumors, Cho levels correlate with degree of malignancy reflecting cellularity. Increased Cho may be seen in infarction (from gliosis or ischemic damage to myelin) or inflammation (glial proliferation). For this reason, Cho is considered to be nonspecific.

Lactate

The Lac peak is difficult to visualize in the normal brain. The peak of Lac is a doublet at 1.33 ppm, which projects above the baseline on short/long TE acquisition and inverts below the baseline at TE of 135 to 144 milliseconds.

A small peak of Lac is visible in some physiologic states such as newborn brains during the first hours of life.[8] Lac is a product of anaerobic glycolysis, so its concentration increases under anaerobic metabolism such as cerebral hypoxia, ischemia, seizures, and metabolic disorders (especially mitochondrial ones). Increased Lac signals also occur with macrophage accumulation (eg, acute inflammation). Lac also accumulates in tissues with poor washout such as cysts, normal-pressure hydrocephalus, and necrotic and cystic tumors.[7]

Lipids

Lipids are components of cell membranes not visualized with long TE because of their very short relaxation time. There are 2 peaks of lipids: methylene protons at 1.3 ppm and methyl protons at 0.9 ppm.[9] These peaks are absent in the normal brain, but presence of lipids may result from improper voxel selection, causing voxel contamination from adjacent fatty tissues (eg, fat in subcutaneous tissue, scalp, and diploic space).

Lipid peaks can be seen when there is cellular membrane breakdown or necrosis, such as in metastases or primary malignant tumors.

Myoinositol

Myo is a simple sugar assigned at 3.56 ppm. Myo is considered a glial marker because it is primarily synthesized in glial cells, almost only in astrocytes. It is also the most important osmolyte in astrocytes. Myo may represent a product of myelin degradation. Elevated Myo occurs with proliferation of glial cells or with increased glial-cell size, as found in inflammation. Myo is elevated in gliosis, astrocytosis, and Alzheimer disease (AD).[7,9]

Alanine

Ala is an amino acid that has a doublet centered at 1.48 ppm. This peak is located above the baseline in spectra obtained with short/long TE and inverts below the baseline on acquisition using TE of 135 to 144 milliseconds. Its peak may be obscured by Lac (at 1.33 ppm). The function of Ala is uncertain, but it plays a role in the citric acid cycle.[7] Increased concentration of Ala may occur in defects of oxidative metabolism.[9] In tumors, an elevated level of Ala is specific for meningiomas (**Fig. 7**).

Glutamate-glutamine

Glx has complex peaks from glutamate, glutamine, and γ-aminobutyric acid assigned at 2.05 to 2.50 ppm. These metabolite peaks are difficult to separate at 1.5 T. Glutamate is an important excitatory neurotransmitter and also plays a role in the redox cycle.[7,9] Elevated concentration of glutamine are found in a few diseases such as hepatic encephalopathy.[5,9]

Regional Variations of the Spectra

Metabolite peaks may differ slightly according to the brain region being studied. Studies have shown differences between the spectra of white and gray matter and between supratentorial and infratentorial structures. Nevertheless, no significant asymmetries of metabolite spectra between the left and right hemispheres or between genders have been found.[10,11]

In specific quantitative techniques, the concentration of NAA in gray matter is higher than that in white matter. For clinical purposes, concentrations of NAA in both gray and white matter are not significantly different. Most studies have found higher Cho levels in white matter than in gray matter, whereas the Cr level is higher in gray matter.[6,12–14] There are some frontal-occipital variations too. The clearest difference is a caudal decrease in Cho in the cortex.[15,16] Regional variations of Glx and Myo have been studied less than those of NAA, Cho, and Cr. One study[17] found higher Glx levels in gray matter than in white matter. The regional distribution of Myo is unclear, but tends to be higher in gray matter than in white matter.[17]

Regarding the brainstem and cerebellum, the highest levels of NAA are in the pons.[18] Significantly higher levels of Cho have been found in the cerebellum and pons than in supratentorial regions.[16,18] Cerebellar levels of Cr are also significantly higher than supratentorial levels, whereas low levels of Cr are seen in the pons.[16,18]

^{1}H-MRS of the hippocampus has been studied especially in epilepsy and AD. There are anterior-posterior gradients of metabolites in the hippocampi. The concentration of Cho increases from the posterior to anterior hippocampus, whereas a lower NAA concentration has been found anteriorly.[19,20]

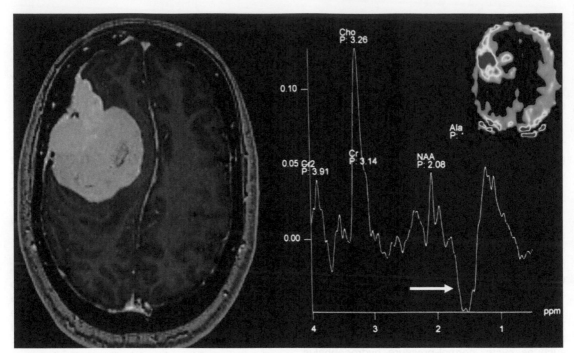

Fig. 7. Extra-axial mass on the right frontal region with enhancement post gadolinium on T1-weighted imaging and hyperperfusion on arterial spin-labeling volume map (*upper right*). An inverted doublet peak is seen at 1.48 ppm at ^{1}H-MRS that corresponds to alanine (*arrow*). High peaks of Cho and low NAA are also depicted. Ala, alanine; Cho, choline; Cr and Cr2, creatine; NAA, *N*-acetylaspartate.

Spectra in Pediatrics

Regardless of the differences in methodology, there are differences in metabolite levels in the developing brain. MR spectra depend on age, and during the first year of life significant changes occur. In general, the spectral pattern in pediatrics is considered to be similar to that of adults when older than 2 years of age, and the concentration of metabolites is practically constant by 4 years of age.[7,21,22] NAA levels are low, whereas levels of Myo and Cho are high at birth. Both gray and white matter show similar patterns. Myo is a prominent metabolite in brain spectra of newborns. As age increases, increased concentration of NAA and decreased concentrations of choline-containing compounds and Myo become evident.[5,7,21] Concentrations of Cr and phosphocreatine are constant and may be used as reference values (**Fig. 8**). An increased concentration of NAA reflects brain maturation, and its concentration correlates with myelination.[6,21] With cerebral maturation, there is also a decrease in the concentration of Cho compounds. A small amount of Lac may be seen in newborn brains.[8] Glutamate and glutamine do not demonstrate significant alterations with age.[21]

According to gestational age, the equation of Kreis and colleagues[22] describes changes in metabolite concentration. With this equation and parameters for a multiexponential model,[21] graphs of metabolite changes with age can be drawn (**Fig. 9**).

Spectra in the Elderly

^{1}H-MRS studies of elderly brains are less consistent than those of pediatric brains. Some studies have found a reduced concentration of NAA with aging, which suggests a decrease in neuronal mass.[7,23,24] By contrast, other studies have found relatively stable concentrations of NAA in older groups but increased Cho and/or Cr.[14,25] A systematic review of ^{1}H-MRS in healthy aging summarized the findings of ^{1}H-MRS in aging in that they are varied. Most studies have reported no changes in metabolites with advanced age. However, some data suggest lower NAA and higher Cho and Cr with increasing age.[26] Disagreement of the studies could be due to the use of different techniques (eg, evaluation of different brain regions and atrophy correction). Different study populations may also affect results.

CLINICAL APPLICATION
Brain Tumors

Brain tumors are currently the main application of ^{1}H-MRS. This technique is usually used as

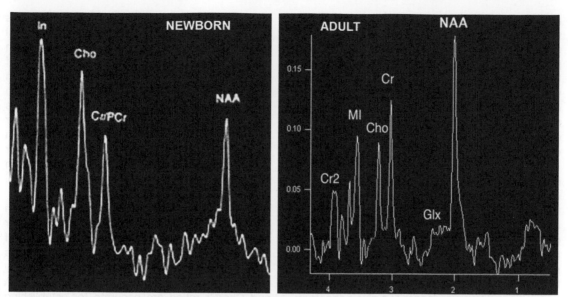

Fig. 8. Normal spectra in newborn (*left*) demonstrate high levels of myoinositol (Myo) and Cho but low NAA compared with the normal spectra in an adult (*right*). Cho, choline; CrPcr, creatine/phosphocreatine; Cr and Cr2, creatine; Glx, glutamate-glutamine; In, Myo; MI, Myo; NAA, *N*-acetylaspartate.

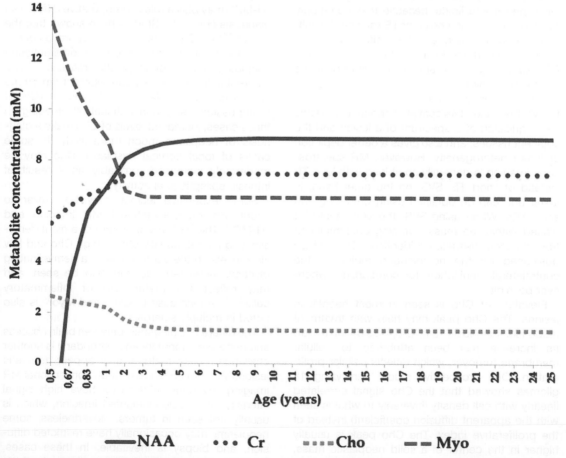

Fig. 9. Changes in metabolite concentrations with age calculated by the equation of Kries and colleagues and the parameters of Dezortova and Hajek. Cho, choline; Cr, creatine; Myo, myoinositol; NAA, *N*-acetylaspartate.

a complement to conventional MR imaging, along with other advanced techniques such as perfusion. Combined with conventional MR imaging, proton MR spectra may improve diagnosis and treatment of brain tumors. ^{1}H-MRS may help with differential diagnosis, histologic grading, degree of infiltration, tumor recurrence, and response to treatment, mainly when radionecrosis develops, and is indistinguishable from tumor by conventional MR imaging.

An important decision regarding analysis of intracranial masses concerns which ^{1}H-MRS technique to use. Different ^{1}H-MRS parameters may be varied to optimize the results, the most relevant of which is TE.[27] Short TE allows for recognition of more peaks than does long TE, which may be important for the differential diagnosis of brain masses and for grading tumors. Myo is a marker for low-grade gliomas, only seen on short-TE acquisitions. However, longer TEs give a spectrum with a limited number of peaks, making it easier to analyze. Long TEs varying from 135 to 140 milliseconds also invert peaks of Lac and Ala. This inversion is important for differentiating between these peaks and lipids, because they commonly overlap. Hence, the choice of TE may be difficult, and one solution is to acquire 2 different spectra using both short and long TEs. In clinical practice, 2 ^{1}H-MRS acquisitions are rarely feasible because of time constraints.

MR spectroscopy imaging is usually preferable to SVS because of its spatial distribution. It allows the acquisition of a spectrum of a lesion and the adjacent tissues, and also gives a better depiction of tumor heterogeneity. However, MR spectroscopy imaging is generally combined with long TE instead of short TE. SVS, on the other hand, is faster and can be obtained using both long and short TEs. When using SVS, the VOI should be placed within the mass, avoiding contamination from adjacent tissues. An identical VOI must be positioned on the homologous region of the contralateral hemisphere for comparison, whenever possible.

Elevation of Cho is seen in most neoplastic lesions. The Cho peak may help with treatment response, diagnosis, and progression of tumor. Its increase has been attributed to cellular membrane turnover, which reflects cellular proliferation. One prospective study[28] analyzing 18 gliomas showed that the Cho signal correlated linearly with cell density (inversely to what is seen with the apparent diffusion coefficient) instead of the proliferative index. The Cho peak is usually higher in the center of a solid neoplastic mass, and decreases peripherally. The Cho signal is consistently low in necrotic areas.

Another ^{1}H-MRS feature seen in brain tumors is decreased NAA. This metabolite is a neuronal marker, and its reduction denotes destruction and displacement of normal tissue. Absence of NAA in an intra-axial tumor generally implies an origin outside of the central nervous system (metastasis) or a highly malignant tumor that has destroyed all neurons in that location. The Cr signal, on the other hand, is slightly variable in brain tumors, and changes according to tumor type and grade. The typical ^{1}H-MRS spectrum for a brain tumor is one of a high level of Cho, low NAA, and minor changes in Cr (Fig. 10).

Cho elevation is usually evidenced by an increase in Cho/NAA or Cho/Cr ratios, rather than its absolute concentration. Estimation of absolute Cho concentration, although possible, is susceptible to many errors because many assumptions are required. Therefore, Cho/NAA and Cho/Cr ratios are accurate for establishing Cho levels in brain neoplasms.

When faced with intracranial expansive lesions, conventional MR imaging with or without perfusion may lead to a reliable diagnosis. In doubtful cases, ^{1}H-MRS may play a role in preoperative differential diagnosis (Table 2). Studies have shown that the use of ^{1}H-MRS in specific cases improves accuracy and the level of confidence in differentiating neoplastic from nonneoplastic masses.[29] The differentiation of a low-grade glioma from stroke or focal cortical dysplasia (Fig. 11) may be difficult or impossible using conventional MR imaging. In these cases, increased levels of Cho make a diagnosis of neoplasm much more likely. In some cases of focal cortical dysplasia, Cho may be moderately increased, probably as a result of intrinsic epileptic ictal activity.[30]

Some expansive lesions may be similar to neoplasms on conventional MR imaging and ^{1}H-MRS. The ^{1}H-MRS spectrum of a giant demyelinating plaque usually shows high Cho and low NAA levels. In the acute stage of a demyelinating disease, increased Lac can also be seen, and may reflect the metabolism of inflammatory cells.[31,32] An increase in Glu[33] and Myo[34] is also noted in multiple sclerosis.

The differential diagnosis between brain abscess and neoplasms (primary and secondary) is another challenge. These features may appear as cystic lesions with rim enhancement on conventional MR imaging. Pyogenic abscesses have high signal intensity on diffusion-weighted imaging, which is usually not seen in tumors. Nevertheless, some neoplasms may occasionally have restricted diffusion, and biopsy is inevitable. In these cases, ^{1}H-MRS may help to establish a diagnosis. If the VOI is positioned in the enhancing area, presence

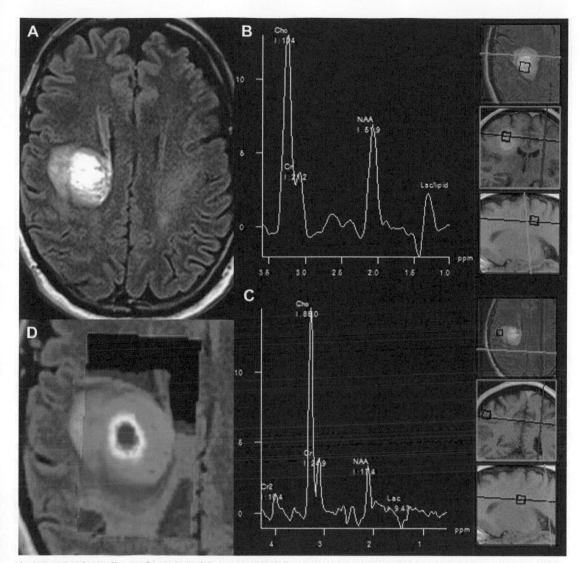

Fig. 10. Histologically confirmed glioblastoma. Axial fluid-attenuated inversion recovery (FLAIR) MR image (*A*) shows a lesion with high signal intensity in a posterior region of the right frontal lobe. ¹H-MRS with long TE demonstrates increase in Cho peak and decrease in NAA peak inside the lesion (*B*) and in the surrounding tissue (*C*), representing tumor infiltration. Lactate and lipids are also present. Color metabolite map (*D*) also demonstrates abnormal Cho/Cr ratio. Cho, choline; Cr and Cr2, creatine; Lac, lactate; NAA, *N*-acetylaspartate.

of Cho favors a neoplasm.[35] If the VOI is positioned in the cystic area of a lesion, abscess and tumor both demonstrate a high Lac peak. Nonetheless, the presence of acetate, succinate, and amino acids such as valine, Ala, and leucine in the core of the lesion has high sensitivity for pyogenic abscess (**Fig. 12**).[36,37] These peaks are not seen in tumors. It is important to be aware that in patients with pyogenic brain abscess who are under antibiotic therapy, these peaks may be absent.

¹H-MRS can also help in the differentiation of high-grade gliomas from solitary metastasis. Both lesions show the same ¹H-MRS pattern, with high Cho and low NAA. However, the high

signal intensity on T2-weighted imaging seen in the perilesional area demonstrates an elevated Cho/Cr ratio only in high-grade gliomas (see **Fig. 10**).[38] This feature is consistent with the pathologic findings of infiltrating tumor cells in areas of edema not seen in metastases.

Gliomas, the most common and the most studied lesions among neuroepithelial tumors, originate from glial cells (eg, astrocytes or oligodendrocytes). Gliomas have an infiltrative nature, resulting in neuronal cell damage and decreased NAA. Cohen and colleagues[39] found decreased whole-brain NAA in patients with glial tumors beyond the main tumor. This significant whole-brain NAA depletion

Table 2
¹H-MRS changes in tumors and other lesions

	Cho	NAA	Lac	Lip	Myo	Glu	Suc	Acet	Ala	Aa
Low-grade tumor	↑	↓			↑					
High-grade tumor	↑	↓	↑	↑						
Metastasis	↑	Absent[a]	↑	↑						
Oligodendroglioma	↑	↓	↑[b]							
Meningioma	↑	Absent							↑	
Gliomatosis cerebri	↑	↓								
Lymphoma	↑	Absent[a]		↑						
Radionecrosis	↓	↓	↑	↑						
Abscess	N	↓	↑	↑				↑	↑	↑
Demyelination	↑	↓	↑[c]	↑	↑	↑[c]				

Abbreviations: ↑, increased peak; ↓, reduced peak; Aa, amino acids; Acet, acetate; Ala, alanine; Cho, choline; Glu, glutamine; Lac, lactate; Lip, lipids; Myo, myoinositol; N, normal peak; NAA, N-acetylaspartate; Suc, succinate.
 [a] NAA is absent in the core of the tumor, but may be present where it infiltrates brain parenchyma or with voxel bleeding.
 [b] The presence of lactate depends on the grade of the tumor.
 [c] Lac and Glu are increased only in the early stage of the disease.

may reflect extensive tumor infiltration in the normal-appearing brain on MR imaging. One quantitative ¹H-MRS study[40] found a correlation between the percentage of tumor infiltration from the ¹H-MRS–guided biopsy samples and changes in NAA, Cho, and Cho/NAA ratio in corresponding voxels. Absolute concentration of NAA decreased, whereas absolute concentration of Cho and the Cho/NAA ratio increased with degree of tumor infiltration.

Astrocytomas can be classified into low grade (grades I and II, benign) and high grade (grades III and IV, malignant). High-grade gliomas (anaplastic gliomas or grade III, and glioblastoma multiforme or grade IV) have higher Cho and lower NAA than low-grade gliomas. Elevated Cho correlates with cellular proliferation and density. Although several studies in one systematic review[41] have reported that ¹H-MRS can accurately differentiate between low-grade and high-grade gliomas, the results of glioma grading using ¹H-MRS vary widely. Such wide variations may be attributed to different methods and metabolites overlapping between different tumor grades. Statistically significantly higher Cho/Cr, Cho/NAA, and relative cerebral blood volume (rCBV) have been reported in high-grade in comparison with low-grade gliomas,[42] although threshold values of metabolite ratios for grading of gliomas are not well established. Cho/Cr is the most frequently used ratio. Some institutions use a threshold value of 2.0 for Cho/Cr to differentiate low-grade from high-grade gliomas, whereas some use a cutoff value of 2.5.

As described earlier, lipid and Lac peaks are absent under normal conditions. Lipid peak indicates necrosis in malignant tumors. Lac, a product of anaerobic glucolysis, accumulates in necrotic portions of tumors. The presence of lipids and Lac correlates with necrosis in high-grade gliomas. Compared with high-grade gliomas, low-grade gliomas show higher Myo levels,[43,44] which may be due to a low mitotic index in low-grade gliomas and, thus, fewer mitogens (substances that trigger cell mitosis). Some mitogens can influence the metabolism of phosphatidylinositol, and Myo is also involved in the formation of phosphatidylinositol. Thus, lack of activation of phosphatidylinositol metabolism results in Myo accumulation. Howe and colleagues[44] concluded that high Myo was characteristic of grade II astrocytomas.

On serial ¹H-MRS, malignant degeneration of gliomas can be detected using percentage signal change in Cho. Tedeschi and colleagues[45] have demonstrated that interval percentage changes in Cho intensity in stable gliomas and progressive gliomas (malignant degeneration or recurrent disease) is less than 35 and more than 45, respectively. Interval increased Cho/Cr or Cho/NAA is suggestive of malignant progression.

Gliomatosis cerebri is a distinct entity of glial tumors. This rare disease is characterized by diffuse infiltration of glial-cell neoplasm throughout the brain. Gliomatosis cerebri has various histologic subtypes (astrocytoma, oligodendroglioma, or mixed glioma). The World Health Organization (WHO) classification denotes grades II, III, and IV gliomatosis cerebri[46]; therefore, patients with this

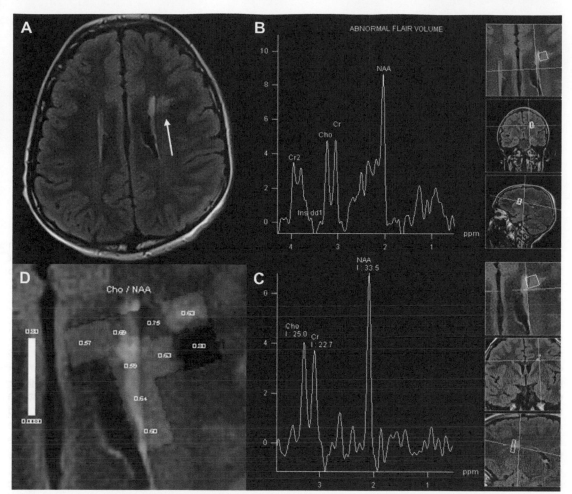

Fig. 11. A 10-year-old boy with intractable seizures. (*A*) FLAIR image shows focal high signal intensity in the white matter of the centrum semiovale of the left frontal lobe (*arrow*) and overlying blurry gray matter–white matter junction. ^{1}H-MRS images with TE = 35 milliseconds (*B*) and TE = 144 (*C*) demonstrate normal Cho and NAA peaks. Color metabolite map (*D*) demonstrates normal Cho/NAA ratio. These findings are suggestive of a cortical dysplasia with adjacent abnormal white matter. Cho, choline; Cr and Cr2, creatine; Ins dd1, myoinositol.

tumor have a widely variable prognosis. Marked elevation of Myo and Cr has been found in gliomatosis cerebri, and this may be attributed to glial activation rather than glial proliferation[47] because the Cho level is moderately elevated, suggesting low density of glial cells.

Oligodendroglioma is a subgroup of gliomas that has a better response to treatment (chemosensitive) and better prognosis than glioblastoma. This distinct tumor is divided into two groups according to the WHO classification: grades II and III.[48] It originates from oligodendrocytes but often contains a mixed population of cells, particularly astrocytes. Loss of genes in chromosomes 1p and 19q is a characteristic genetic alteration of most oligodendrogliomas. On dynamic contrast-enhanced MR perfusion, low-grade oligodendrogliomas may demonstrate

high rCBV because they contain a dense network of branching capillaries.[49] Thus several oligodendrogliomas can be misinterpreted as high-grade tumors because of their high rCBV, which contributes to decreasing the reliability of rCBV in differentiating high-grade and low-grade gliomas. Among the low-grade gliomas, low-grade oligodendrogliomas also exhibit significantly higher rCBV on dynamic-contrast MR perfusion.[50] In subgroups of the oligodendroglial tumors, MR imaging studies have found that contrast enhancement is not suggestive of anaplasia as it is in astrocytomas. One study showed that rCBV was not significantly different between low-grade and high-grade oligodendroglimas,[51] in contrast to another study[52] showing rCBV to differ significantly between the low and high grades.

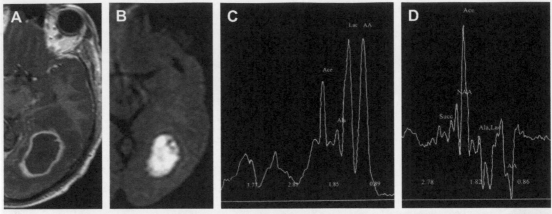

Fig. 12. Parenchymal pyogenic abscess presenting as lesion with rim enhancement after gadolinium injection on T1-weighted imaging (*A*) and high signal diffusion on diffusion-weighted imaging (*B*). ¹H-MRS images with short TE (*C*) and long TE (*D*) show high levels of acetate (Ace), alanine (Ala), lactate (Lac), succinate (Succ), and amino acids (AA). The VOI was positioned in the core of the lesion.

The results of ¹H-MRS studies in oligodendrogliomas are more consistent than those of MR perfusion studies. Similarly to astrocytomas, ¹H-MRS of oligodendrogliomas demonstrates significantly higher Cho, Cho/Cr ratio, and a higher incidence of Lac and lipids in high-grade than in low-grade tumors.[51–53] Nevertheless, low-grade oligodendrogliomas may show highly elevated Cho, mimicking high-grade tumors, because these low-grade tumors can have high cellular density but absent endothelial proliferation and necrosis.[52] Apart from higher rCBV, the level of glutamine plus glutamate is significantly higher in low-grade oligodendrogliomas than in low-grade astrocytomas, and may help to distinguish these tumors from each other.[53]

Accurate grading of gliomas based on ¹H-MRS alone may be difficult. On combining ¹H-MRS with conventional and other advanced MR imaging techniques such as perfusion MR imaging, grading becomes more precise. Some features of tumors on conventional MR imaging (eg, contrast enhancement, surrounding edema, signal heterogeneity, necrosis, hemorrhage, and midline crossing) and perfusion MR imaging (high rCBV) suggest a high grade. ¹H-MRS is complementary and helpful for glioma grading. High-grade gliomas demonstrate marked elevation of Cho, decreased NAA, and presence of Lac and lipids. Myo is high in low-grade gliomas and decreases with increasing grades of tumors.

An important issue regarding postradiation therapy in patients with brain tumors is differentiation between recurrent brain tumor and radiation injury/change, particularly when new contrast-enhancing lesions are seen in previously operated and/or irradiated regions. Many studies have found that Cho/Cr and/or Cho/NAA ratios are significantly higher in recurrent tumor (or predominantly tumor) than in radiation injury (**Fig. 13**).[54–57]

One study[57] reported that the Lac/Cr ratio was significantly higher in recurrent tumor than in radiation injury, whereas the lipid/Cr ratio was significantly lower in recurrent tumor than in radiation injury. Another study showed that the Lac or lipid signal alone was not helpful in differentiating these 2 conditions.[56] Rabinov and colleagues[54] have also demonstrated no correlation between the signal intensity of lipids and the histopathology, but they observed that the signal intensity of Lac in 2 patients with enhancing areas corresponded to recurrent tumor. It is probable that the amount of lipids may be higher in an area of radiation changes than in tumor recurrence, whereas Lac may be found in recurrent tumor, but both lipids and Lac cannot differentiate these conditions.

Infections

Distinguishing brain abscesses from necrotic brain tumors can be difficult on computed tomography or conventional MR imaging; these can appear as rim-enhancing lesions. Although pyogenic brain abscesses show restricted diffusion and brain tumors usually do not show the restriction, in some instances neoplasms may have restricted diffusion. ¹H-MRS may be helpful for establishing the diagnosis. In pyogenic abscess, typical ¹H-MRS spectra of the enhancing rim demonstrate a decrease in NAA and Cr levels but no change or a slight decrease in Cho level.[58,59] In one study,[35] maximum Cho/Cr, Cho/NAA, and Cho/Cho ratios in glioblastomas multiforme were significantly higher than in brain abscesses; thus, an increased Cho level specifies brain tumors.

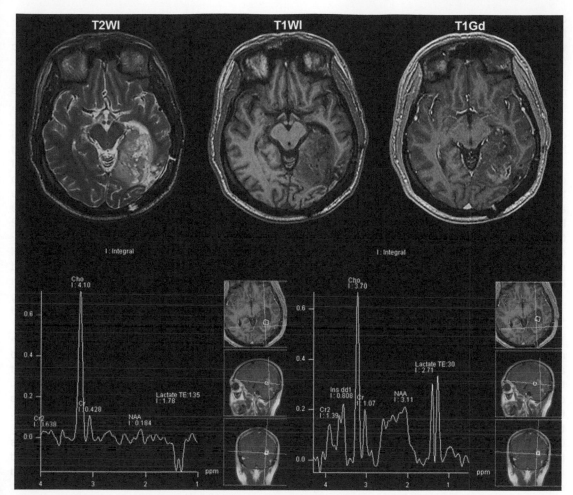

Fig. 13. Glioblastoma multiforme in deep portions of the left temporal and occipital lobes previously treated with surgery and radiotherapy. An area of irregular and patchy contrast enhancement is seen on the region of prior surgery that could correspond to tumor recurrence or treatment-induced changes. ¹H-MRS image shows high peak of Cho (and high Cho/Cr) and low NAA in all voxels of the grid (2 are shown), a pattern that is consistent with tumor recurrence. The presence of lactate could reflect tumor ischemia, but may be seen after treatment and thus its meaning is not clear. After treatment, the presence of lactate may signify treatment-induced necrosis and not high histologic grade. Cho, choline; Cr and Cr2, creatine; NAA, N-acetylaspartate; T1Gd, T1-weighted with gadolinium; T1WI, T1-weighted; T2WI, T2-weighted.

Spectra of the cystic portion of necrotic tumor or abscess cavity show a Lac peak and may show lipid signals, therefore Lac and lipid peaks are nonspecific.[35,37] By contrast, abscess demonstrates elevation of acetate, succinate, and some amino acids (eg, valine, leucine, and Ala), which are specific spectra and are not seen in the neoplasms.[35–37] However, there are 2 situations that one must be aware of. First, the resonances of acetate, succinate, and amino acids may be absent in an abscess under effective antibiotic therapy. Second, in aerobic bacterial abscesses, acetate is usually not present. Moreover, typical spectra of anaerobic bacterial abscesses (acetate, succinate, and amino acids) do not exist in

Staphylococcus aureus abscess, which is one of the aerobic bacterial abscesses.[35] Therefore, interpretation of ¹H-MRS spectra of the enhancing rim along with the spectra of cystic components of the rim-enhancing lesions could differentiate anaerobic and aerobic bacterial abscesses, and necrotic brain tumors from each other.

Another challenge is discriminating between toxoplasmosis and lymphoma in human immunodeficiency virus infection. Both can have the appearance of rim-enhancing lesions. Lymphoma typically demonstrates restricted diffusion; however, toxoplasmosis has a variation of the diffusion and may overlap with that of the lymphoma.[60] Typical MR perfusion of lymphoma shows elevation of rCBV, whereas toxoplasmosis does not. Positive findings using single-photon emission computed tomography and positron emission tomography (PET) are found in lymphoma.[61] On ^{1}H-MRS, lymphoma has an elevated Cho level. Toxoplasmosis shows lipid and Lac peaks, but these peaks are rather nonspecific and can be found in the necrotic portion of lymphoma.[61] A moderate decrease in NAA and a moderate increase in Cho have been documented in toxoplasmosis as well.[62]

Herpes simplex encephalitis is the most common encephalitis, which has typical distribution of brain involvement at the hippocampus and cortex of temporal, frontobasal, and insular lobes.[63] ^{1}H-MRS shows marked reduction of NAA and NAA/Cr ratio, and elevation of Cho and Cho/Cr ratio at the involved region, which reflect neuronal loss and gliosis and correlate with histopathologic findings.[63–65]

Inborn Error of Metabolism

The diagnosis of an inborn error of metabolism is always challenging and is mainly based on clinical and laboratory findings, evolution, and genetic tests. Brain MR imaging may help to narrow the differential diagnosis, avoid expensive genetic tests, or even establish a final diagnosis. Because these disorders are caused by inherited enzymatic defects, concentrations of some metabolites may be abnormally low or high. Metabolites with a very small concentration in brain tissue are not depicted on ^{1}H-MRS. In these cases, the changes in the spectrum usually correspond to a general abnormality, such as demyelination or ischemia. For some diseases, however, ^{1}H-MRS may identify a specific biomarker that helps in the diagnosis.[66]

Disorders that have specific ^{1}H-MRS patterns may manifest as an increase, decrease, or absence of particular metabolites. Specific biomarkers can be seen in phenylketonuria (phenylalanine), Canavan disease (NAA), nonketotic hyperglycinemia (glycine), creatine deficiency (Cr), and maple syrup urine disease (branched-chain amino acids and keto acids).[67]

Phenylalanine is an α-amino acid that is assigned at 7.36 ppm and can be used for the diagnosis of phenylketonuria, follow-up of treatment, and evolution of the disease. ^{1}H-MRS is usually not needed because early diagnosis is made by neonatal screening tests, and response to treatment can be monitored by phenylalanine blood levels and neuropsychological tests.

An increase in NAA signal is characteristic of Canavan disease (a disorder caused by a defect of the enzyme aspartoacylase that results in NAA accumulation in the brain) in a child with diffusely abnormal white matter and macrocephaly. However, a high peak at 2.03 ppm is also noted in Salla disease, a rare autosomal recessive free sialic acid storage disorder.[68] This latter disease accumulates acetylneuraminic acid (NANA), which resonates at the same frequency as NAA. In patients diagnosed with Pelizaeus-Merzbacher disease, the NAA peak may also be elevated.

Nonketotic hyperglycinemia is an autosomal recessive disease that manifests mainly during the neonatal period. There is accumulation of glycine in the brain, and this metabolite shows up in ^{1}H-MRS as a peak at 3.55 ppm. Of importance is that Myo resonates at 3.56 ppm, therefore these peaks overlap. However, glycine has a higher T2 value, and is seen with both short-TE and long-TE sequences.[66] Thus ^{1}H-MRS is an important tool for diagnosing nonketotic hyperglycinemia, and long-TE studies must be acquired. ^{1}H-MRS can also be used for monitoring the disease, correlating more with the clinical findings than levels of blood and cerebrospinal fluid glycine.

Maple syrup urine disease is an aminoacidopathy with accumulation of branched-chain α-keto and amino acids. These metabolites resonate at 0.9 ppm, a region that is usually attributed to lipids. Lac may also be present. In Cr deficiency there is a severe reduction in the Cr peak. In both diseases, ^{1}H-MRS may help with diagnosis and treatment.

All mitochondrial diseases caused by disorders of pyruvate metabolism, disorders of fatty acid oxidation, or defects of the respiratory chain and may show Lac elevation on ^{1}H-MRS. However, this finding is nonspecific and Lac is not always present. Nonetheless, in mitochondrial disorders an abnormal Lac peak may be present when the VOI is positioned in normal brain parenchyma on MR imaging and in the ventricles.[69,70] Therefore, even if the findings of ^{1}H-MRS are nonspecific, they may be useful in the evaluation of mitochondrial disorders.

Dementia

Dementia is a clinical diagnosis in patients with a decline in memory and cognitive function. MR imaging may play an important role in ruling out neurologic disorders that may clinically present with dementia, such as subdural hematomas, tumors, and multiple cerebral infarctions. The most common causes of dementia, however, are AD, dementia with Lewy bodies, and vascular dementia. Although there are clinical criteria to differentiate these pathologic subtypes of dementia, pathologic studies have shown that such criteria are not accurate. Therefore, specific imaging neuromarkers may help in the differential diagnosis.

In patients with dementia, ^{1}H-MRS may aid in the differential diagnosis and progression of the disease.[71] AD is associated with neuronal damage, particularly in the limbic cortical regions. In the end stages of the disease, primary sensorimotor and neuronal cortices are also involved. ^{1}H-MRS shows a reduction on NAA/Cr ratio and elevation of Myo/Cr ratio, especially in paralimbic cortical regions (posterior cingulate gyri).[72,73] The higher level of Myo is thought to be associated with gliosis.[74]

Mild cognitive impairment (MCI) is established as a transitional state between the cognitive changes of normal aging and AD.[75] Patients with MCI have memory loss, but still do not meet criteria for AD; however, they usually have AD pathology. This condition is suitable for early therapeutic intervention. ^{1}H-MRS depicts high Myo/Cr levels in the parietal lobes of these patients. NAA/Cr is either mildly decreased or normal.

^{1}H-MRS measurements of NAA and Myo levels are also a marker for progression of clinical disease, and correlate with dementia severity and neuropsychological cognitive function. A study comparing antemortem ^{1}H-MRS and neuropathologic criteria for AD demonstrated a strong association between NAA/Myo levels and disease progression.[76]

Seizures

Localization of the focus of an epileptogenic seizure relies on the combination of many different techniques, such as video-electroencephalography (EEG), neuropsychological assessment, and PET. MR imaging may also be useful in detecting the epileptic focus. MR imaging is usually performed in patients with recent-onset or recurring focal seizures. Underlying structural abnormalities, such as cortical dysplasia and tumors, are depicted on MR imaging and may be the cause of focal epilepsy. However, in some patients with focal epilepsy, MR imaging does not show any structural abnormality. The role of ^{1}H-MRS is to help characterize and localize the epileptogenic focus, especially when studying patients with refractory focal epilepsy and without clear MR imaging abnormalities.

Temporal lobe epilepsy (TLE) is the most common cause of focal epilepsy. Hippocampal sclerosis is responsible for most cases of TLE. The characteristic MR imaging findings are hippocampal increased T2-weighted signal, reduced volume, and architectural distortion. The accuracy of MR imaging to detect abnormalities in TLE is controversial. Studies[77,78] have indicated a high reliability in the diagnosis of hippocampal sclerosis using MR imaging, with sensitivity of up to 90% and specificity up to 70%. However, other studies

showed that approximately 20% of patients with TLE have no findings on MR imaging.[79]

^{1}H-MRS may help to distinguish the side of the focus in some cases of TLE, particularly in patients with normal brain MR imaging.[71,80] A reduction in NAA concentration and NAA/Cho + Cr ratio is the typical abnormality of TLE, and is a reflection of neuronal damage.[81] Increased Cho and Myo signals may also be present, and are believed to be caused by gliosis. However, the specificity of the abnormal concentration of the metabolites on ^{1}H-MRS is unknown. Abnormalities on ^{1}H-MRS have been seen in both temporal lobes in patients with TLE.[71,79] Moreover, metabolic changes were also found in other areas distant to the seizure focus, probably due to widespread effects of seizures.[71] These ^{1}H-MRS abnormalities in distant areas may reverse after surgery.[82]

SUMMARY

MR spectroscopy offers a noninvasive means of assessing in vivo brain metabolites that shed light on cellular concentrations, cell function and dysfunction, cellular energetics, presence of ischemia, and presence of necrosis, among others. Studies obtained at higher field strengths are evolving toward sampling of smaller tissue volumes, greater SNR, and higher metabolic spatial resolution. From the clinical standpoint MR spectroscopy is useful in various disorders, as described in this review. However, to be valid and significant the results of MR spectroscopy should always be correlated with their imaging counterparts.

REFERENCES

1. Duyn JH, Moonen CT. Fast proton spectroscopic imaging of human brain using multiple spin-echoes. Magn Reson Med 1993;30:409–14.

2. Duyn JH, Gillen J, Sobering G, et al. Multisection proton MR spectroscopic imaging of the brain. Radiology 1993;188:277–82.

3. Posse S, DeCarli C, Le Bihan D. Three-dimensional echoplanar MR spectroscopic imaging at short echo times in the human brain. Radiology 1994; 192:733–8.

4. Ethofer T, Mader I, Seeger U, et al. Comparison of longitudinal metabolite relaxation times in different regions of the human brain at 1.5 and 3 Tesla. Magn Reson Med 2003;50:1296–301.

5. Fayed N, Olmos S, Morales H, et al. Physical basis of magnetic resonance spectroscopy and its application to central nervous system diseases. Am J Appl Sci 2006;3:1836–45.

6. Hajek M, Dezortova M. Introduction to clinical in vivo MR spectroscopy. Eur J Radiol 2008;67:185–93.

7. Soares DP, Law M. Magnetic resonance spectroscopy of the brain: review of metabolites and clinical applications. Clin Radiol 2009;64:12–21.

8. Mullins ME. MR spectroscopy: truly molecular imaging; past, present and future. Neuroimaging Clin N Am 2006;16:605–18.

9. van der Graaf M. In vivo magnetic resonance spectroscopy: basic methodology and clinical applications. Eur Biophys J 2010;39:527–40.

10. Charles HC, Lazeyras F, Krishnan KR, et al. Proton spectroscopy of human brain: effects of age and sex. Prog Neuropsychopharmacol Biol Psychiatry 1994;18:995–1004.

11. Nagae-Poetscher LM, Bonekamp D, Barker PB, et al. Asymmetry and gender effect in functionally lateralized cortical regions: a proton MRS imaging study. J Magn Reson Imaging 2004;19:27–33.

12. Hetherington HP, Mason GF, Pan JW, et al. Evaluation of cerebral gray and white matter metabolite differences by spectroscopic imaging at 4.1T. Magn Reson Med 1994;32:565–71.

13. Kreis R, Ernst T, Ross BD. Absolute quantitation of water and metabolites in the human brain. II. Metabolite concentrations. J Magn Reson B 1993;102:9–19.

14. Soher BJ, van Zijl PC, Duyn JH, et al. Quantitative proton MR spectroscopic imaging of the human brain. Magn Reson Med 1996;35:356–63.

15. Degaonkar MN, Pomper MG, Barker PB. Quantitative proton magnetic resonance spectroscopic imaging: regional variations in the corpus callosum and cortical gray matter. J Magn Reson Imaging 2005;22:175–9.

16. Pouwels PJ, Frahm J. Regional metabolite concentrations in human brain as determined by quantitative localized proton MRS. Magn Reson Med 1998; 39:53–60.

17. Baker EH, Basso G, Barker PB, et al. Regional apparent metabolite concentrations in young adult brain measured by (1)H MR spectroscopy at 3 Tesla. J Magn Reson Imaging 2008;27:489–99.

18. Jacobs MA, Horská A, van Zijl PC, et al. Quantitative proton MR spectroscopic imaging of normal human cerebellum and brain stem. Magn Reson Med 2001; 46:699–705.

19. Arslanoglu A, Bonekamp D, Barker PB, et al. Quantitative proton MR spectroscopic imaging of the mesial temporal lobe. J Magn Reson Imaging 2004;20:772–8.

20. Vermathen P, Laxer KD, Matson GB, et al. Hippocampal structures: anteroposterior N-acetylaspartate differences in patients with epilepsy and control subjects as shown with proton MR spectroscopic imaging. Radiology 2000;214:403–10.

21. Dezortova M, Hajek M. (1)H MR spectroscopy in pediatrics. Eur J Radiol 2008;67:240–9.

22. Kreis R, Ernst T, Ross BD. Development of the human brain: In vivo quantification of metabolite and water content with proton magnetic resonance spectroscopy. Magn Reson Med 1993;30:424–37.

23. Christiansen P, Toft P, Larsson HB, et al. The concentration of N-acetyl aspartate, creatine + phosphocreatine, and choline in different parts of the brain in adulthood and senium. Magn Reson Imaging 1993;11:799–806.

24. Lim KO, Spielman DM. Estimating NAA in cortical gray matter with applications for measuring changes due to aging. Magn Reson Med 1997;37:372–7.

25. Chang L, Ernst T, Poland RE, et al. In vivo proton magnetic resonance spectroscopy of the normal aging human brain. Life Sci 1996;58:2049–56.

26. Haga KK, Khor YP, Farrall A, et al. A systemic review of brain metabolite changes, measured with (1)H magnetic resonance spectroscopy, in healthy aging. Neurobiol Aging 2009;30:353–63.

27. Majós C, Julià-Sapé M, Alonso J, et al. Brain tumor classification by proton MR spectroscopy: comparison of diagnostic accuracy at short and long TE. AJNR Am J Neuroradiol 2004;10:1696–704.

28. Gupta, Rakesh K. Relationships between choline magnetic resonance spectroscopy, apparent diffusion coefficient and quantitative histopathology in human glioma. Journal of Neuro-oncology 2000; 50(3):215–26.

29. Majós C, Aguilera C, Alonso J, et al. Proton MR spectroscopy improves discrimination between tumor and pseudotumoral lesion in solid brain masses. AJNR Am J Neuroradiol 2009;30(3):544–51.

30. Vuori K, Kankaanranta L, Häkkinen AM, et al. Lowgrade gliomas and focal cortical developmental malformations: differentiation with proton MR spectroscopy. Radiology 2004;230(3):703–8.

31. Bitsch A, Bruhn H, Vougioukas V, et al. Inflammatory CNS demyelination: histopathologic correlation with in vivo quantitative proton MR spectroscopy. AJNR Am J Neuroradiol 1999;20(9):1619–27.

32. De Stefano N, Filippi M, Miller D, et al. Guidelines for using proton MR spectroscopy in multicenter clinical MS studies. Neurology 2007;69(20):1942–52.

33. Srinivasan R, Sailasuta N, Hurd R, et al. Evidence of elevated glutamate in multiple sclerosis using magnetic resonance spectroscopy at 3 T. Brain 2005;128(Pt 5):1016–25.

34. Fernando KT, McLean MA, Chard DT, et al. Elevated white matter myo-inositol in clinically isolated syndromes suggestive of multiple sclerosis. Brain 2004;127(Pt 6):1361–9.

35. Lai PH, Weng HH, Chen CY, et al. In vivo differentiation of aerobic brain abscesses and necrotic glioblastomas multiforme using proton MR spectroscopic imaging. AJNR Am J Neuroradiol 2008;29(8):1511–8.

36. Grand S, Passaro G, Ziegler A, et al. Necrotic tumor versus brain abscess: importance of amino acids detected at ^{1}H MR spectroscopy–initial results. Radiology 1999;213(3):785–93.

37. Lai PH, Ho JT, Chen WL, et al. Brain abscess and necrotic brain tumor: discrimination with proton MR spectroscopy and diffusion-weighted imaging. AJNR Am J Neuroradiol 2002;23(8):1369–77.

38. Law M, Cha S, Knopp EA, et al. High-grade gliomas and solitary metastases: differentiation by using perfusion and proton spectroscopic MR imaging. Radiology 2002;222(3):715–21.

39. Cohen BA, Knopp EA, Rusinek H, et al. Assessing global invasion of newly diagnosed glial tumors with whole-brain proton MR spectroscopy. AJNR Am J Neuroradiol 2005;26(9):2170–7.

40. Stadlbauer A, Gruber S, Nimsky C, et al. Preoperative grading of gliomas by using metabolite quantification with high-spatial-resolution proton MR spectroscopic imaging. Radiology 2006;238(3):958–69.

41. Hollingworth W, Medina LS, Lenkinski RE, et al. A systematic literature review of magnetic resonance spectroscopy for the characterization of brain tumors. AJNR Am J Neuroradiol 2006;27(7):1404–11.

42. Law M, Yang S, Wang H, et al. Glioma grading: sensitivity, specificity, and predictive values of perfusion MR imaging and proton MR spectroscopic imaging compared with conventional MR imaging. AJNR Am J Neuroradiol 2003;24(10):1989–98.

43. Castillo M, Smith JK, Kwock L. Correlation of myoinositol levels and grading of cerebral astrocytomas. AJNR Am J Neuroradiol 2000;21(9):1645–9.

44. Howe FA, Barton SJ, Cudlip SA, et al. Metabolic profiles of human brain tumors using quantitative in vivo ^{1}H magnetic resonance spectroscopy. Magn Reson Med 2003;49(2):223–32.

45. Tedeschi G, Lundbom N, Raman R, et al. Increased choline signal coinciding with malignant degeneration of cerebral gliomas: a serial proton magnetic resonance spectroscopy imaging study. J Neurosurg 1997;87(4):516–24.

46. Taillibert S, Chodkiewicz C, Laigle-Donadey F, et al. Gliomatosis cerebri: a review of 296 cases from the ANOCEF database and the literature. J Neurooncol 2006;76(2):201–5.

47. Galanaud D, Chinot O, Nicoli F, et al. Use of proton magnetic resonance spectroscopy of the brain to differentiate gliomatosis cerebri from low-grade glioma. J Neurosurg 2003;98(2):269–76.

48. David NL, Hiroko O, Otmar D, et al. The 2007 WHO Classification of Tumours of the Central Nervous System. Acta Neuropathol 2007;114(2):97–109.

49. Lev MH, Ozsunar Y, Henson JW, et al. Glial tumor grading and outcome prediction using dynamic spin-echo MR susceptibility mapping compared with conventional contrast-enhanced MR: confounding effect of elevated rCBV of oligodendrogliomas [corrected]. AJNR Am J Neuroradiol 2004;25(2):214–21.

50. Cha S, Tihan T, Crawford F, et al. Differentiation of low-grade oligodendrogliomas from low-grade astrocytomas by using quantitative blood-volume measurements derived from dynamic susceptibility contrast-enhanced MR imaging. AJNR Am J Neuroradiol 2005;26(2):266–73.

51. Xu M, See SJ, Ng WH, et al. Comparison of magnetic resonance spectroscopy and perfusion-weighted imaging in presurgical grading of oligodendroglial tumors. Neurosurgery 2005;56(5):919–26 [discussion: 919–26].

52. Spampinato MV, Smith JK, Kwock L, et al. Cerebral blood volume measurements and proton MR spectroscopy in grading of oligodendroglial tumors. AJR Am J Roentgenol 2007;188(1):204–12.

53. Rijpkema M, Schuuring J, van der Meulen Y, et al. Characterization of oligodendrogliomas using short echo time ^{1}H MR spectroscopic imaging. NMR Biomed 2003;16(1):12–8.

54. Rabinov JD, Lee PL, Barker FG, et al. In vivo 3 T MR spectroscopy in the distinction of recurrent glioma versus radiation effects: initial experience. Radiology 2002;225(3):871–9.

55. Smith EA, Carlos RC, Junck LR, et al. Developing a clinical decision model: MR spectroscopy to differentiate between recurrent tumor and radiation change in patients with new contrast-enhancing lesions. AJR Am J Roentgenol 2009;192(2):W45–52.

56. Weybright P, Sundgren PC, Maly P, et al. Differentiation between brain tumor recurrence and radiation injury using MR spectroscopy. AJR Am J Roentgenol 2005;185(6):1471–6.

57. Zeng QS, Li CF, Liu H, et al. Distinction between recurrent glioma and radiation injury using magnetic resonance spectroscopy in combination with diffusion-weighted imaging. Int J Radiat Oncol Biol Phys 2007;68(1):151–8.

58. Burtscher IM, Holtas S. In vivo proton MR spectroscopy of untreated and treated brain abscesses. AJNR Am J Neuroradiol 1999;20:1049–53.

59. Remy C, Grand S, Lai ES, et al. ^{1}H MRS of human brain abscess in vivo and in vitro. Magn Reson Med 1995;34:508–14.

60. Schroeder PC, Post MJ, Orchatz E, et al. Analysis of the utility of diffusion-weighted MRI and apparent diffusion coefficient values in distinguishing central nervous system toxoplasmosis from lymphoma. Neuroradiology 2006;48:715–20.

61. Pomper MG, Constantinides CD, Barker PB, et al. Quantitative MR spectroscopic imaging of brain lesions in patients with AIDS: correlation with [^{11}C-methyl]thymidine PET and thallium-201 SPECT. Acad Radiol 2002;9:398–409.

62. Ionita C, Wasay M, Balos L, et al. MR imaging in toxoplasmosis encephalitis after bone marrow transplantation: paucity of enhancement despite fulminant disease. AJNR Am J Neuroradiol 2004;25:270–3.

63. Samann PG, Schlegel J, Muller G, et al. Serial proton MR spectroscopy and diffusion imaging findings in HIV-related herpes simplex encephalitis. AJNR Am J Neuroradiol 2003;24:2015–9.

64. Hitosugi M, Ichijo M, Matsuoka Y, et al. Proton MR spectroscopy findings in herpes simplex encephalitis. Rinsho Shinkeigaku 1996;36:839–43.

65. Takanashi J, Sugita K, Ishii M, et al. Longitudinal MR imaging and proton MR spectroscopy in herpes simplex encephalitis. J Neurol Sci 1997;149:99–102.

66. Barker PB, Bizzi A, De Stefano N, et al. Clinical MR spectroscopy. 1st edition. New York: Cambridge University Press; 2010. ISBN 9780521868983.

67. van der Knaap MS, Valk J. Magnetic resonance of myelin disorders. 3rd edition. Heidelberg (Germany): Springer; 2005. ISBN 13:9783540222866.

68. Varho T, Komu M, Sonninen P, et al. A new metabolite contributing to N-acetyl signal in ^{1}H MRS of the brain in Salla disease. Neurology 1999;52(8):1668–72.

69. Bianchi MC, Tosetti M, Battini R, et al. Proton MR spectroscopy of mitochondrial diseases: analysis of brain metabolic abnormalities and their possible diagnostic relevance. AJNR Am J Neuroradiol 2003;24(10): 1958–66.

70. Cross JH, Gadian DG, Connelly A, et al. Proton magnetic resonance spectroscopy studies in lactic acidosis and mitochondrial disorders. J Inherit Metab Dis 1993;16(4):800–11.

71. Gillard JH, Waldman AD, Barker PB. Clinical MR neuroimaging: physiological and functional techniques. 2nd edition. New York: Cambridge University Press; 2010. ISBN 9780521515634.

72. Huang W, Alexander GE, Chang L, et al. Brain metabolite concentration and dementia severity in Alzheimer's disease: a (1)H MRS study. Neurology 2001;57(4):626–32.

73. Miller BL, Moats RA, Shonk T, et al. Alzheimer disease: depiction of increased cerebral myo-inositol with proton MR spectroscopy. Radiology 1993;187(2): 433–7.

74. Ross BD, Bluml S, Cowan R, et al. In vivo MR spectroscopy of human dementia. Neuroimaging Clin N Am 1998;8(4):809–22.

75. Petersen RC, Doody R, Kurz A, et al. Current concepts in mild cognitive impairment. Arch Neurol 2001;58(12):1985–92.

76. Kantarci K, Knopman DS, Dickson DW, et al. Alzheimer disease: postmortem neuropathologic correlates of antemortem ^{1}H MR spectroscopy metabolite measurements. Radiology 2008;248(1): 210–20.

77. Lee DH, Gao FQ, Rogers JM, et al. MR in temporal lobe epilepsy: analysis with pathologic confirmation. AJNR Am J Neuroradiol 1998;19:19–27.

78. Park SW, Chang KH, Kim HD, et al. Lateralizing ability of single-voxel proton MR spectroscopy in hippocampal sclerosis: comparison with MR imaging and positron emission tomography. AJNR Am J Neuroradiol 2001;22:625–31.

79. Connelly A, van Paesschen W, Porter DA, et al. Proton magnetic resonance spectroscopy in MRI-negative temporal lobe epilepsy. Neurology 1998; 51(1):61–6.

80. Doelken MT, Stefan H, Pauli E, et al. (1)H-MRS profile in MRI positive versus MRI negative patients with temporal lobe epilepsy. Seizure 2008;17:490–7.

81. Najm IM, Wang Y, Shedid D, et al. MRS metabolic markers of seizures and seizure-induced neuronal damage. Epilepsia 1998;39(3):244–50.

82. Serles W, Li LM, Antel SB, et al. Time course of postoperative recovery of N-acetyl-aspartate in temporal lobe epilepsy. Epilepsia 2001;42(2):190–7.

Proton Magnetic Resonance Spectroscopy
Technique for the Neuroradiologist

Kim M. Cecil, PhD

KEYWORDS

- Chemical shift • Localization • Metabolite • Spectral dispersion • Shimming • Suppression

KEY POINTS

- Magnetic resonance spectroscopy (MRS) provides information on neuronal and axonal viability, energetics of the cellular structures, and status of the cellular membranes.
- The interpretation of a magnetic resonance (MR) spectrum primarily arises from variations in chemical ratios and/or concentrations, which alter peak area for the endogenous metabolites.
- The single-voxel spectroscopy (SVS) technique provides a cubic-based volume of interest, typically 4 cm^3 to 8 cm^3 in volume.

INTRODUCTION

Proton MRS appeals to many clinicians and scientists because its application in the clinical setting can increase the specificity of MR imaging when implemented with appropriate questions for MRS to answer. Enthusiasm for application of this technique is often diminished, however, due to the complexities of data acquisition, processing, and interpretation. The original expectation of MRS included a concept of disease specificity, meaning MRS would be a technique having distinct patterns for specific disease processes. Unfortunately, only a few disease processes have distinct MRS profiles unique to a particular disorder. Instead, MRS typically reveals the metabolic status of the region sampled. In the brain, MRS provides information content on neuronal/axonal viability, energetics of the cellular structures, and status of the cellular membranes. Yet, by examining the composite MR spectrum, a pattern of disease involvement at a molecular level can complement an imaging examination.

The objective of this article is to provide descriptive concepts of the technique and its application in vivo for a variety of patient populations. Ideally, when appropriately incorporating MRS into the neuroradiologic evaluation, this technique will produce relevant information to radiologists and clinicians for their understanding of adult and pediatric neurologically based disease processes.

TECHNICAL CONCERNS

For readers previously unexposed to the MRS technique, many articles in the literature and textbooks describe the origin, mathematical approaches, and physics of MRS acquisition in the brain.[1–4] Conventional MR imaging systems, with 1.5-T and 3.0-T superconducting magnets, offer suitable magnetic field strengths for performing proton MRS of the brain clinically. For practicing radiologists familiar with MR imaging, there are several technical properties that must be considered for MRS. These include the concepts of chemical shift, spectral dispersion associated with magnetic field strength, shimming, signal suppression, combination schemes for signal processing from phased array coils, sequence approach, and localization sequences.

Funded by: NIH (P50MH077138; R01CA112182; R01ES01559).
Department of Radiology, Pediatrics, Neuroscience and Environmental Health, Cincinnati Children's Hospital Medical Center, MLC 5033, 3333 Burnet Avenue, Cincinnati, OH 45229, USA
E-mail address: kim.cecil@cchmc.org

Neuroimag Clin N Am 23 (2013) 381–392
http://dx.doi.org/10.1016/j.nic.2012.10.003

Chemical Shift

Spectroscopy uses signal intensity, line width, and position to display information from molecules of interest. Multiple chemical regions of the same molecule may contribute distinct signals to the spectrum. Typically, these molecules of interest from the human brain are referred to as *metabolites*. Proton MRS plots hydrogen atom (proton) metabolite signal intensity versus an observation frequency. The protons from the backbone components of the molecule (primarily carbon atoms) can produce peaks (or resonances) when in the MR environment with signal intensity proportional to the relative number of protons. The position of the metabolite peaks on the X axis reflects the local chemical and magnetic environment of the molecule. Shielding factors influence the position of the peak (Fig. 1). The position is described using the parts-per-million (ppm) scale. Because locations in Hertz (Hz) change as field strengths vary, a dimensionless unit is necessary to normalize field strengths. The chemical shift for a given peak location is calculated by dividing the difference in frequency of 2 peaks (with 1 peak defined as the reference) by the operating frequency of the MR scanner. This ppm scale refers the magnetic field strength, which is approximately 10^6, or 1 million, Hz. This allows comparison of a peak location found on the spectrum obtained on a 1.5-T scanner with that found at that location on a different field strength scanner. Examples of this property include the methyl (CH_3-) resonance on the acetyl group of *N*-acetylaspartate (NAA) that appears at 2.0 ppm and the creatine (Cr) *N*-methyl resonance that always appears at 3.0 ppm, regardless if measured on a 1.0-T, 1.5-T, 3-T, or 4-T scanner. In general, the locations of the metabolites are stable, because the brain pH does not change sufficiently to result in a change in peak assignment.

Metabolites with a singlet peak, such as those with NAA and Cr (including phosphocreatine), corresponding to a methyl group do not change chemical shift assignment. Metabolites with adjacent methylene and methine elements may produce a slightly different signal position and appearance at different field strengths; however, this does not occur from a pH change. The signal from methylene and methine groups may split peaks into multiplet patterns. The local chemical and magnetic environment influences the appearance of the peaks and reflects local coupling constants between protons within the molecule. *Myo*-inositol (mI), glutamate (Glu), glutamine (Gln), glucose, and aspartate are a few of the molecules with coupled methylene and methine spin systems visible on clinical proton MRS. For the purpose of this discussion, the only routinely reported metabolite with distinct alterations in its assignment and spectral appearance due to field strength is mI. For MRS performed at 1.5 T, the mI peak normally is distinct, with 4 of the molecule's methine protons magnetically indistinguishable, thereby coresonating at the same location (3.57 ppm). Increased spectral dispersion (discussed later) inherent at higher field strengths, however, produces 2 distinct peaks (at a field strength of 3 T, 3.55 ppm and 3.61 ppm) for the 4 protons, effectively reducing the signal intensity by half. Normal mI levels visually appear lower at higher field strengths, such as 3 T in comparison to 1.5 T. Although some reports have found improved detection of mI at high field strength arising from increased signal-to-noise ratio (SNR), it may be problematic depending on the acquisition conditions.[5] A short echo approach (ie, echo time [TE] $\leq$35 milliseconds [ms]) must be used due to the fast relaxation rate to detect mI.

Benefits and Challenges at Fields of 3 T and Higher: Relaxation Times, Signal-to-Noise Ratio, and Spectral Dispersion

The transition from 1.5 T to 3 T or higher field strengths illustrates some of the fundamental principals of MRS by perturbing properties, such as relaxation rate, SNR, and spectral dispersion. As with MR imaging, the relaxation properties influence the metabolite signal appearance. T1 relaxation reflects the time it takes for the perturbed magnetization to return to equilibrium. T2 relaxation represents the time it takes for dephasing or loss of coherence within the applied field. For the metabolites, T1 relaxation rates lengthen slightly whereas T2 shortens on moving to fields of 3 T or higher compared with 1.5 T. For metabolites (NAA, Cr, and choline [Cho]), the longitudinal relaxation T1 times approximate 1.2 to 1.4 seconds at 1.5 T and increase slightly to 1.2 to 1.6 seconds at 4 T, with Cho the shortest.[6–9] These values have an impact on the repetition time (TR) necessary to conduct the MRS experiment. At least

CH_3F CH_3Cl CH_3Br CH_3I

4.13   2.84   2.45   1.98 ppm

$$\sigma(F) < \sigma(Cl) < \sigma(Br) < \sigma(I)$$

Fig. 1. The influence of the environment on the methyl (CH_3-) group location due to the shielding factor (σ) of the adjacent atom (in this example, fluoride [F], chloride [Cl], bromide [Br], and iodide [I]) or groups of atoms. The adjacent atom influences the position (chemical shift value) on the X axis in parts per million.

5 times the longest T1 value is needed to obtain a fully relaxed experimental condition. For practical purposes, most clinical MRS sites use TR times of approximately 2000 ms to balance the signal afforded from decaying metabolites and beginning a new excitation. For transverse relaxation, T2, several common metabolites have values of approximately 270 ms to 480 ms at 1.5 T and 150 ms to 210 ms at 3 T, 140 ms to 185 ms at 4 T, with Cr values the shortest.[7,9] These 3 primary metabolites are observed at long TEs greater than 135 ms. Other metabolites generally have much shorter T2 values, thus requiring TEs of approximately 35 ms or less (discussed later). The protocols used must consider the relaxation properties of the metabolites and how the field strength influences them.

Acquiring proton MRS data at 3 T compared with 1.5 T should provide a significant benefit with an increase in SNR, which can then be applied for increased speed of acquisition (temporal resolution), spatial resolution (smaller voxel sizes with equivalent SNR to lower field), or some hybrid of speed and voxel size. This increase has been found, however, to be approximately 20% for short TE (20 ms) and approaching 100% for long-echo single-voxel proton MRS.[9] At short TEs, it seems that the peaks acquired at 3 T are wider than those at 1.5 T. With any increase in magnetic field strength, there is a decrease in metabolite T2* relaxation times, resulting in increased metabolite line widths.[10] Other postprocessing factors also influence the overall appearance of the peaks (ie, spectral apodization, also known as line broadening) (Fig. 2). The improved resolution afforded from increased field strength is accomplished with increased spectral dispersion (ie, the spectrum is dispersed or spread apart because the frequency

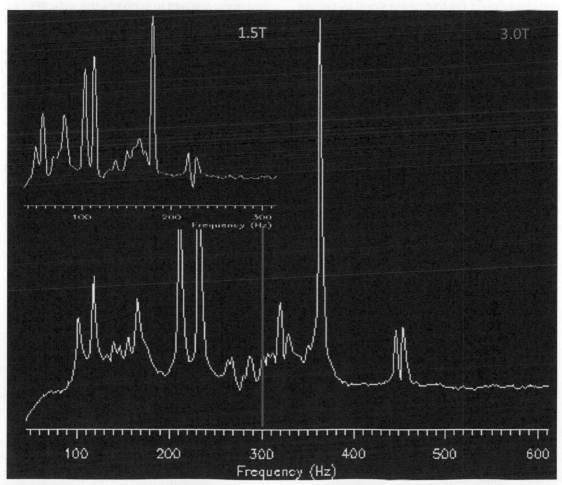

Fig. 2. Illustration of field strength effects on spectral dispersion. Both spectra were obtained using a water-based phantom, with lactate, NAA, Glu, Cr, Cho, and mI included with the water location set at 0 Hz. For the spectrum below obtained at 3 T, metabolites within the spectrum appear from 100 Hz to 600 Hz. (*Insert*) A spectrum obtained at 1.5 T demonstrates the metabolites within the spectrum appearing from 100 Hz to 300 Hz.

between peaks is greater at higher field strength) (**Fig. 3**). The ability to distinguish where one peak begins and ends is improved. For instance, the fat and water peaks are separated by 220 Hz at 1.5 T but 440 Hz at 3 T, with the Cr and Cho peaks appearing further apart at 3 T than at 1.5 T.

Shimming

Shimming is the process of homogenizing the magnetic field by applying direct current offsets to gradient coils (usually found as first-order shim coils on clinical MR imaging systems and higher-order shims on research MR imaging systems) via automated software packages provided by the system manufacturers or research groups (an example is FastMap[11]). Shimming can be conducted on the raw time domain signal or the frequency (post–Fourier transformed) signal. Shimming is performed to enhance the sensitivity and resolution of the metabolite signal by narrowing the peak widths and increasing the SNR (**Fig. 4**). Shimming also allows for improved water suppression, because a narrower water peak is more easily nulled because the center frequency can be optimized. Single-voxel spectra are less susceptible to the effects of large variations in magnetic field inhomogeneity. Thus, it is easier to shim on a small, 8 cm³, volume compared with an entire region, slice, or volume. Regions of interest in spectroscopic imaging or multivoxel spectroscopy acquisitions are more difficult to shim, because distortions in the magnetic field arise from tissue-air, tissue-bone, tissue-cerebrospinal fluid (CSF), and other interfaces and have large magnetic susceptibility differences because the tissues are magnetized differently. A compromise in homogeneity is inherent across the volume of interest for spectroscopic imaging because the shimming algorithm balances the need for higher shim settings around the sinus and frontal lobes compared with regions in the cerebrum away from ventricles, bone, and so forth.

Suppression

Briefly, proton MRS requires suppression of signals from water and fat. Water has a concentration level of approximately 80 M whereas most metabolites of interest are at the 1-mM to 10-mM level. Water suppression is implemented using pulse sequences, such as chemically selective saturation (CHESS[12]), Water suppression Enhanced through T1 effects (WET),[13] Variable Pulse power and Optimied Relaxation delays (VAPOR),[14] and so forth. The most commonly implemented sequence on clinical MR scanners, CHESS, has 3 narrow, frequency-selective pulses applied along with a dephasing gradient to suppress the water (**Fig. 5**). For fat, signals can be nulled, with the application of a sequence with inversion pulses, or simply avoided with placement of a volume-selective localization pulse sequence (described later) of the region of interest. To further eliminate signal from scalp and sinuses, outer volume suppression uses very selective suppression pulses.[15–17] The outer volume suppression pulses are graphically prescribed using the imaging sequences to guide locations and angles around the scalp by a technologist. Although the very selective suppression pulses can be used with body coil excitation, they have low radiofrequency peak power. These pulses have large bandwidths and sharp transition bands, which minimize chemical shift errors because the edges of the selected volume are better defined, thus minimizing chemical shift misregistration.

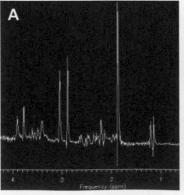 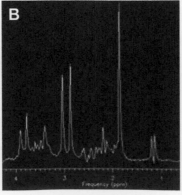 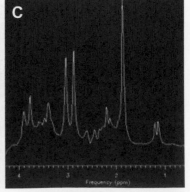

Fig. 3. The effects of line broadening (also referred to as spectral apodization) on a proton spectrum obtained using a water-based phantom, with lactate, NAA, Glu, Cr, Cho, and mI included. (*A*) No line broadening, (*B*) minimal line broadening applied, and (*C*) excessive line broadening applied to the spectra. Note (*C*) the distortion of the baseline.

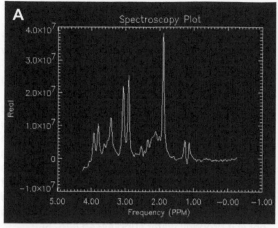
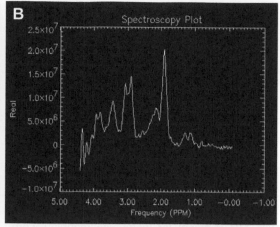

Fig. 4. The effects of shimming on a proton spectrum obtained using a water-based phantom, with lactate, NAA, Glu, Cr, Cho, and mI included. (*A*) Optimized shimming; (*B*) distorted shimming. Note the loss of baseline resolution for Cr (3.0 ppm) and Cho (3.2 ppm).

Also known as chemical shift displacement artifact, misregistration occurs when the signal is excited from metabolites that do not originate from exactly the same volume. This arises due to the variation in chemical shift within a spectrum, because the metabolites on one end of the spectrum experience different excitation profiles from the other. The localization pulse sequence selection strongly influences this artifact with a stimulated echo-based approach minimizing displacement.

Approaches and Localization

The easiest clinical approach for proton spectroscopic analysis is known as single-volume element (voxel) proton MR spectroscopy (SVS). In its basic

form on clinical MR imaging scanners, the SVS technique uses either a spin-echo (point-resolved spectroscopy [PRESS])–based or stimulated echo (stimulated echo acquisition mode [STEAM])–based volume-selective localization pulse sequence providing a cubic-based volume of interest, typically 4 cm^3 to 8 cm^3 in volume. Crusher field gradient pulses are applied to remove signals (free induction decays from a single pulse and spin echoes generated from 2 pulses) arising from outside of the voxel. As the name implies, SVS is limited to a single acquisition in a given region. Although the SVS technique does not interrogate multiple regions of interest simultaneously, it does afford good signal to noise and homogenous peaks due to a limited region of interest for shimming

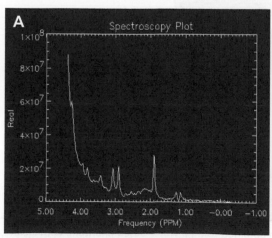
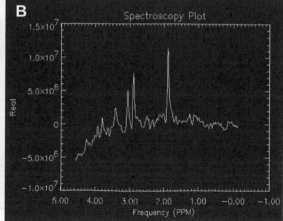

Fig. 5. The effects of water suppression on a proton spectrum obtained using a water-based phantom, with lactate, NAA, Glu, Cr, Cho, and mI included. (*A*) Undersuppressed, nonoptimized spectrum; (*B*) oversuppressed spectrum with over-rotation of the third CHESS pulse.

within a few minutes of scan time. Magnetic resonance spectroscopic imaging (MRSI) (also known as multivoxel spectroscopy) generates spectra from a larger number of usually smaller-sized voxels with broader anatomic coverage providing a choice of single slices and multiple slices in multiple dimensions and orientations. Volumes of interest are much larger and are also usually obtained using PRESS localization. The MRSI spectra can be transformed into color maps yielding metabolite images. Historically, long acquisition times, complicated postprocessing, poor homogeneity across the regions of interest sampled, partial volume effects with signal contamination from outside a voxel, and low resolution (on comparison with MR imaging) for metabolite mapping were significant limitations for the early implementation of MRSI. Recent advances provide improved accuracy in localization, speed, and resolution for spectroscopic imaging. The technical development of fast spectroscopic imaging continues to focus on implementing k-space sampling strategies (ellipsoid k-space encoding, echo planar

spectroscopic imaging, spiral spectroscopic imaging, and parallel imaging reconstruction, such as SENSitivity Encoding (SENSE)) for spectroscopic acquisition without artifacts from eddy currents, especially for short TEs, and spectral aliasing effects in spectral fitting due to limitations in gradient rise times.[2]

During the prescan, several steps are performed to optimize the scanner, including identifying the center of the water frequency, shimming the region of interest, and setting the power for applying the pulses in the localization and suppression sequences. If power levels for the pulses are not properly set, the voxel or region of interest sampled does not match what was graphically prescribed nor is it properly water suppressed (**Fig. 6**).

Another challenge is devising the optimal methods for combining metabolite signals from multiple channels afforded from parallel techniques while preserving sensitive phase information. Spectra from each coil can be combined with weighting factors, such as deriving from the first point of the unsuppressed water-free

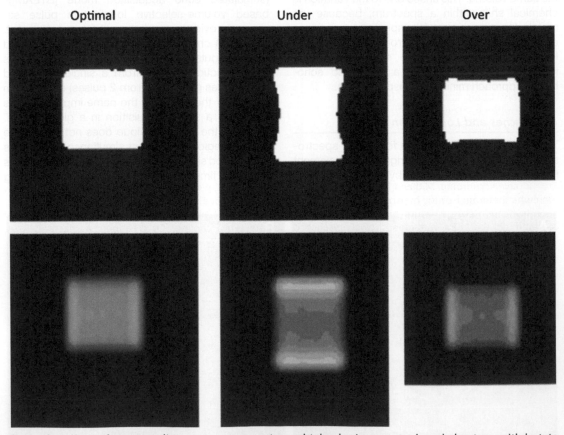

Fig. 6. The effects of power scaling on a proton spectrum obtained using a water-based phantom, with lactate, NAA, Glu, Cr, Cho, and mI included. The optimization of pulse power during prescan optimizes localization and water suppression. When values are not optimized, the voxel location can be distorted. Two window scalings are displayed in this figure. Optimal, Under and Over refer to power scaling for voxel delineation.

induction decay signal from each coil, or other schemes, such as SENSE sensitivity encoding for fast MR imaging,[18] and nonparametric, semiparametric, and parametric processing tools with available prior knowledge.[19]

POSTPROCESSING

In clinical settings, metabolite ratios are often used both for SVS or MRSI rather than obtaining absolute metabolite concentrations due to variations in magnetic field homogeneity, radiofrequency coil homogeneity and patient loading, susceptibility of tissues, composition of tissues, and changes in the receiver gain, which are not easily accounted for given the time constraints of imaging a patient in a typical clinical MR imaging scanner. Often the internal Cr signal is used as the reference metabolite, because both Cr and phosphocreatine are sampled on proton MRS. Although it is recognized that many pathologies (neoplasms, infarcts, and metabolic diseases) may have alterations in the Cr and phosphocreatine concentration, Cr is among the primary 3 metabolites (NAA, Cr, and Cho) the most consistent for the majority of conditions.

Each MR imaging manufacturer supplies software on the scanner or workstation that uses various algorithms to treat the raw data with zero-filling, line broadening, eddy current corrections; Fourier transformation; phasing; baseline correction; peak fitting; and intensity and area approximations. These software packages are either fully automated, with no selection of parameters, or semiautomated, requiring a technologist to select a postprocessing protocol where parameters can be modified. These software packages are acceptable postprocessing for clinical MRS within an institution or for comparison with similar scanners. If more rigorous determinations of concentration are necessary, however, there are other widely recognized software packages that work with data from the major clinical MR imaging vendors. Linear combination of modeled spectra[20] (LCModel) is a commercially available software package that compares a library of model spectra with the user's proton MRS data in frequency domain (meaning data are analyzed after Fourier transformation). The model spectra in the LCModel library are obtained from either in vitro solutions of individual metabolites using the same field strength, pulse sequence, and other general parameters or via computer simulations.[21] This software allows for the entire spectrum to be modeled simultaneously. Vendor software usually performs fitting on individual peaks independent of the relationship with other peaks from the same molecule within the spectrum. With the known concentrations from the model metabolite solutions, the LCModel software can be thought of as mixing and matching various combinations of the pure metabolite spectra to fit a user's spectral data. This software allows concentration estimates to be generated almost instantaneously but requires extra off-line processing with extracting the raw spectral data and exporting to a separate workstation, because the software is not usually installed on the scanner.

Although LCModel can fit short-echo and long-echo spectra, a freely downloadable software package, known as jMRUI, can provide spectral processing of long-echo proton MRS data in the time domain (meaning data are decay signals measured in seconds before Fourier transformation).[22,23] With jMRUI, user data are fitted using prior knowledge of frequencies, line widths, coupling patterns, and so forth. The software allows editing of unwanted signals, such as artifacts or water. LCModel and jMRUI provide not only signal intensity estimates but also a measure of the quality of the fitting with the Cramér-Rao lower bound as an error estimate. Although these software packages are improvements over vendor-supplied software, they do not fully obtain absolute concentrations. Users often report the levels of a metabolite in institutional units. This could mean the output from LCModel untouched or treated with additional corrections, such as CSF correction, relaxation rate corrections, tissue composition, and so forth. The literature provides details about performing additional corrections for proton MRS quantification.[24–26] The author reminds readers not to be discouraged if only vendor-supplied software is available. Qualitative and semiquantitative interpretation of MRS is usually sufficient to support a diagnosis. At the same time, monitoring certain therapeutic responses requires a more rigorous, research style of quantitation.

INTERPRETATION

The interpretation of an MR spectrum primarily arises from variations in chemical ratios and/or concentrations, which alter peak area for the endogenous metabolites, and the appearance of pathologic metabolites (lactate, alanine, and so forth) and exogenous compounds (ie, propanediol and mannitol) if administered.

The 3 main metabolite entities, NAA, Cr, and Cho, are commonly observed independent of TE and standard localization technique. The key metabolites observed with proton MRS are discussed according to their spectral locations (relative to water located at 4.7 ppm) with their known roles briefly described further later.

The NAA Resonance

NAA and *N*-acetylaspartylglutamate (NAAG) appear at 2.0 ppm. NAA comprises a majority of the NAA resonance found on neurospectroscopy. Regional variations of NAA and NAAG, the other primary component of the resonance, have been reported.[27] NAA is second only to Glu as the most abundant free amino acid in the adult brain.[28] Although discovered by Tallan in 1956, the function of this amino acid is not fully known.[29,30] Studies in the developing rat brain show that NAA is synthesized in the mitochondria from aspartate and acetyl coenzyme A.[31] After transport across the mitochondrial membrane, it is cleaved in the cytosol by aspartoacylase into aspartate and acetate.[32] This suggests NAA may function as a transporter of acetyl groups across the mitochondrial membrane for lipogenesis during development.[33] NAA is almost exclusively localized to neurons, however. It is found in cell cultures of oligodendroglia progenitors but absent from mature glial cells, CSF, and blood.[34,35]

Studies[36] indicate other possible roles for NAA:

1. NAA may operate as neuronal osmolyte, serving as a cotransport substrate for a molecular water pump removing excess water from neurons.
2. NAA plays a role in neuronal energy metabolism of mitochondria and specific brain fatty acids.
3. NAA provides a reservoir for Glu.[37]
4. NAA serves as a substrate for NAAG biosynthesis.

NAAG, a dipeptide derivative of NAA and Glu, is the most abundant brain peptide. With a concentration of approximately 1 mM, NAAG is found in neurons, oligodendrocytes, and microglia. NAAG signals astrocytes about the state of neurostimulation of the neurons' changing requirements for vascular energy supplies and metabolic waste removal.

The NAA resonance is widely regarded as a marker for neuronal injury and death.[38] A majority of pathologic conditions and diseases demonstrate reduced NAA. A leukodystrophy in which NAA is elevated is Canavan disease. NAA accumulation in the mitochondria arises when a genetic defect affects aspartoacylase, which is responsible for transporting NAA into the cytosol. It may also be elevated in Pelizaeus-Merzbacher disease, Salla disease, and hypermetabolic conditions. There is one reported incidence of a patient without brain NAA.[39]

The Cr Resonance

Cr and phosphocreatine appear at 3.0 ppm and 3.9 ppm. For interested readers, Wyss and Kaddurah-Daouk[40] published a comprehensive review of Cr and creatinine metabolism. Cr and phosphocreatine are compounds involved in the regulation of cellular energy metabolism. Phosphocreatine serves as a reserve for high-energy phosphates in the cytosol of muscle and neurons and buffers cellular ATP/ADP reservoirs.[41] The enzyme, creatine kinase, converts Cr to phosphocreatine using ATP. Although regarded as an internal standard, it has been demonstrated in certain pathologies, such as stroke, tumor, and head injury, to be reduced as well as absent in Cr deficiency syndromes.

The Cho Resonance

Cho compounds—choline, acetylcholine, phosphocholine, cytidine diphosphate choline, and glycerophosphocholine composite—appear at 3.2 ppm. MRS detects the trimethylammonium residues of choline itself and mobile Cho-containing compounds. Changes in the Cho level are inherently linked to membrane biochemistry. Cho is regarded as a product of myelin breakdown. Cell proliferation associated with tumor growth is responsible for the elevation in Cho observed by proton MRS. Mobile Cho-containing compounds contribute to the Cho signal. These primarily include the intracellular pools of the membrane precursor phosphocholine, membrane breakdown product GPC (glycerophosphocholine), and a small portion (5%) of free Cho for an approximate total observable Cho concentration approximating 1 mM to 2 mM. Although phosphatyidylcholine is a major membrane constituent produced in all cells, it does not contribute significantly to the observable Cho signal. For white matter diseases, elevations of the resonance reflect the precursors of myelin synthesis as well as the degradation products on myelin degradation and/or destruction. Increased Cho levels observed in tumors arise from increased cellular density and proliferation of membrane phospholipids.[42]

On short-echo MRS (TE 35 ms or less), elevations of lipids, macromolecules, neurotransmitters, mI, and lactate can be appreciated in vivo because these metabolites have short T2 values at commonly encountered field strengths (1.5 T, 3 T, and 4 T).

The mI Resonance

mI, mI-monophosphate, and glycine appear at 3.5 ppm. mI is important because it may relate to intracellular sodium content and glial activation. Changes in mI levels have been correlated with osmolarity conditions in the brain.[43] The mI resonance at 3.5 ppm is largely comprised of mI

(5 mM concentration in the brain) along with mI-monophosphate and the α-protons of glycine.[44] In the brain, mI is also believed primarily located in glial cells and absent from neurons.[34] Elevations of mI may be attributed to gliosis and reactive astrocytosis in certain pathologies.

The Amino Acid Peaks

Gln, Glu, γ-aminobutyric acid (GABA), and aspartate form a composite set of peaks between 2.2 ppm and 2.6 ppm with additional components at 3.6 ppm. In addition, glucose (Glc) has peaks at 3.43 ppm and 3.80 ppm. Glu is a neurotransmitter and is the most abundant amino acid in the human brain. Gln is found primarily in cerebral astrocytes. Gln is the primary derivative for Glu. Increases in the composite of Glu and Gln (referred to as GLX) are indications of destructive processes. Glc dominates the fuel supply for brain in accordance with blood flow. Increases in Glc concentration have been reported in cases of diabetes mellitus and hypoxic encephalopathy. GABA is an important inhibitory neurotransmitter derived from Glu via decarboxylation with its ultimate source considered Gln.

The Lipid, Acetate and Macromolecular Protein Peaks

Lipids have broad multiple peaks at 0.8 ppm and 1.3 ppm, which include acetate and macromolecular proteins. Macromolecules have multiple peaks centered at 0.9 ppm, 2.05 ppm, and 3.0 ppm. Lipids are shown to be elevated, as are lactate and alanine in a variety of tumors. The significance of the macromolecule peaks is less certain, but changes in the levels are associated with stroke, multiple sclerosis, and tumors.[45] Membrane changes may be reflected by alterations in lipid levels. In neonatal rats, macromolecule peaks were present before myelination occurred. In the pediatric brain, regions sampled before myelination demonstrate elevated lipid signals.

The Lactate Resonance

The lactate resonance is a doublet at 1.3 ppm. The lactate resonance, demonstrated in proton MR spectroscopy, represents the endpoint of anaerobic glycolysis. In pathologies, such as stroke, high-grade tumors, and abscess, this finding is consistent with understanding of each of the biochemical processes taking place in the body. The presence of lactate in low-grade tumors without regions of necrosis and other metabolic disorders, however, is explained as alterations in metabolism to provide alternative energetic pathways. It is sometimes necessary to differentiate lactate from lipid/macromolecule peaks in short-echo MRS studies. The interaction of the lactate methyl and methine proton peaks (occurs at 7 Hz), referred to as J-coupling, provides for a distinct double-peak (doublet) pattern and location indicative of lactate in long-echo proton MRS studies. Using long TEs, such as 144 ms and 288 ms (multiples of 1/7 Hz), lactate can be distinguished from lipid signals. Sampling with a TE of 144 ms inverts the resonance below the baseline due to spin or J-coupling. Although this distinguishes the lactate doublet peak from macromolecules and lipids, the signal intensity is diminished, which is especially problematic in low concentrations (approximately 5 mM or less) and within some technical circumstances (ie, errors in pulse generation and reception).[46] The doublet peak emerges above the baseline at a TE of 288 ms. The peak should primarily represent lactate. Technical issues with signal transmission and reception may cause the doublet to be asymmetric. Shimming problems may broaden the signal so as to smooth the doublet. At a TE of 288 ms, if the signal arises from lipids, it should correspond anatomically with high signal from fat on imaging; otherwise, it likely represents lactate. The appearance of lactate is pathologic because it classically represents anaerobic glycolysis. Lactate signal may also possibly reflect mitochondrial impairment as an inflammatory response and macrophage infiltration depending on the condition.

Contrast-enhanced sequences are frequently a vital component of MR imaging studies, especially in neoplastic and infectious diseases. If proton MRS can be performed before contrast administration, the likelihood of diagnostic spectra is improved over MRS obtained after contrast administration. Gadolinium-based contrast agents that quickly accumulate in a lesion can broaden line widths to the degree where the spectra are not diagnostic. In a study of adult brain tumors, however, in which proton MRS was acquired both before and after contrast administration, a blinded review failed to show a significant difference in the MR spectroscopic diagnosis related to the presence of contrast. Individual ratios changed pre versus post contrast administration; however, no systemic change was appreciated in the study. Thus, MRS should not be abandoned if the only option is to obtain spectra after contrast administration.

NORMAL DEVELOPMENT

During the first 2 to 3 years of brain development, metabolite levels vary primarily due to the myelination process.[47] Defining normal metabolite concentration levels is heavily dependent on the

MRS technique and operating parameters. Most sites either develop their own normative databases or rely on the literature and the work of others because automated MRS acquisition protocols allow MRS acquisitions to be more closely replicated between sites. In both adult and pediatric settings, differences in metabolite levels are also found between gray and white matter as well as between the different lobes of the brain (frontal vs occipital).[48]

NORMAL AGING

During the last decades of life (>60 years), there is an observable and region-specific reduction in brain tissue volume with age. With this volume loss, metabolite changes are expected with the typical aging process. Haga and colleagues[49] reviewed the literature for studies evaluating healthy aging with proton MRS. Beginning with 231 potentially relevant studies, a meta-analysis identified, from 4 studies with extractable metabolite data, a decrease in frontal NAA levels approaching significance and significant increases in parietal Cho and Cr levels. The investigators identified the need for large-scale studies with rigorous approaches for defining healthy participants, and advanced processing approaches such as performing tissue segmentation and reporting absolute metabolite concentrations in multiple brain regions.

PROTOCOLS
Diffuse Disorders, Disorders Without Focal Lesions: Location and Echo Times

Diffuse disorders, especially those without focal lesions, can be assessed using either SVS or MRSI approaches. The choice should be based on the available software, skill, and experience of the technologists at the institution for the given approach.

A standard MRS location sampled for gray matter assessment in infants and children includes the left basal ganglia composed of the caudate, internal capsule, globus pallidus, and putamen, with minimal inclusion of the thalamus. As children become adolescents, iron deposition within the basal ganglia widens the spectral peaks, which may affect quantitation. At this point, the standard MRS location is often across the hemispheres within the parasagittal cortex of the occipital or parietal lobes.

A standard location chosen to assess myelination and white matter disorders is the frontal lobe for pediatric populations. Sampling within this region inevitably has some gray matter involvement. For practical purposes, all of the metabolite

levels, other than Cho, remain unaffected with this mixture of composition. In adults, sampling within the centrum semiovale is appropriate. A key pitfall of these locations is the inclusion of the lateral ventricles, which results in a selective decrease in the Cr signal. This change artificially elevates metabolite ratios.

If radiologists were asked to perform only one MR imaging sequence to evaluate a patient, a variety of opinions would be expressed. For spectroscopists, the same analogy is found when asking which one TE should be acquired within an MRS examination. Short-echo MRS affords many more metabolites, which ultimately are useful in diagnosis. The baseline, however, is not as flat as the MRS acquired with long-echo sequences. Thus, the spectral fitting and interpretation are more complex. The flatter baseline is also a key reason why MRSI usually uses long-echo pulse sequences. The long-echo sequence is primarily heralded for its ability to demonstrate lactate peaks. To answer the question of which echo to use if only one is allowed, the short-echo MRS is the preferred approach by the author of this article, especially for SVS studies, because useful changes in the peaks with short T2 values are often found that are absent on long-echo studies.

Focal Lesions

Sampling within focal lesions is straightforward; however, there are some pitfalls to be aware of in the process. Again, the SVS or MRSI approach and choice of TE are site dependent. For most scenarios, the ideal protocol uses a short-echo SVS sequence followed by a long-echo sequence, either a 144-ms or 288-ms TE MRSI with inclusion of the focal lesion, adjacent parenchyma, and, when possible, the contralateral hemisphere. This approach provides for a full complement of metabolite sampling, determining lesion extent and providing an internal comparison. Focal lesions that are very small or likely need reproducible follow-up over time (such as a demyelinating lesion) should be studied with an MRSI approach because this method is not as technically demanding with respect to precise voxel positioning because it can allow for voxel shifting in postprocessing procedures and produce very small voxel sizes. If MRSI is not in use at a site, SVS is usually performed with voxel dimensions of approximately 1.5 cm per side (a total volume of 4–8 cm^3 should be maintained, so 1 voxel dimension could potentially be as small as 1 cm whereas others are 2 cm or larger). Although partial voluming with unaffected parenchyma adjacent to the focal lesion may occur, significant changes in Cho or other metabolite levels can usually be appreciated, especially if a separate reference SVS is acquired in the contralateral hemisphere at an equivalent symmetric location.

In some pediatric patients with cerebral abscess, sampling within the core of the lesion can be accomplished to visualize succinate, acetate, valine, and other amino acids. In adults, however, the central core of an abscess is usually necrotic. Cerebral abscess and regions with large necrotic portions, such as high-grade gliomas, can be technically challenging due to large lipid peaks altering shimming and quantification of other metabolites. For qualitative assessment, the Y-axis scale of the spectrum is usually automatically matched to visualize the height of the largest peak. (Some manufacturers provide a scale for qualitative comparison, but others do not.) In a necrotic pathology, the lipid peak often becomes the largest peak in the spectrum.

SUMMARY

The goal of this article is to explain the principals behind proton MRS in a practical fashion. Understanding the principals behind proton MRS can provide exceptional benefit to neuroradiologists when MRS is applied in the clinical setting.

REFERENCES

1. Drost DJ, Riddle WR, Clarke GD. Proton magnetic resonance spectroscopy in the brain: report of AAPM MR Task Group #9. Med Phys 2002;29(9): 2177–97.
2. Zhu H, Barker PB. MR spectroscopy and spectroscopic imaging of the brain. Methods Mol Biol 2011;711:203–26.
3. Di Costanzo A, Trojsi F, Tosetti M, et al. High-field proton MRS of human brain. Eur J Radiol 2003; 48(2):146–53.
4. Tran T, Ross B, Lin A. Magnetic resonance spectroscopy in neurological diagnosis. Neurol Clin 2009; 27(1):21–60, xiii.
5. Srinivasan R, Vigneron D, Sailasuta N, et al. A comparative study of myo-inositol quantification using LCmodel at 1.5 T and 3.0 T with 3 D 1H proton spectroscopic imaging of the human brain. Magn Reson Imaging 2004;22(4):523–8.
6. Kreis R. Issues of spectral quality in clinical 1H-magnetic resonance spectroscopy and a gallery of artifacts. NMR Biomed 2004;17(6):361–81.
7. Posse S, Cuenod CA, Risinger R, et al. Anomalous transverse relaxation in 1H spectroscopy in human brain at 4 Tesla. Magn Reson Med 1995;33(2):246–52.
8. Hetherington HP, Mason GF, Pan JW, et al. Evaluation of cerebral gray and white matter metabolite differences by spectroscopic imaging at 4.1T. Magn Reson Med 1994;32(5):565–71.
9. Barker PB, Hearshen DO, Boska MD. Single-voxel proton MRS of the human brain at 1.5T and 3.0T. Magn Reson Med 2001;45(5):765–9.
10. Bartha R, Drost DJ, Menon RS, et al. Comparison of the quantification precision of human short echo time (1)H spectroscopy at 1.5 and 4.0 Tesla. Magn Reson Med 2000;44(2):185–92.
11. Gruetter R. Automatic, localized in vivo adjustment of all first- and second-order shim coils. Magn Reson Med 1993;29(6):804–11.
12. Haase A, Frahm J, Hanicke W, et al. 1H NMR chemical shift selective (CHESS) imaging. Phys Med Biol 1985;30(4):341–4.
13. Ogg RJ, Kingsley PB, Taylor JS. WET, a T1- and B1-insensitive water-suppression method for in vivo localized 1H NMR spectroscopy. J Magn Reson B 1994;104(1):1–10.
14. Tkac I, Starcuk Z, Choi IY, et al. In vivo 1H NMR spectroscopy of rat brain at 1 ms echo time. Magn Reson Med 1999;41(4):649–56.
15. Duyn JH, Gillen J, Sobering G, et al. Multisection proton MR spectroscopic imaging of the brain. Radiology 1993;188(1):277–82.
16. Tran TK, Vigneron DB, Sailasuta N, et al. Very selective suppression pulses for clinical MRSI studies of brain and prostate cancer. Magn Reson Med 2000; 43(1):23–33.
17. Osorio JA, Xu D, Cunningham CH, et al. Design of cosine modulated very selective suppression pulses for MR spectroscopic imaging at 3T. Magn Reson Med 2009;61(3):533–40.
18. Pruessmann KP, Weiger M, Scheidegger MB, et al. SENSE: sensitivity encoding for fast MRI. Magn Reson Med 1999;42(5):952–62.
19. Sandgren N, Stoica P, Frigo FJ, et al. Spectral analysis of multichannel MRS data. J Magn Reson 2005; 175(1):79–91.
20. Provencher SW. Automatic quantitation of localized in vivo 1H spectra with LCModel. NMR Biomed 2001;14(4):260–4.
21. Provencher SW. Estimation of metabolite concentrations from localized in vivo proton NMR spectra. Magn Reson Med 1993;30(6):672–9.
22. Naressi A, Couturier C, Devos JM, et al. Java-based graphical user interface for the MRUI quantitation package. MAGMA 2001;12(2–3):141–52.
23. Naressi A, Couturier C, Castang I, et al. Java-based graphical user interface for MRUI, a software package for quantitation of in vivo/medical magnetic resonance spectroscopy signals. Comput Biol Med 2001;31(4):269–86.

24. Barantin L, Le Pape A, Akoka S. A new method for absolute quantitation of MRS metabolites. Magn Reson Med 1997;38(2):179–82.

25. Henriksen O. In vivo quantitation of metabolite concentrations in the brain by means of proton MRS. NMR Biomed 1995;8(4):139–48.

26. Soher BJ, van Zijl PC, Duyn JH, et al. Quantitative proton MR spectroscopic imaging of the human brain. Magn Reson Med 1996;35(3):356–63.

27. Pouwels PJ, Frahm J. Differential distribution of NAA and NAAG in human brain as determined by quantitative localized proton MRS. NMR Biomed 1997;10: 73–8.

28. Matalon R, Michals K, Sebesta D, et al. Aspartoacylase deficiency and N-acetylaspartic aciduria in patients with Canavan disease. Am J Med Genet 1988;29(2):463–71.

29. Tallan HH, Moore S, Stein WH. N-acetyl-L-aspartic acid in brain. J Biol Chem 1956;219:257–64.

30. Tallan HH. Studies on the distribution of N-acetyl-L-aspartic acid in brain. J Biol Chem 1956;224:41–5.

31. Benuck M, D'Adamo JA. Acetyl transport mechanisms. Metabolism of N-acetyl-L-aspartic acid in the non-nervous tissues of the rat. Biochim Biophys Acta 1968;152(3):611–8.

32. D'Adamo AF Jr, Smith JC, Woiler C. The occurrence of N-acetylaspartate amidohydrolase (Aminoacylase II) in the developing rat. J Neurochem 1973; 20:1275–8.

33. Austin SJ, Connelly A, Gadian DG, et al. Localized 1H NMR spectroscopy in Canavan's disease: a report of two cases. Magn Reson Med 1991;19:439–45.

34. Brand A, Richter-Landsberg C, Leibfritz D. Multinuclear NMR studies on the energy metabolism of glial and neuronal cells. Dev Neurosci 1993;15(3–5): 289–98.

35. Urenjak J, Williams SR, Gadian DG, et al. Specific expression of N-acetylaspartate in neurons, oligodendrocyte- type-2 astrocyte progenitors, and immature oligodendrocytes in vitro. J Neurochem 1992;59(1):55–61.

36. Moffett JR, Tieman SB, Weinberger DR, et al. N-Acetylaspartate: a unique neuronal molecule in the central nervous system. New York: Springer; 2006.

37. Clark JF, Doepke A, Filosa JA, et al. N-acetylaspartate as a reservoir for glutamate. Med Hypotheses 2006;67(3):506–12.

38. Birken DL, Oldendorf WH. N-acetyl-L-aspartic acid: a literature review of a compound prominent in 1H-NMR spectroscopic studies of brain. Neurosci Biobehav Rev 1989;13(1):23–31.

39. Martin E, Capone A, Schneider J, et al. Absence of N-acetylaspartate in the human brain: impact on neurospectroscopy? Ann Neurol 2001;49(4):518–21.

40. Wyss M, Kaddurah-Daouk R. Creatine and creatinine metabolism. Physiol Rev 2000;80(3):1107–213.

41. Miller B. A review of chemical issues in 1H NMR spectroscopy: N-Acetyl-L-aspartate, creatine and choline. NMR Biomed 1991;4:47–52.

42. Stork C, Renshaw PF. Mitochondrial dysfunction in bipolar disorder: evidence from magnetic resonance spectroscopy research. Mol Psychiatry 2005;10(10): 900–19.

43. Lee J, Arcinue E, Ross B. Organic osmolytes in the brain of an infant with hypernatremia. N Engl J Med 1994;331:439–42.

44. Ross BD. Biochemical considerations in 1H spectroscopy. Glutamate and glutamine; Myo-inositol and related metabolites. NMR Biomed 1991;4:59–63.

45. Petroff OA, Pleban LA, Spencer DD. Symbiosis between in vivo and in vitro NMR spectroscopy: the creatine, N-acetylaspartate, glutamate, and GABA content of the epileptic human brain. Magn Reson Imaging 1995;13(8):1197–211.

46. Lange T, Dydak U, Roberts TP, et al. Pitfalls in lactate measurements at 3T. AJNR Am J Neuroradiol 2006; 27(4):895–901.

47. Kreis R, Ernst T, Ross BD. Development of the human brain: in vivo quantification of metabolite and water content with proton magnetic resonance spectroscopy. Magn Reson Med 1993;30(4):424–37.

48. Pouwels PJ, Frahm J. Regional metabolite concentrations in human brain as determined by quantitative localized proton MRS. Magn Reson Med 1998; 39:53–60.

49. Haga KK, Khor YP, Farrall A, et al. A systematic review of brain metabolite changes, measured with 1H magnetic resonance spectroscopy, in healthy aging. Neurobiol Aging 2009;30(3):353–63.

Magnetic Resonance Spectroscopy in Common Dementias

Kejal Kantarci, MD, MS

KEYWORDS

- Magnetic resonance spectroscopy • Dementias • Alzheimer's disease • *N*-Acetylaspartate
- Mild cognitive impairment

KEY POINTS

- Neurodegenerative dementia is characterized by elevated myoinositol and decreased *N*-acetylaspartate (NAA) levels.
- The increase in myoinositol seems to precede decreasing NAA levels in Alzheimer's disease.
- NAA/*myo*-inositol ratio in the posterior cingulate gyri decreases with increasing burden of Alzheimer's disease pathologic conditions.
- Proton magnetic resonance spectroscopy (^{1}H MRS) is sensitive to the pathophysiologic processes associated with the risk of dementia in patients with mild cognitive impairment.
- Although significant progress has been made in improving the acquisition and analysis techniques in ^{1}H MRS, translation of these technical developments to clinical practice have not been effective because of the lack of standardization for multisite applications and normative data and an insufficient understanding of the pathologic basis of ^{1}H MRS metabolite changes.

INTRODUCTION

Aging is the primary risk factor for dementia. With increasing life expectancy and the aging populations around the world, dementia is becoming a significant public health problem of the century. The most common pathologic condition underlying dementia in older adults is Alzheimer's disease (AD). Cerebrovascular disease and Lewy body disease pathologic conditions are other common causes of dementia in the elderly, and in many instances AD is also present in patients with dementia with Lewy bodies (DLB) and vascular dementia. A relatively less common type of dementia is frontotemporal lobar degeneration, which tends to affect younger individuals compared with other dementia pathologies. The focus of this article is potential role of proton magnetic resonance spectroscopy (^{1}H MRS) in these common dementias.

MRS IN AD

Initial MRS studies in AD were limited to phosphorous magnetic resonance spectroscopy (^{31}P MRS) revealing alterations in membrane phospholipid metabolism.[1–4] In 1992, Klunk and colleagues[4] demonstrated the decrease in the neuronal metabolite *N*-acetylaspartate (NAA) on ^{1}H MRS using perchloric acid extracts from brains from persons with AD. Soon after, an in vivo MRS study revealed elevated *myo*-inositol/creatine (mI/Cr) levels in patients with AD along with decreased NAA/Cr.[5] Further investigations in patients with AD confirmed this finding (**Fig. 1**).[6–17] Many of these early studies also revealed that the increase in mI/Cr and

Grant Support: Dr Kantarci's research program is supported by National Institutes of Health grants R01 AG40042, P50 AG16574/Project1, and R21 NS066147.
Division of Neuroradiology, Department of Radiology, Mayo Clinic, 200 First Street Southwest, Rochester, MN 55905, USA
E-mail address: kantarci.kejal@mayo.edu

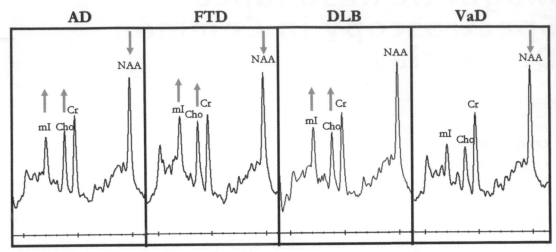

Fig. 1. Posterior cingulate gyrus voxel ^{1}H MRS findings in common dementia syndromes. AD, Alzheimer's disease; DLB, dementia with Lewy bodies; FTD, frontotemporal dementia; VaD, vascular dementia.

decrease in NAA/Cr in AD were not associated with a change in Cr using absolute quantification methods.[10,11,14,18–21] For this reason. Cr is commonly used as an internal reference in MRS studies of AD to account for individual and acquisition related variability. There have been conflicting reports on choline (Cho) levels in AD. Some studies found elevated Cho or Cho/Cr levels,[8,9,12] whereas others found no changes in Cho or Cho/Cr levels in AD.[10,13,19,20] Decreased glutamate plus glutamine levels have been found in several studies of AD.[22,23]

Regional alterations of ^{1}H MRS metabolites in patients with AD seem to be widespread,[8,24] involving the parietal,[25,26] medial and lateral temporal,[7,20,27] and frontal lobes.[17,25] Furthermore, decreases in NAA or NAA/Cr correlate with dementia severity,[6,28] cognitive function,[29,30] and behavioral and psychiatric symptoms,[31,32] indicating that NAA is a marker for AD severity on various clinical features.

Most of the ^{1}H MRS studies in AD have used single-voxel ^{1}H MRS. Choice of the single-voxel ^{1}H MRS region for detecting and monitoring metabolite levels in AD depends on both the pathophysiology of AD and the technical considerations. The neurofibrillary pathologic conditions of AD and associated neuronal loss involve medial temporal lobes earlier and more severely than other regions of the brain. Although ^{1}H MRS from the medial temporal lobe or hippocampus yields spectra of reasonable quality using long echo times (TE = 130–272 milliseconds), it may be more difficult to achieve MR spectra of consistent quality from the hippocampus using short echo times required for quantification of the ml peak (TE <35 milliseconds).[33,34] At 4 T using

adiabatic selective refocusing for localization and TE of 46 milliseconds, it was possible to measure decreased glutamate levels from the hippocampus in AD.[35] Another region that is commonly investigated in single voxel MRS studies of AD is the posterior cingulate gyrus voxel. Posterior cingulate gyrus is severely involved with the β-amyloid (Aβ) pathologic condition of AD[36] and ^{18}F fluorodeoxyglucose positron emission tomography (PET) studies suggest that the synaptic activity is reduced in this region very early in the disease process such as in cognitively normal carriers of the *APOE ε4* allele who are at a higher risk for AD than noncarriers.[37,38] Recently, it was demonstrated that posterior cingulate gyrus is the hub for the resting state connectivity networks on task-free functional MRI, which are affected by AD early in the disease course.[39] It is possible to consistently obtain acceptable-quality short-echo time MR spectra from the posterior cingulate gyrus voxel for quantification of ml levels, which is critical for longitudinal evaluations and multisite studies.[34]

Human tissue studies in transgenic mouse models of AD have provided some insight into the pathologic underpinnings of decreased NAA and glutamate levels and increased ml levels, which closely resemble the metabolic abnormalities observed in patients with AD.[40–44] For example, lower NAA and glutamate levels were associated with Aβ plaque load in mice with *PS2APP* mutation.[44] Magic angle spinning ^{1}H MRS in superior temporal cortex tissue from patients with AD showed a correlation between NAA concentration and neuronal density.[41] Recently, an in vivo ^{13}carbon (^{13}C)-MRS and ^{1}H MRS study suggested a link between increased glial or microglial activation and mI elevation in AD.[45]

Our investigation of pathologic correlates of MRS metabolite changes in 54 cases with varying degrees of AD pathologic conditions demonstrated that both NAA/Cr and mI/Cr levels measured antemortem are associated with the pathologic classification of AD severity.[46] Whereas mI/Cr ratio was elevated at earlier stages of pathologic involvement (ie, intermediate likelihood AD), NAA/Cr levels were decreased only at the late stage of pathologic involvement (ie, high likelihood AD). A combined ratio of the 2 metabolites as the NAA/mI, however, revealed the strongest association with pathologic

severity, suggesting that both NAA and mI provide complementary information on AD pathologic conditions (**Fig. 2**).

Longitudinal MRS studies in patients with AD demonstrate gradually decreasing NAA, NAA/Cr, and NAA/mI levels compared with controls.[47–49] The changes in NAA and NAA/Cr also correlate with the cognitive decline.[48,50] Although the data are limited, no study has yet reported a longitudinal increase in mI or mI/Cr levels in patients with AD. The reasons may be 2-fold: (1) lower reliability of mI quantification compared with NAA[48,51,52] and (2) stage of the AD pathologic process. If the elevation of mI is an early event in the pathologic

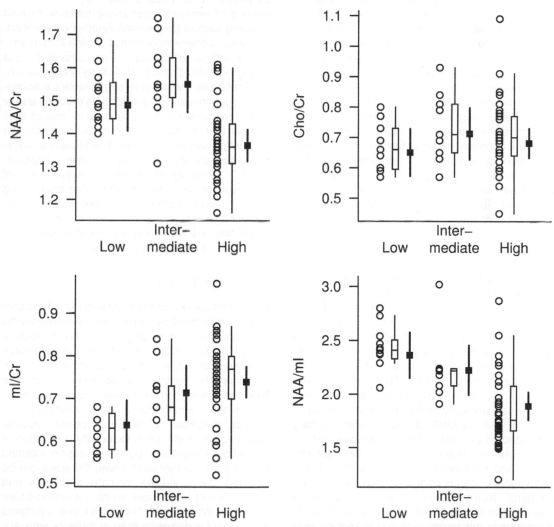

Fig. 2. Posterior cingulate gyrus voxel ^{1}H MRS findings by pathologic diagnosis of AD. The pathologic diagnosis of AD is classified as a low, intermediate, and high likelihood of AD. For each pathologic diagnosis, the plot shows individual values, a box plot of the distribution, and the estimated mean and 95% CI for the mean. The strongest association was observed with the NAA/mI ratio ($R_N^2 = 0.40$). (*From* Kantarci K, Knopman DS, Dickson DW, et al. Alzheimer disease: postmortem neuropathologic correlates of antemortem 1H MR spectroscopy metabolite measurements. Radiology 2008;248:210–20; with permission.)

progression of AD, it is possible that a plateau is reached in the ml elevation toward the later stages of the pathologic process, which remains to be investigated.

The applications of MRS as a biomarker for treatment response in clinical trials have been limited to single-site studies. The change in NAA/Cr correlated with the change on the Alzheimer's Disease Assessment Scale, cognitive part scores during a cholinesterase inhibitor treatment trial.[53] Short-term or temporary increases in NAA/Cr and Glu/Cr was observed in cholinesterase inhibitor–treated AD patients versus placebo[54–56] and one trial found no effect on NAA/Cr ratio but found a decrease in Cho/Cr and ml/Cr ratios in the hippocampus, albeit in the absence of cognitive response.[57] Overall, MRS seems to be a feasible biomarker in single-site clinical trials in AD. Efforts to extend these applications to multisite clinical trials are under way.[33,51] Larger sample sizes may be needed for MRS compared with structural MRI measurements (eg, hippocampal volumes) to detect a similar effect size.[49] However, effect sizes of a single treatment may differ among imaging markers of different pathophysiologic processes. For example, a treatment that improves neuronal function may dramatically improve NAA levels but not significantly alter atrophy rates. Therefore, effects of the intervention should be considered when comparing imaging markers of different biologic sensitivity on sample size and power.

MRS IN DLB

The presence of Lewy bodies in substantia nigra is the pathologic feature of Parkinson's disease. Although cortical Lewy bodies can occasionally be detected in Parkinson's disease, cortical Lewy bodies presenting with dementia is recognized as DLB, a distinct neurodegenerative disease with established clinical and pathologic criteria.[58] DLB is frequently accompanied by AD in patients with dementia.[59] Lewy body pathologic condition by itself is less common than the mixed (AD and DLB) type.[60] In our ^{1}H MRS series, patients clinically diagnosed as probable DLB have normal NAA/Cr levels, whereas patients with AD, vascular dementia, and frontotemporal dementia have lower NAA/Cr levels than normal, in the posterior cingulate gyri.[61] Normal NAA/Cr levels in the posterior cingulate gyri in patients with DLB suggest integrity of neurons in this region, which is in keeping with the preserved neuronal numbers found in the neocortex of DLB patients at autopsy.[60] Normal neocortical NAA or NAA/Cr levels may be useful in distinguishing patients with DLB from those with other dementia syndromes. Reduced NAA/Cr

has been detected in the hippocampi of patients with DLB[62]; however, many patients with DLB may have hippocampal atrophy because of the presence of concomitant neurofibrillary tangle pathologic conditions of AD,[63] making it hard to determine whether the low NAA/Cr levels in DLB is associated with the coexistent AD pathologic conditions. One study found reduced white matter NAA/Cr in patients with DLB compared with the control group, suggesting white matter involvement in DLB.[64] The white matter involvement in DLB was later confirmed with diffusion tensor imaging studies.[65,66]

We found elevated Cho/Cr in the posterior cingulate gyri of patients with DLB (see **Fig. 1**). Elevation of Cho in DLB and AD may be the consequence of increased membrane turnover caused by dying back of the neuropil. Another explanation, however, is down-regulation of choline acetyltransferase activity, which may be responsible for this change in both AD and DLB. Activity of choline acetyltransferase, the enzyme responsible for acetylcholine synthesis from free Cho, is reduced earlier and more severely in the disease course of DLB than in that of AD.[67] Furthermore, patients with DLB who were treated with cholinesterase inhibitors have shown substantial cognitive improvement,[68] revealing the functional significance of acetylcholine deficiency in DLB. The finding that Cho/Cr levels decrease with cholinergic agonist treatment in AD[69] raises the possibility that Cho/Cr levels may be a biomarker of therapeutic efficacy in both AD and DLB treatment trials.

MRS IN VASCULAR DEMENTIA

Cerebrovascular disease is another common pathologic condition observed in patients with dementia in autopsy series. In most cases, however, vascular pathologic conditions coexist with the pathologic conditions of AD, and a pure vascular pathologic condition is relatively uncommon.[70] Vascular lesions are more common in patients with dementia than in the normal elderly.[71] In a patient with the clinical diagnosis of AD and cerebrovascular disease, the challenge is to identify how much, if any, of the 2 pathologic conditions are contributing to dementia, so that appropriate therapies can be planned. MRS studies indicate that NAA and NAA/Cr levels are reduced in patients with vascular dementia. White matter NAA/Cr is lower in patients with vascular dementia than in patients with AD, reflecting the white matter ischemic damage in vascular dementia with respect to the cortical degenerative pathologic conditions in AD.[72,73] NAA levels are further decreased in patients with stroke who have cognitive impairment compared with those who are cognitively normal even in regions remote from the infarction, suggesting NAA/Cr is a marker for neuronal dysfunction that may extend beyond the region of infarct.[74] Cortical mI/Cr levels on the other hand are normal in patients with vascular dementia (see **Fig. 1**).[61,75,76] Because mI/Cr is elevated in patients with AD, mI/Cr may help identify the presence of AD in a demented patient with cerebrovascular disease. Studies that include histopathologic confirmation are necessary to clarify the role of mI/Cr in differential diagnosis of vascular dementia, mixed dementia (vascular dementia and AD), and AD.

MRS IN FRONTOTEMPORAL LOBAR DEGENERATION

MRS metabolite changes in frontotemporal dementia are similar to the changes encountered in AD: lower NAA/Cr and higher mI/Cr than normal (see **Fig. 1**).[21,77,78] NAA/Cr is lower and mI/Cr is higher in the frontal cortex of patients with frontotemporal dementia than in patients with early AD, suggesting that regional ^{1}H MRS measurements may help differentiate neurodegenerative disorders that display regionally specific involvement.[18,79] It should be noted, however, that although regional differences may be prominent during early stages of the pathologic process in neurodegenerative diseases, these differences may be lost as neurodegenerative pathologic conditions involve most of the cerebral cortex in later stages.[61,77]

Frontotemporal dementia with parkinsonism linked to chromosome 17 is an autosomal dominant tauopathy that is linked to mutations in the gene encoding for the microtubule-associated protein tau (*MAPT*) on chromosome 17.[80–83] Mutations in *MAPT* result in filamentous accumulation of hyperphosphorylated tau in neurons and glia leading to neurodegeneration and atrophy.[84–86] Progressive accumulation of filamentous tau and subsequent neuronal death is central to the pathogenesis of many neurodegenerative diseases, including AD, and may begin years before the onset of clinical symptoms. We recently demonstrated ^{1}H MRS metabolite abnormalities in presymptomatic carriers of mutations in the gene encoding for *MAPT* on chromosome 17. The severity of ^{1}H MRS and MRI abnormalities was associated with the proximity to the estimated age of symptom onset. NAA/mI ratio was fully outside of the control range in presymptomatic *MAPT* mutation carriers who had 5 years to reach estimated age of symptom onset or who were past the estimated age of symptom onset, indicating the presence of ^{1}H MRS metabolite abnormalities related to neurodegeneration, years before the onset of symptoms and atrophy in *MAPT* mutation carriers (**Fig. 3**).

MRS IN MILD COGNITIVE IMPAIRMENT AND OTHER AD RISK GROUPS

There are no proven treatments for AD pathologic conditions; however, current efforts to arrest or slow disease progression generate the prospect for preventive interventions.[87] There is considerable interest in early diagnosis by identifying individuals with cognitive difficulties who eventually progress to dementia from those who are aging with normal cognitive function.[88] Mild cognitive impairment (MCI) was established on clinical grounds to identify symptomatic individuals who do not meet the criteria for dementia.[89] Most people with MCI develop dementia in the future.

The progression of AD pathophysiologic processes starts decades before the clinical diagnosis of AD and the earliest cognitive impairments occur in the memory domain.[90] The syndrome of amnestic MCI represents this prodromal phase in the progression of AD.[89] More recently, the construct of MCI has been broadened to include individuals with impairments in nonamnestic cognitive domains such as attention/executive, language, or visuospatial processing domains.[91] The clinical presentation of this broadened definition of MCI is heterogeneous. Both the amnestic and nonamnestic subtypes of MCI may present with involvement of a single cognitive domain or multiple cognitive domains. It is clear from several independent studies that most people with the amnestic form of MCI who progress to dementia in the future develop AD.[92–98] People with nonamnestic MCI on average have more vascular comorbidity and infarctions and a higher prevalence of extrapyramidal features, mood disorders, and behavioral symptoms than do people with amnestic MCI.[99,100] The cause of MCI is also heterogeneous. A variety of early stage dementia-associated pathophysiologic processes such as AD, cerebrovascular disease and Lewy body pathologic conditions have been identified in patients with MCI at autopsy.[101–104] Many of these pathologies coexist in MCI[103] and require different therapeutic strategies. Furthermore, patients with MCI do not develop dementia at similar rates.[105,106] The heterogeneity of MCI warrants development of noninvasive biomarkers that can predict the rate of future progression to different dementias, for early diagnosis and treatment with potential disease-specific preventive interventions.

Early ^{1}H MRS studies in MCI included individuals who had impairments in memory function (ie, amnestic MCI).[8,29,107,108] Most patients with

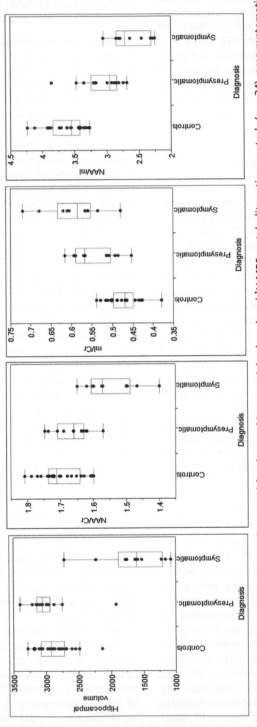

Fig. 3. Box plots show the hippocampal volumes (corrected for the total intracranial volume) and ¹H MRS metabolite ratios: controls (n = 24), presymptomatic (n = 14), and symptomatic (n = 10) *MAPT* mutation carriers. (*From* Kantarci K, Boeve BF, Wszolek ZK, et al. MRS in presymptomatic MAPT mutation carriers: a potential biomarker for tau-mediated pathology. Neurology 2010;75:771–8; with permission.)

amnestic MCI develop AD in the future, and many of these individuals have early AD pathologic conditions.[95] In keeping with this, the ¹H MRS findings in amnestic MCI are similar to but milder than the findings in AD.[8,29,108] However, there are distinct groupwise differences in MRI and ¹H MRS findings between amnestic MCI and nonamnestic MCI subtypes. Patients with amnestic MCI tend to have smaller hippocampal volumes and elevated mI/Cr ratios compared with patients with nonamnestic MCI and cognitively normal controls. On the other hand, nonamnestic MCI patients have normal hippocampal volumes and normal mI/Cr ratios, but a greater proportion of these patients have cortical infarctions compared with the amnestic MCI patients.[99] Both hippocampal atrophy and elevated mI/Cr are sensitive markers of early AD pathologic conditions, and the severity of these abnormalities correlates with the pathologic severity of AD.[46,109–114] For this reason, hippocampal atrophy and elevated mI/Cr most likely represent a higher frequency of early AD pathologic conditions in patients with amnestic MCI compared with nonamnestic MCI. On the contrary, normal hippocampal volumes and mI/Cr ratios in the nonamnestic MCI subtype suggest that other pathologic conditions, in addition to AD, underlie nonamnestic MCI. A higher prevalence of cortical infarctions on MRI and a history of transient ischemic attack and stroke in nonamnestic MCI patients suggest that cerebrovascular disease is one of the pathologic contributors to nonamnestic MCI.

The pathologic and clinical heterogeneities of MCI require multimodality imaging markers that are sensitive to the various dementia-related pathophysiologic processes for early diagnosis in patients with MCI. The most common dementia-related pathologic conditions observed in MCI are AD, cerebrovascular disease, and DLB.[102–104] Lesions that are associated with cerebrovascular disease on MRI include infarctions and white matter hyperintensities on T2-weighted images. These cerebrovascular lesions are more common in patients with MCI compared with cognitively normal older adults.[99] An MR marker that is highly sensitive to the pathophysiologic processes of AD (specifically, the neurofibrillary tangle pathologic condition–associated neurodegeneration early in the disease course) is hippocampal atrophy.[112,114] Both cortical infarctions[115] and hippocampal atrophy[116] are predictors of dementia risk in MCI.

There is evidence that ¹H MRS is sensitive to the pathophysiologic processes associated with the risk of dementia in patients with MCI.[117,118] Decreased NAA/Cr ratio in the posterior cingulate gyrus voxel is associated with an increased risk of

dementia in patients with MCI.[115] Furthermore, posterior cingulate gyrus voxel NAA/Cr levels decline with time in patients with MCI who progress to an AD diagnosis.[48] ¹H MRS is complementary in predicting future progression to dementia in MCI when considered with other strong predictors of dementia risk in MCI such as hippocampal volumes and cortical infarctions. Decreased posterior cingulate gyrus NAA/Cr increases the risk of progression to dementia in patients with MCI with hippocampal atrophy, and the risk of dementia increases even further if cortical infarctions are present in a patient with MCI (**Fig. 4**).[115] The complementary role of multimodality imaging markers in predicting the risk of dementia in MCI is consistent with cross-sectional studies showing the added value of ¹H MRS and hippocampal volumes for discriminating cognitively impaired but nondemented individuals from cognitively

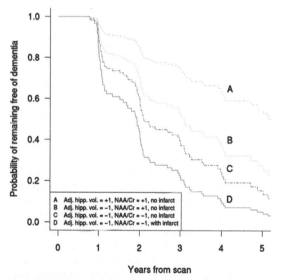

Fig. 4. Multiple MR markers of underlying dementia pathologies improve the ability to identify patients with prodromal dementia over a single MR marker. Estimates of the probability of remaining free of dementia for 4 patient groups with increasingly negative prognoses. Group A has adjusted hippocampal volume and NAA/Cr 1 SD greater than MCI average and no cortical infarctions. Group B has adjusted hippocampal volume 1 SD less than MCI average with NAA/Cr 1 SD greater than MCI average and no cortical infarctions. Group C has adjusted hippocampal volume and NAA/Cr both 1 SD less than MCI average and no cortical infarctions. Group D has adjusted hippocampal volume and NAA/Cr both 1 SD less than MCI average and cortical infarctions. (*From* Kantarci K, Weigand SD, Przybelski SA, et al. Risk of dementia in MCI: combined effect of cerebrovascular disease, volumetric MRI, and 1H MRS. Neurology 2009;72:1519–25; with permission.)

normal subjects[108] and distinguishing patients with AD from those who are cognitively normal.[119] Furthermore, hippocampal volumes and NAA/Cr levels are independent and complementary predictors of verbal memory on neuropsychometric testing in nondemented older adults, demonstrating that verbal memory depends on both structural and metabolic integrity of the hippocampus.[120]

Recently, the diagnostic criteria for AD and MCI were revised by 2 separate work groups charged by the National Institute on Aging and Alzheimer's Association.[121–123] A third work group was charged to define the preclinical stage of AD in light of the evidence that the pathophysiologic process of AD begins decades before the diagnosis of clinical dementia.[90] The changes in most well-validated imaging biomarkers have been hypothetically modeled for the 3 clinical stages of AD (ie, preclinical AD, MCI, and AD). According to this hypothetical model, the accumulation of Aβ pathologic conditions imaged with PET amyloid ligands or measured with cerebrospinal fluid Aβ-42 levels precedes the change in imaging markers of neurodegeneration associated with the neurofibrillary tangle pathologic conditions of AD such as hippocampal atrophy on MRI.[124] The model that emerged from evidence on well-validated imaging biomarkers will be critical for tracking disease progression and for assessment of primary and secondary preventive interventions in individuals at the preclinical and MCI stages of AD.

Several well-validated imaging biomarkers exist for various pathologic features of the early AD pathologic conditions such as increased Aβ load on PET, atrophy on structural MRI, or glucose metabolic reductions on PET. However, there are other features of AD pathologic conditions for which a well-validated biomarker does not exist. For example, there is no widely accepted biomarker for glial or microglial activation. The glial metabolite mI quantified with ^{1}H MRS may potentially be useful as a biomarker for glial activation in neurodegenerative diseases including AD.

Cross-sectional studies indicate that mI/Cr is elevated in MCI and mild AD even in the absence of a decrease in NAA/Cr.[6,8,107] Our data for a pathologic condition–confirmed sample of older adults with a range of AD pathologic conditions additionally showed that the mI/Cr elevation is associated with an intermediate likelihood (ie, an earlier stage) of AD pathologic conditions, whereas the decrease in NAA/Cr is associated with a higher likelihood (ie, a later stage) of AD pathologic conditions (see Fig. 2).[46] Furthermore, mI/Cr levels increase in the predementia phase of Down syndrome[15,125] and in presymptomatic individuals with familial dementia,[126,127] even in the absence of structural MRI and NAA/Cr changes.[127] The mI peak consists of glial metabolites that are responsible for osmoregulation.[128,129] MI levels correlate with glial proliferation in inflammatory central nervous system demyelination.[130] Because the dense-cored amyloid deposits in AD are surrounded by clusters of microglia and astrocytes,[131] it is thought that the elevation of the mI peak is related to glial proliferation and microglial activation in AD.[45,132] A significant correlation between mI/Cr levels and amyloid load measured with Pittsburgh Compound-B PET imaging was found in a population-based sample of 311 cognitively normal older adults (Fig. 5).[133] It is possible that the mI/Cr levels are associated with the microglial and glial activations that surround the senile amyloid plaques. However, an ^{1}H MRS–histology correlation study in a mouse model of spinocerebellar ataxia type 1 found elevated mI/Cr levels even in the absence of gliosis.[134] Based on limited evidence, it is not possible to attribute elevation in mI solely to glial activation in neurodegenerative diseases. Although there is evidence that mI/Cr elevation is an early marker in sporadic AD, familial AD, and frontotemporal lobar degeneration even before cognitive impairment, loss of neuronal integrity, and atrophy, histologic confirmation is needed to better understand the pathologic basis of mI/Cr elevation in MCI.

MCI is a clinically and pathologically heterogeneous disorder. MRS may potentially provide information on the underlying pathologic situations in patients with MCI that is not available from other imaging biomarkers. Data from cognitively normal older adults and cognitively normal adults at risk for familial dementia suggest that MRS may be useful as a biomarker for preclinical pathologic processes and for potentially assessing the response to preventive interventions.

FUTURE PERSPECTIVES

Although significant progress has been made in improving the acquisition and analysis techniques in ^{1}H MRS, translation of these technical developments into clinical practice has not been effective. The main reasons for ineffective translation of technology into clinical practice or patient-oriented research are (1) a lack of standardization for multisite applications and normative data and (2) insufficient understanding the pathologic basis of ^{1}H MRS metabolite changes. Advances on these grounds would further increase the impact of ^{1}H MRS as a biomarker for the early pathologic involvement in neurodegenerative diseases and in turn increase the use ^{1}H MRS in clinical practice.

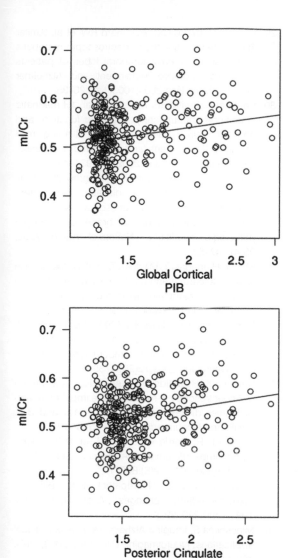

Fig. 5. Association between posterior cingulate myo-inositol to creatine (ml/Cr) ratio and beta-amyloid load as measured with Pittsburgh compound-B(PIB) retention on positron emission tomography retention: scatter plots demonstrate the association between log-transformed global cortical PIB retention ratio and ml/Cr (*top*) and between log-transformed posterior cingulate cortical PIB retention ratio and ml/Cr (*bottom*). (*From* Kantarci K, Lowe V, Przybelski SA, et al. Magnetic resonance spectroscopy, beta-amyloid load, and cognition in a population-based sample of cognitively normal older adults. Neurology 2011;77: 951–8; with permission.)

REFERENCES

1. Brown GG, Levine SR, Gorell JM, et al. In vivo 31P NMR profiles of Alzheimer's disease and multiple subcortical infarct dementia. Neurology 1989; 39(11):1423–7.

2. Pettegrew JW, Moossy J, Withers G, et al. 31P nuclear magnetic resonance study of the brain in Alzheimer's disease. J Neuropathol Exp Neurol 1988;47(3):235–48.

3. Pettegrew JW, Panchalingam K, Moossy J, et al. Correlation of phosphorus-31 magnetic resonance spectroscopy and morphologic findings in Alzheimer's disease. Arch Neurol 1988;45(10):1093–6.

4. Klunk WE, Panchalingam K, Moossy J, et al. N-acetyl-L-aspartate and other amino acid metabolites in Alzheimer's disease brain: a preliminary proton nuclear magnetic resonance study. Neurology 1992;42(8):1578–85.

5. Miller BL, Moats RA, Shonk T, et al. Alzheimer disease: depiction of increased cerebral myo-inositol with proton MR spectroscopy. Radiology 1993;187(2):433–7.

6. Huang W, Alexander GE, Chang L, et al. Brain metabolite concentration and dementia severity in Alzheimer's disease: a (1)H MRS study. Neurology 2001;57(4):626–32.

7. Jessen F, Block W, Traber F, et al. Proton MR spectroscopy detects a relative decrease of N-acetylaspartate in the medial temporal lobe of patients with AD. Neurology 2000;55(5):684–8.

8. Kantarci K, Jack CR Jr, Xu YC, et al. Regional metabolic patterns in mild cognitive impairment and Alzheimer's disease: a 1H MRS study. Neurology 2000;55(2):210–7.

9. Meyerhoff DJ, MacKay S, Constans JM, et al. Axonal injury and membrane alterations in Alzheimer's disease suggested by in vivo proton magnetic resonance spectroscopic imaging. Ann Neurol 1994;36(1):40–7.

10. Moats RA, Ernst T, Shonk TK, et al. Abnormal cerebral metabolite concentrations in patients with probable Alzheimer disease. Magn Reson Med 1994;32(1):110–5.

11. Mohanakrishnan P, Fowler AH, Vonsattel JP, et al. Regional metabolic alterations in Alzheimer's disease: an in vitro 1H NMR study of the hippocampus and cerebellum. J Gerontol A Biol Sci Med Sci 1997;52(2):B111–7.

12. Pfefferbaum A, Adalsteinsson E, Spielman D, et al. In vivo spectroscopic quantification of the N-acetyl moiety, creatine, and choline from large volumes of brain gray and white matter: effects of normal aging. Magn Reson Med 1999;41(2):276–84.

13. Rose SE, de Zubicaray GI, Wang D, et al. A 1H MRS study of probable Alzheimer's disease and normal aging: implications for longitudinal monitoring of dementia progression. Magn Reson Imaging 1999;17(2):291–9.

14. Schuff N, Capizzano AA, Du AT, et al. Selective reduction of N-acetylaspartate in medial temporal and parietal lobes in AD. Neurology 2002;58(6): 928–35.

15. Shonk T, Ross BD. Role of increased cerebral myo-inositol in the dementia of Down syndrome. Magn Reson Med 1995;33(6):858–61.

16. Rai GS, McConnell JR, Waldman A, et al. Brain proton spectroscopy in dementia: an aid to clinical diagnosis. Lancet 1999;353(9158):1063–4.

17. Christiansen P, Toft P, Larsson HB, et al. The concentration of N-acetyl aspartate, creatine + phosphocreatine, and choline in different parts of the brain in adulthood and senium. Magn Reson Imaging 1993;11(6):799–806.

18. Ernst T, Chang L, Melchor R, et al. Frontotemporal dementia and early Alzheimer disease: differentiation with frontal lobe H-1 MR spectroscopy. Radiology 1997;203(3):829–36.

19. Parnetti L, Tarducci R, Presciutti O, et al. Proton magnetic resonance spectroscopy can differentiate Alzheimer's disease from normal aging. Mech Ageing Dev 1997;97(1):9–14.

20. Schuff N, Amend D, Ezekiel F, et al. Changes of hippocampal N-acetyl aspartate and volume in Alzheimer's disease. A proton MR spectroscopic imaging and MRI study. Neurology 1997;49(6):1513–21.

21. Shonk TK, Moats RA, Gifford P, et al. Probable Alzheimer disease: diagnosis with proton MR spectroscopy. Radiology 1995;195(1):65–72.

22. Antuono PG, Jones JL, Wang Y, et al. Decreased glutamate + glutamine in Alzheimer's disease detected in vivo with (1)H-MRS at 0.5 T. Neurology 2001;56(6):737–42.

23. Hattori N, Abe K, Sakoda S, et al. Proton MR spectroscopic study at 3 Tesla on glutamate/glutamine in Alzheimer's disease. Neuroreport 2002;13(1):183–6.

24. Tedeschi G, Bertolino A, Lundbom N, et al. Cortical and subcortical chemical pathologic conditions in Alzheimer's disease as assessed by multislice proton magnetic resonance spectroscopic imaging. Neurology 1996;47(3):696–704.

25. Schuff N, Amend DL, Meyerhoff DJ, et al. Alzheimer disease: quantitative H-1 MR spectroscopic imaging of frontoparietal brain. Radiology 1998;207(1):91–102.

26. Zhu X, Schuff N, Kornak J, et al. Effects of Alzheimer disease on fronto-parietal brain N-acetyl aspartate and myo-inositol using magnetic resonance spectroscopic imaging. Alzheimer Dis Assoc Disord 2006;20(2):77–85.

27. Frederick BB, Satlin A, Yurgelun-Todd DA, et al. In vivo proton magnetic resonance spectroscopy of Alzheimer's disease in the parietal and temporal lobes. Biol Psychiatry 1997;42(2):147–50.

28. Kwo-On-Yuen PF, Newmark RD, Budinger TF, et al. Brain N-acetyl-L-aspartic acid in Alzheimer's disease: a proton magnetic resonance spectroscopy study. Brain Res 1994;667(2):167–74.

29. Chantal S, Braun CM, Bouchard RW, et al. Similar 1H magnetic resonance spectroscopic metabolic pattern in the medial temporal lobes of patients with mild cognitive impairment and Alzheimer disease. Brain Res 2004;1003(1–2):26–35.

30. Kantarci K, Smith GE, Ivnik RJ, et al. 1H magnetic resonance spectroscopy, cognitive function, and apolipoprotein E genotype in normal aging, mild cognitive impairment and Alzheimer's disease. J Int Neuropsychol Soc 2002;8(7):934–42.

31. Sweet RA, Panchalingam K, Pettegrew JW, et al. Psychosis in Alzheimer disease: postmortem magnetic resonance spectroscopy evidence of excess neuronal and membrane phospholipid pathologic conditions. Neurobiol Aging 2002;23(4):547–53.

32. Shinno H, Inagaki T, Miyaoka T, et al. A decrease in N-acetylaspartate and an increase in myoinositol in the anterior cingulate gyrus are associated with behavioral and psychological symptoms in Alzheimer's disease. J Neurol Sci 2007;260(1–2):132–8.

33. Jessen F, Gur O, Block W, et al. A multicenter (1)H-MRS study of the medial temporal lobe in AD and MCI. Neurology 2009;72(20):1735–40.

34. Kantarci K, Reynolds G, Petersen RC, et al. Proton MR spectroscopy in mild cognitive impairment and Alzheimer disease: comparison of 1.5 and 3 T. AJNR Am J Neuroradiol 2003;24(5):843–9.

35. Rupsingh R, Borrie M, Smith M, et al. Reduced hippocampal glutamate in Alzheimer disease. Neurobiol Aging 2011;32(5):802–10.

36. Braak H, Braak E. Neuropathological staging of Alzheimer-related changes. Acta Neuropathol 1991;82(4):239–59.

37. Minoshima S. Imaging Alzheimer's disease: clinical applications. Neuroimaging Clin N Am 2003;13(4):769–80.

38. Reiman EM, Caselli RJ, Yun LS, et al. Preclinical evidence of Alzheimer's disease in persons homozygous for the epsilon 4 allele for apolipoprotein E [see comment]. N Engl J Med 1996;334(12):752–8.

39. Buckner RL, Andrews-Hanna JR, Schacter DL. The brain's default network: anatomy, function, and relevance to disease. Ann N Y Acad Sci 2008;1124:1–38.

40. Chen SQ, Wang PJ, Ten GJ, et al. Role of myo-inositol by magnetic resonance spectroscopy in early diagnosis of Alzheimer's disease in APP/PS1 transgenic mice. Dement Geriatr Cogn Disord 2009;28(6):558–66.

41. Cheng LL, Newell K, Mallory AE, et al. Quantification of neurons in Alzheimer and control brains with ex vivo high resolution magic angle spinning proton magnetic resonance spectroscopy and stereology. Magn Reson Imaging 2002;20(7):527–33.

42. Dedeoglu A, Choi JK, Cormier K, et al. Magnetic resonance spectroscopic analysis of Alzheimer's

disease mouse brain that express mutant human APP shows altered neurochemical profile. Brain Res 2004;1012(1–2):60–5.

43. Marjanska M, Curran GL, Wengenack TM, et al. Monitoring disease progression in transgenic mouse models of Alzheimer's disease with proton magnetic resonance spectroscopy. Proc Natl Acad Sci U S A 2005;102(33):11906–10.

44. von Kienlin M, Kunnecke B, Metzger F, et al. Altered metabolic profile in the frontal cortex of PS2APP transgenic mice, monitored throughout their life span. Neurobiol Dis 2005;18(1):32–9.

45. Sailasuta N, Harris K, Tran T, et al. Minimally invasive biomarker confirms glial activation present in Alzheimer's disease: a preliminary study. Neuropsychiatr Dis Treat 2011;7:495–9.

46. Kantarci K, Knopman DS, Dickson DW, et al. Alzheimer disease: postmortem neuropathologic correlates of antemortem 1H MR spectroscopy metabolite measurements. Radiology 2008;248(1):210–20.

47. Adalsteinsson E, Sullivan EV, Kleinhans N, et al. Longitudinal decline of the neuronal marker N-acetyl aspartate in Alzheimer's disease. Lancet 2000;355(9216):1696–7.

48. Kantarci K, Weigand SD, Petersen RC, et al. Longitudinal 1H MRS changes in mild cognitive impairment and Alzheimer's disease. Neurobiol Aging 2007;28(9):1330–9.

49. Schott JM, Frost C, MacManus DG, et al. Short echo time proton magnetic resonance spectroscopy in Alzheimer's disease: a longitudinal multiple time point study. Brain 2010;133(11):3315–22.

50. Jessen F, Block W, Traber F, et al. Decrease of N-acetylaspartate in the MTL correlates with cognitive decline of AD patients. Neurology 2001;57(5):930–2.

51. Traber F, Block W, Freymann N, et al. A multicenter reproducibility study of single-voxel 1H-MRS of the medial temporal lobe. Eur Radiol 2006;16(5):1096–103.

52. Okada T, Sakamoto S, Nakamoto Y, et al. Reproducibility of magnetic resonance spectroscopy in correlation with signal-to-noise ratio. Psychiatry Res 2007;156(2):169–74.

53. Modrego PJ, Fayed N, Errea JM, et al. Memantine versus donepezil in mild to moderate Alzheimer's disease: a randomized trial with magnetic resonance spectroscopy. Eur J Neurol 2010;17(3):405–12.

54. Krishnan KR, Charles HC, Doraiswamy PM, et al. Randomized, placebo-controlled trial of the effects of donepezil on neuronal markers and hippocampal volumes in Alzheimer's disease. Am J Psychiatry 2003;160(11):2003–11.

55. Modrego PJ, Pina MA, Fayed N, et al. Changes in metabolite ratios after treatment with rivastigmine in Alzheimer's disease: a nonrandomised controlled trial with magnetic resonance spectroscopy. CNS Drugs 2006;20(10):867–77.

56. Penner J, Rupsingh R, Smith M, et al. Increased glutamate in the hippocampus after galantamine treatment for Alzheimer disease. Prog Neuropsychopharmacol Biol Psychiatry 2010;34(1):104–10.

57. Bartha R, Smith M, Rupsingh R, et al. High field (1)H MRS of the hippocampus after donepezil treatment in Alzheimer disease. Prog Neuropsychopharmacol Biol Psychiatry 2008;32(3):786–93.

58. McKeith IG, Dickson DW, Lowe J, et al. Diagnosis and management of dementia with Lewy bodies: third report of the DLB Consortium. Neurology 2005;65(12):1863–72.

59. Hamilton RL. Lewy bodies in Alzheimer's disease: a neuropathological review of 145 cases using alpha-synuclein immunohistochemistry. Brain Pathol 2000;10(3):378–84.

60. Gomez-Isla T, Growdon WB, McNamara M, et al. Clinicopathologic correlates in temporal cortex in dementia with Lewy bodies. Neurology 1999;53(9):2003–9.

61. Kantarci K, Petersen RC, Boeve BF, et al. 1H MR spectroscopy in common dementias. Neurology 2004;63(8):1393–8.

62. Xuan X, Ding M, Gong X. Proton magnetic resonance spectroscopy detects a relative decrease of N-acetylaspartate in the hippocampus of patients with dementia with Lewy bodies. J Neuroimaging 2008;18(2):137–41.

63. Kantarci K, Ferman TJ, Boeve BF, et al. Focal Atrophy on MRI and neuropathologic classification of dementia with lewy bodies. Neurology 2012;79(6):553–60.

64. Molina JA, Garcia-Segura JM, Benito-Leon J, et al. Proton magnetic resonance spectroscopy in dementia with Lewy bodies. Eur Neurol 2002;48(3):158–63.

65. Firbank MJ, Blamire AM, Krishnan MS, et al. Diffusion tensor imaging in dementia with Lewy bodies and Alzheimer's disease. Psychiatry Res 2007;155(2):135–45.

66. Kantarci K, Avula R, Senjem ML, et al. Dementia with Lewy bodies and Alzheimer disease: neurodegenerative patterns characterized by DTI. Neurology 2010;74(22):1814–21.

67. Tiraboschi P, Hansen LA, Alford M, et al. Early and widespread cholinergic losses differentiate dementia with Lewy bodies from Alzheimer disease. Arch Gen Psychiatry 2002;59(10):946–51.

68. McKeith IG, Grace JB, Walker Z, et al. Rivastigmine in the treatment of dementia with Lewy bodies: preliminary findings from an open trial. Int J Geriatr Psychiatry 2000;15(5):387–92.

69. Satlin A, Bodick N, Offen WW, et al. Brain proton magnetic resonance spectroscopy (1H-MRS) in

Alzheimer's disease: changes after treatment with xanomeline, an M1 selective cholinergic agonist. Am J Psychiatry 1997;154(10):1459–61.

70. Holmes C, Cairns N, Lantos P, et al. Validity of current clinical criteria for Alzheimer's disease, vascular dementia and dementia with Lewy bodies. Br J Psychiatry 1999;174:45–50.

71. Schneider JA, Arvanitakis Z, Bang W, et al. Mixed brain pathologies account for most dementia cases in community-dwelling older persons. Neurology 2007;69(24):2197–204.

72. Kattapong VJ, Brooks WM, Wesley MH, et al. Proton magnetic resonance spectroscopy of vascular- and Alzheimer-type dementia. Arch Neurol 1996;53(7):678–80.

73. MacKay S, Meyerhoff DJ, Constans JM, et al. Regional gray and white matter metabolite differences in subjects with AD, with subcortical ischemic vascular dementia, and elderly controls with 1H magnetic resonance spectroscopic imaging. Arch Neurol 1996;53(2):167–74.

74. Ross AJ, Sachdev PS, Wen W, et al. 1H MRS in stroke patients with and without cognitive impairment. Neurobiol Aging 2005;26(6):873–82.

75. Waldman AD, Rai GS, McConnell JR, et al. Clinical brain proton magnetic resonance spectroscopy for management of Alzheimer's and sub-cortical ischemic vascular dementia in older people. Arch Gerontol Geriatr 2002;35(2):137–42.

76. Shiino A, Watanabe T, Shirakashi Y, et al. The profile of hippocampal metabolites differs between Alzheimer's disease and subcortical ischemic vascular dementia, as measured by proton magnetic resonance spectroscopy. J Cereb Blood Flow Metab 2012;32(5):805–15.

77. Garrard P, Schott JM, MacManus DG, et al. Posterior cingulate neurometabolite profiles and clinical phenotype in frontotemporal dementia. Cogn Behav Neurol 2006;19(4):185–9.

78. Kantarci K. 1H magnetic resonance spectroscopy in dementia. Br J Radiol 2007;80(Spec No 2):S146–52.

79. Mihara M, Hattori N, Abe K, et al. Magnetic resonance spectroscopic study of Alzheimer's disease and frontotemporal dementia/Pick complex. Neuroreport 2006;17(4):413–6.

80. Boeve BF, Hutton M. Refining frontotemporal dementia with parkinsonism linked to chromosome 17: introducing FTDP-17 (MAPT) and FTDP-17 (PGRN). Arch Neurol 2008;65(4):460–4.

81. Hutton M, Lendon CL, Rizzu P, et al. Association of missense and 5'-splice-site mutations in tau with the inherited dementia FTDP-17. Nature 1998; 393(6686):702–5.

82. Rademakers R, Cruts M, van Broeckhoven C. The role of tau (MAPT) in frontotemporal dementia and related tauopathies. Hum Mutat 2004;24(4):277–95.

83. Foster NL, Wilhelmsen K, Sima AA, et al. Frontotemporal dementia and parkinsonism linked to chromosome 17: a consensus conference. Conference participants. Ann Neurol 1997;41(6):706–15.

84. Ingram DA, Wenning MJ, Shannon K, et al. Leukemic potential of doubly mutant Nf1 and Wv hematopoietic cells. Blood 2003;101(5):1984–6.

85. Whitwell JL, Jack CR Jr, Boeve BF, et al. Voxel-based morphometry patterns of atrophy in FTLD with mutations in MAPT or PGRN. Neurology 2009;72(9):813–20.

86. Bunker JM, Kamath K, Wilson L, et al. FTDP-17 mutations compromise the ability of tau to regulate microtubule dynamics in cells. J Biol Chem 2006; 281(17):11856–63.

87. Sperling RA, Jack CR Jr, Aisen PS. Testing the right target and right drug at the right stage. Sci Transl Med 2011;3(111):111cm133.

88. Thal LJ, Kantarci K, Reiman EM, et al. The role of biomarkers in clinical trials for Alzheimer disease. Alzheimer Dis Assoc Disord 2006;20(1):6–15.

89. Petersen RC, Doody R, Kurz A, et al. Current concepts in mild cognitive impairment. Arch Neurol 2001;58(12):1985–92.

90. Sperling RA, Aisen PS, Beckett LA, et al. Toward defining the preclinical stages of Alzheimer's disease: recommendations from the National Institute on Aging-Alzheimer's Association workgroups on diagnostic guidelines for Alzheimer's disease. Alzheimers Dement 2011;7(3):280–92.

91. Petersen RC. Mild cognitive impairment as a diagnostic entity. J Intern Med 2004;256(3):183–94.

92. Bennett DA, Wilson RS, Schneider JA, et al. Natural history of mild cognitive impairment in older persons. Neurology 2002;59(2):198–205.

93. Bowen J, Teri L, Kukull W, et al. Progression to dementia in patients with isolated memory loss. Lancet 1997;349(9054):763–5.

94. Flicker C, Ferris SH, Reisberg B. Mild cognitive impairment in the elderly: predictors of dementia. Neurology 1991;41(7):1006–9.

95. Jicha GA, Parisi JE, Dickson DW, et al. Neuropathologic outcome of mild cognitive impairment following progression to clinical dementia. Arch Neurol 2006;63(5):674–81.

96. Meyer JS, Xu G, Thornby J, et al. Is mild cognitive impairment prodromal for vascular dementia like Alzheimer's disease? Stroke 2002;33(8):1981–5.

97. Morris JC, Storandt M, Miller JP, et al. Mild cognitive impairment represents early-stage Alzheimer disease. Arch Neurol 2001;58(3):397–405.

98. Petersen RC, Smith GE, Waring SC, et al. Mild cognitive impairment: clinical characterization and outcome [Erratum appears in Arch Neurol 1999;56(6):760]. Arch Neurol 1999;56(3):303–8.

99. Kantarci K, Petersen RC, Przybelski SA, et al. Hippocampal volumes, proton magnetic resonance

spectroscopy metabolites, and cerebrovascular disease in mild cognitive impairment subtypes. Arch Neurol 2008;65(12):1621–8.

100. Mariani E, Monastero R, Ercolani S, et al. Vascular risk factors in mild cognitive impairment subtypes. Findings from the ReGAl project. Dement Geriatr Cogn Disord 2007;24(6):448–56.

101. Bennett DA, Schneider JA, Bienias JL, et al. Mild cognitive impairment is related to Alzheimer disease pathologic conditions and cerebral infarctions. Neurology 2005;64(5):834–41.

102. Petersen RC, Parisi JE, Dickson DW, et al. Neuropathologic features of amnestic mild cognitive impairment. Arch Neurol 2006;63(5):665–72.

103. Schneider JA, Arvanitakis Z, Leurgans SE, et al. The neuropathology of probable Alzheimer disease and mild cognitive impairment. Ann Neurol 2009;66(2):200–8.

104. Molano J, Boeve B, Ferman T, et al. Mild cognitive impairment associated with limbic and neocortical Lewy body disease: a clinicopathological study. Brain 2010;133(Pt 2):540 56.

105. Busse A, Hensel A, Guhne U, et al. Mild cognitive impairment: long-term course of four clinical subtypes. Neurology 2006;67(12):2176–85.

106. Fischer P, Jungwirth S, Zehetmayer S, et al. Conversion from subtypes of mild cognitive impairment to Alzheimer dementia. Neurology 2007;68(4):288–91.

107. Catani M, Cherubini A, Howard R, et al. (1)H-MR spectroscopy differentiates mild cognitive impairment from normal brain aging. Neuroreport 2001;12(11):2315–7.

108. Chao LL, Schuff N, Kramer JH, et al. Reduced medial temporal lobe N-acetylaspartate in cognitively impaired but nondemented patients. Neurology 2005;64(2):282–9.

109. Barkhof F, Polvikoski TM, van Straaten EC, et al. The significance of medial temporal lobe atrophy: a postmortem MRI study in the very old. Neurology 2007;69(15):1521–7.

110. Bobinski M, Wegiel J, Tarnawski M, et al. Relationships between regional neuronal loss and neurofibrillary changes in the hippocampal formation and duration and severity of Alzheimer disease. J Neuropathol Exp Neurol 1997;56(4):414–20.

111. Gosche KM, Mortimer JA, Smith CD, et al. Hippocampal volume as an index of Alzheimer neuropathology: findings from the Nun Study. Neurology 2002;58(10):1476–82.

112. Jack CR Jr, Dickson DW, Parisi JE, et al. Antemortem MRI findings correlate with hippocampal neuropathology in typical aging and dementia. Neurology 2002;58(5):750–7.

113. Zarow C, Vinters HV, Ellis WG, et al. Correlates of hippocampal neuron number in Alzheimer's disease and ischemic vascular dementia. Ann Neurol 2005;57(6):896–903.

114. Jagust WJ, Zheng L, Harvey DJ, et al. Neuropathological basis of magnetic resonance images in aging and dementia. Ann Neurol 2008;63(1):72–80.

115. Kantarci K, Weigand SD, Przybelski SA, et al. Risk of dementia in MCI: combined effect of cerebrovascular disease, volumetric MRI, and 1H MRS. Neurology 2009;72(17):1519–25.

116. Jack CR Jr, Petersen RC, Xu YC, et al. Prediction of AD with MRI-based hippocampal volume in mild cognitive impairment. Neurology 1999;52(7):1397–403.

117. Martinez-Bisbal MC, Arana E, Marti-Bonmati L, et al. Cognitive impairment: classification by 1H magnetic resonance spectroscopy. Eur J Neurol 2004;11(3):187–93.

118. Metastasio A, Rinaldi P, Tarducci R, et al. Conversion of MCI to dementia: role of proton magnetic resonance spectroscopy. Neurobiol Aging 2006;27(7):926–32.

119. Westman E, Wahlund LO, Foy C, et al. Magnetic resonance imaging and magnetic resonance spectroscopy for detection of early Alzheimer's disease. J Alzheimers Dis 2011;26(Suppl 3):307–19.

120. Zimmerman ME, Pan JW, Hetherington HP, et al. Hippocampal neurochemistry, neuromorphometry, and verbal memory in nondemented older adults. Neurology 2008;70(18):1594–600.

121. Albert MS, DeKosky ST, Dickson D, et al. The diagnosis of mild cognitive impairment due to Alzheimer's disease: recommendations from the National Institute on Aging-Alzheimer's Association workgroups on diagnostic guidelines for Alzheimer's disease. Alzheimers Dement 2011;7(3):270–9.

122. Jack CR Jr, Albert MS, Knopman DS, et al. Introduction to the recommendations from the National Institute on Aging-Alzheimer's Association workgroups on diagnostic guidelines for Alzheimer's disease. Alzheimers Dement 2011;7(3):257–62.

123. McKhann GM, Knopman DS, Chertkow H, et al. The diagnosis of dementia due to Alzheimer's disease: recommendations from the National Institute on Aging-Alzheimer's Association workgroups on diagnostic guidelines for Alzheimer's disease. Alzheimers Dement 2011;7(3):263–9.

124. Jack CR Jr, Knopman DS, Jagust WJ, et al. Hypothetical model of dynamic biomarkers of the Alzheimer's pathological cascade. Lancet Neurol 2010;9(1):119–28.

125. Huang W, Alexander GE, Daly EM, et al. High brain myo-inositol levels in the predementia phase of Alzheimer's disease in adults with Down's syndrome: a 1H MRS study. Am J Psychiatry 1999;156(12):1879–86.

126. Godbolt AK, Waldman AD, MacManus DG, et al. MRS shows abnormalities before symptoms in familial Alzheimer disease. Neurology 2006;66(5):718–22.

127. Kantarci K, Boeve BF, Wszolek ZK, et al. MRS in presymptomatic MAPT mutation carriers: a potential biomarker for tau-mediated pathologic conditions. Neurology 2010;75(9):771–8.

128. Brand A, Richter-Landsberg C, Leibfritz D. Multinuclear NMR studies on the energy metabolism of glial and neuronal cells. Dev Neurosci 1993; 15(3–5):289–98.

129. Urenjak J, Williams SR, Gadian DG, et al. Proton nuclear magnetic resonance spectroscopy unambiguously identifies different neural cell types. J Neurosci 1993;13(3):981–9.

130. Bitsch A, Bruhn H, Vougioukas V, et al. Inflammatory CNS demyelination: histopathologic correlation with in vivo quantitative proton MR spectroscopy. AJNR Am J Neuroradiol 1999;20(9):1619–27.

131. Dickson DW. The pathogenesis of senile plaques. J Neuropathol Exp Neurol 1997;56(4): 321–39.

132. Ross BD, Bluml S, Cowan R, et al. In vivo MR spectroscopy of human dementia. Neuroimaging Clin N Am 1998;8(4):809–22.

133. Kantarci K, Lowe V, Przybelski SA, et al. Magnetic resonance spectroscopy, beta-amyloid load, and cognition in a population-based sample of cognitively normal older adults. Neurology 2011;77(10): 951–8.

134. Oz G, Nelson CD, Koski DM, et al. Noninvasive detection of presymptomatic and progressive neurodegeneration in a mouse model of spinocerebellar ataxia type 1. J Neurosci 2010;30(10): 3831–8.

The Use of Magnetic Resonance Spectroscopy in the Evaluation of Epilepsy

Paul A. Caruso, MD[a],*, Jason Johnson, MD[a], Ron Thibert, MD[b], Otto Rapalino[a], Sandra Rincon[a], Eva-Maria Ratai, PhD[a,c]

KEYWORDS

- ^{1}H MR spectroscopy • Epilepsy • Inborn error of metabolism • Focal cortical dysplasia

KEY POINTS

- Magnetic resonance spectroscopy (MRS) is indicated in the imaging protocol of the patient with epilepsy to screen for metabolic derangements such as inborn errors of metabolism and to characterize masses that may be equivocal on conventional magnetic resonance imaging for dysplasia versus neoplasia.
- Single-voxel MRS with an echo time of 35 milliseconds may be used for this purpose as a quick screening tool in the epilepsy imaging protocol.
- MRS is useful in the evaluation of both focal and generalized epilepsy.

INTRODUCTION

This article concerns the use of proton magnetic resonance (MR) spectroscopy (^{1}H MRS) in the evaluation of the patient with epilepsy. It is a practical "why, how to, and when" article. It is written in 3 parts to address 3 questions that arise when the neuroimager evaluates a patient with epilepsy.

Why do MRS? This first part addresses the question of whether MRS is indicated in the evaluation of the patient with epilepsy. It is addressed to the radiologist, faced with a requisition to perform MR imaging for a patient with epilepsy, who often needs to ask the referring clinician to add an order for MRS for the same patient. It answers the question, "Is there evidence that MRS is indicated in this setting?" The term "conventional MR imaging" is used to distinguish those sequences such as anatomic T1- and T2-weighted and susceptibility-weighted images and functional sequences such as diffusion-weighted or diffusion tensor imaging that we routinely perform for MR evaluation of the patient with epilepsy.

How to do MRS in the patient with epilepsy? This second part addresses MRS technique. It is written for the radiologist, spectroscopist, or MR imaging technologist who is at the scanner console with a patient on the table and considers the parameters to enter into the MR unit.

When, in what clinical-imaging setting, *can MRS help you* to diagnose or manage the patient with epilepsy? This third part addresses the question of interpretation and exemplifies the use of MRS by the use of cases. It is written for the radiologist or spectroscopist who is trying to interpret the semiologic, conventional MR imaging, and MRS data combined to diagnose or manage the patient.

a Division of Neuroradiology, Department of Radiology, Harvard Medical School, Massachusetts General Hospital, Boston, MA 02114, USA; b Epilepsy Service, Department of Neurology, Harvard Medical School, Massachusetts General Hospital, Boston, MA 02114, USA; c Athinoula A. Martinos Center for Biomedical Imaging, Harvard Medical School, Massachusetts General Hospital, Boston, MA 02129, USA
* Corresponding author. Division of Neuroradiology, Department of Radiology, Massachusetts General Hospital, 55 Fruit Street, Boston, MA 02114.
E-mail address: pcaruso@partners.org

Neuroimag Clin N Am 23 (2013) 407–424
http://dx.doi.org/10.1016/j.nic.2012.12.012
1052-5149/13/$ – see front matter © 2013 Published by Elsevier Inc.

PART I: WHY DO MRS?

In our practice, many clinicians who refer patients for MR imaging of the brain for evaluation for epilepsy do not initially request MRS. When we ask clinicians to add a requisition for MRS, 2 questions are usually raised:

"Is there evidence that MRS is going to make a difference for my patient?"

"Is it covered by my patient's insurance, and, if not, who will pay for it?"

The answer to the first question requires knowledge of the evidence in favor of the diagnostic yield of MRS, reviewed later.

The answer to the second question requires a practical billing strategy. Consideration of reimbursement for MRS is simply imaging *realpolitik* for any radiologist interested in sustaining a clinical MRS practice. It is our experience that without a consensus institutional policy on the reimbursement for MRS, the MRS component of the practice is at risk of shutting down under the weight of negative feedback from rejected insurance claims.

"Is there clear evidence that MRS is going to make a difference for my patient?"

The evidence in favor of an indication for MRS is best understood in the context of the broader consideration of the role of neuroimaging in the evaluation of the patient with epilepsy. The first goal of neuroimaging in the evaluation of the patient with epilepsy is etiologic triage. When a patient seizes, the goal of imaging is to detect certain treatable epileptogenic lesions, such as tumors, hemorrhage, vascular malformations, or inborn errors of metabolism, that would indicate involvement of the neurosurgical, neurointerventional, or metabolism and genetic services. From the perspective of the managing epileptologist, the initial goal of imaging is to determine if other clinical services need to be involved in the care of the patient.

Triage

In this initial triage phase of imaging, MRS is indicated for the following:

1. Screening for metabolic derangements that may occur from seizure or from certain metabolic disorders that may present with seizures such as mitochondrial disorders and creatine (Cr) deficiencies (**Figs. 1** and **2**).
2. The characterization of masses detected by conventional MR imaging as neoplasm versus dysplasia (**Fig. 3**).

Screening for metabolic derangements

Seizure alone and inborn errors of metabolism that may cause seizure can produce metabolic derangements that may be detectable by MRS and may be missed by conventional MR imaging (see **Figs. 1** and **2**). During seizure, the metabolic demands of brain cells can exceed the supply of oxygen and nutrients to the brain tissue undergoing elevated electrical activity, and this metabolic disturbance can be detected by MRS, including the abnormal accumulation of lactate and the reduction in *N*-acetyl aspartate (NAA).[1]

Parikh and colleagues[2] reviewed the records of 429 patients admitted to a pediatric epilepsy unit during the course of 1 year and found that of the 85 patients who had undergone metabolic testing, 11% had known inborn errors of metabolism. In addition, the 2002 Amalfi conference provides a clear consensus recommendation that screening for inborn errors of metabolism should be performed in the initial workup.[3] MRS fits squarely into this imperative for screening.[4]

In many inborn errors of metabolism that may cause seizures, MRS can characterize further those abnormal findings seen on conventional MR imaging (**Fig. 4**); however, the indication for the inclusion of MRS in the initial imaging protocol becomes more clear when one considers that MRS may diagnose certain metabolic disorders that commonly result in seizures (eg, mitochondrial disorders and Cr deficiency), when conventional MR imaging may be insensitive or nondiagnostic.[5,6] Mitochondrial disorders are important considerations in the evaluation of the patient with epilepsy; in a review of 429 children admitted to a major pediatric epilepsy center in 2005, of the 85 patients with metabolic testing and without prior diagnosis, Parikh and colleagues[2] found metabolic evidence of mitochondrial dysfunction in 28% of cases. Epilepsy, conversely, occurs frequently in mitochondrial disorders; Khurana and colleagues[7] evaluated 38 patients with mitochondrial disorders and found that 61% had seizures. In mitochondrial disorders, moreover, seizures may be the presenting finding: Canofoglia and colleagues[8] reviewed 31 patients with mitochondrial encephalopathies and found that seizures were the presenting feature in 53% of patients. Mitochondrial disorders may exhibit considerable epileptic phenotypic heterogeneity and may present with partial or generalized epilepsy.[9] MRS, moreover, may reveal metabolites, in voxels placed over areas that appear normal on conventional MR imaging sequences. Cristina Bianchi and colleagues,[5] for example, studied 15 patients with mitochondrial disorders and found that MRS voxels placed methodically over white or gray matter that appeared normal on conventional

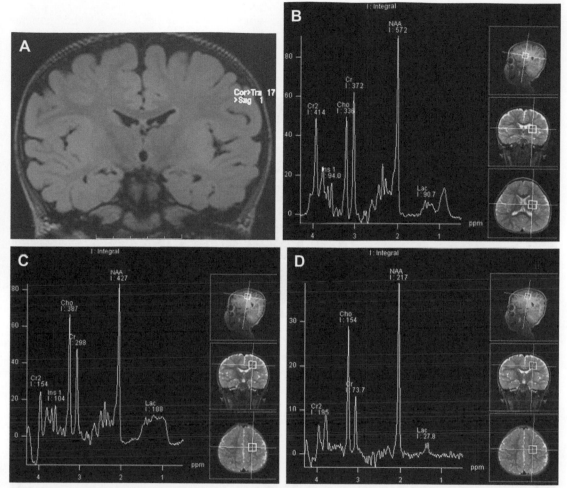

Fig. 1. MRS raises concern for a metabolic derangement and seizure when the conventional MR images appear normal. A 2-year-old boy underwent MR imaging and MRS for evaluation for global developmental delay and had not, previous to the MR imaging/MRS, manifested clinically recognized seizures. (*A*) The conventional 3-T MR imaging was normal and showed normal hippocampi and basal ganglia. (*B*) ^{1}H MRS obtained at TE of 35 milliseconds over the left basal ganglia as a screening tool for metabolic derangement showed a peak at 1.3 ppm equivocal for lactate versus lipid. This finding then prompted additional SV MRS at TE 35 over the left frontal white matter first at TE of 35 milliseconds (*C*) and then at TE of 288 milliseconds (*D*) that confirmed the abnormal lactate and distinguished it definitively from lipid. Based on the MRS findings, the boy underwent EEG that was interpreted as diffusely abnormal because of the presence of frequent bursts of high-amplitude generalized 3- to 4-Hz spike-and-wave activity.

imaging showed abnormal metabolites. They found reduced choline (Cho) in 80% of normal-appearing cerebellar white matter, 67% of normal-appearing peritrigonal white matter, and 60% of normal cortical gray matter. Cristina Bianchi and colleagues[5] also found reduced NAA/Cr ratios in 93% of normal-appearing cerebellum and in 87% of normal-appearing cortex, and in many cases, they found an abnormal small peak at 0.9 parts per million (ppm) that they attributed to amino acids. Abnormal lactate was often detected over abnormal-appearing brain but was also found in 2 patients over normal-appearing brain.[5] In 3 patients

in whom conventional MR imaging was interpreted as completely normal, MRS detected reduced Cho, NAA, and peaks at 0.9 ppm.[5] These findings suggest that MRS is indicated as a screen for mitochondrial disorders even in MR imaging of normal-appearing brain.

Cr disorders are also important considerations in the evaluation of the patient with epilepsy. Cr is an important metabolite for central nervous system function.[10] Two inherited enzymatic defects (L-arginine-glycine amidinotransferase [*AGAT*] and guanidinoacetate methyltransferase [*GAMT*]) and one inherited defect in Cr transport (*SLC6A8*) have

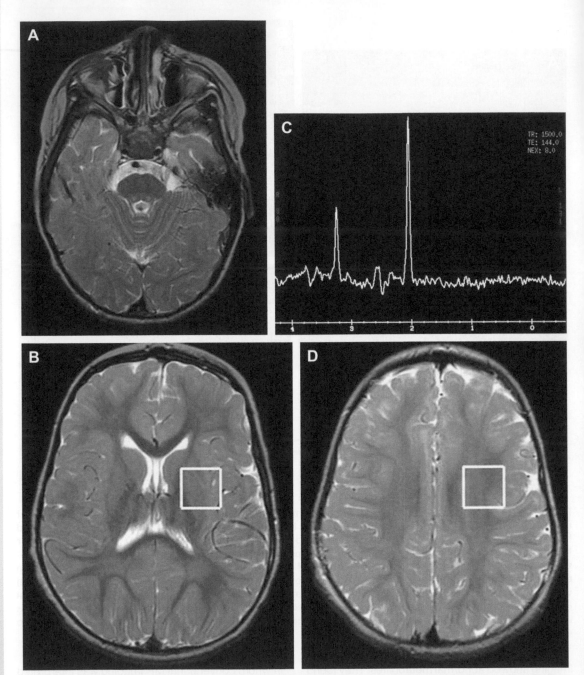

Fig. 2. MRS shows an inborn error of metabolism (Cr transport deficiency) when the conventional MR images are nonspecific. A 3-year-old boy with language delay (not speaking) and history of multiple generalized reportedly febrile seizures underwent MR imaging and MRS. (A) The conventional MR imaging showed two 3-mm nonspecific hyperintensities deep to the facial colliculi and was otherwise normal. (B, C) ^{1}H MRS at 1.5 T and TE of 144 milliseconds showed conspicuous absence of the normal Cr resonance at 3.0 ppm. (D, E) ^{1}H MRS obtained over the left fontal white matter at TE of 144 milliseconds confirms absence of the Cr peak. Serologic testing showed low levels of Cr and guanidinoacetate consistent with arginine:glycine amidinotransferase (AGAT) deficiency. (F) Normal level of central nervous system Cr after 3 months of Cr replacement therapy.

been characterized that result in a deficiency of cerebral Cr.[10] Cr deficiency may present with epilepsy or developmental delay.[11] Arias and colleagues[12] reviewed 1600 patients with mental retardation, autism, and/or epilepsy and found the prevalence of Cr transporter deficiency prevalence to be 0.25% (4 of 1600 cases). Of the 14 patients with global developmental delay who

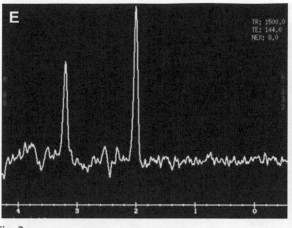

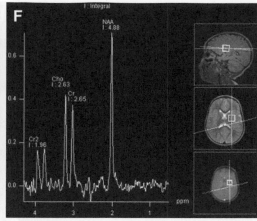

Fig. 2.

Neumeyer and colleagues[6] studied, moreover, 2 had Cr transporter deficiency diagnosed by MRS, and in both of these cases, MR imaging showed only nonspecific T2 hyperintensity in the periventricular white matter.

Medical Management

Once the goal of etiologic triage has been met, however, neuroimaging, not only MRS but also MR imaging, magnetoencephalography, and positron emission tomography, has a minor role in the initial management of the new patient with epilepsy. Management decisions are based principally on semiologic and electroencephalographic (EEG) findings. Although the detection of a gliotic scar or unequivocal malformation of cortical development may be of interest to the clinician, such data are "kept in consideration" or followed, whereas a trial of antiepileptic drugs (AEDs) is initiated.

Some studies have suggested a role for MRS as a biomarker for response to AEDs. Campos and colleagues,[13] for example, studied 25 patients with temporal lobe epilepsy (TLE) who responded to first-line AEDs and 21 patients with TLE who did not respond. The authors found a statistically significantly lower NAA/Cr ratio in the hippocampi of the nonresponders. Although certainly of interest, it is the authors' experience that such findings, initially, are not yet considered to be actionable, in that they do not practically influence the choice of AED or duration of the trial of AED therapy and do not per se justify the inclusion of MRS into the imaging protocol.

Presurgical Evaluation

If, however, the patient becomes refractory to medical therapy and the patient is considered for surgical management, MR Imaging and MRS reemerge as tools in the evaluation. Although the indication for MRS in this phase again certainly includes the detection of inborn errors of metabolism that may have been missed during the initial triage phase, the indication for MRS in this phase is based more on the reevaluation of lesions that may have been characterized initially as a dysplasia (eg, for evidence of neoplasia) (Fig. 5) or, as mentioned later, in confirmation of laterality of the epileptogenic nidus.

MRS for lateralization of the epileptogenic nidus in TLE

During persurgical planning for epilepsy surgery, localization of the epileptogenic nidus can be seen as a process of triangularization among seizure semiology, EEG findings, and imaging. A patient may be considered a surgical candidate if the seizure semiology, EEG findings, and imaging cohere (ie, if the lesion suggested by imaging would expectedly produce the seizure semiology showed clinically and if the lesion seen on imaging corresponds anatomically to the electrographic maxima seen on EEG).

In the specific semiologic setting of TLE, when this process of triangularization fails, some investigators have proposed, as detailed later, that MRS may play an adjunct role in the presurgical evaluation of medically refractory TLE.[14,15] Cendes and colleagues,[14] for example, performed ^{1}H MRS and MR volumetric analyses of the temporal lobes in 100 patients with medically refractory TLE. Using reduced NAA/Cr ratios as a marker of neuronal loss, they found that MRS alone agreed with the lateralization determined by EEG in 86% of patients, better than MR imaging volumetry alone (83%), and that MRS was abnormal in 12 patients

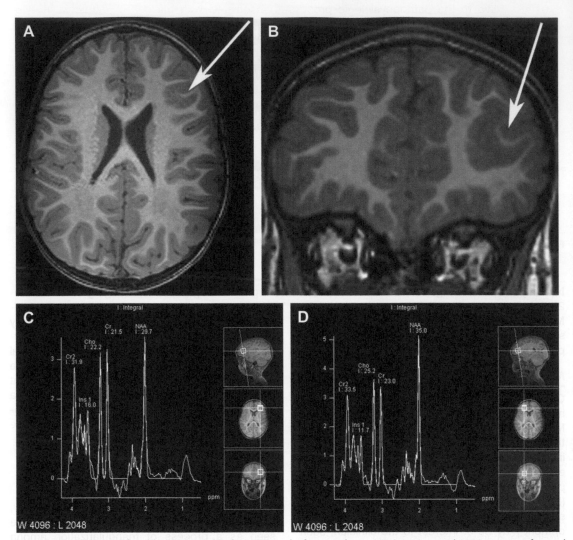

Fig. 3. MRS confirms a focal lesion as a dysplasia instead of a neoplasm. MR imaging and MRS were performed for evaluation of a 2-year-old boy with focal seizure semiology consisting of right head turn and eye deviation and staring, which evolved to tonic seizures with bilateral arm raising. EEG showed nearly continuous spikes with slow-wave discharges in the left frontal region F3/Fp1. Axial (*A*) and coronal reformats (*B*) from an MPRAGE show asymmetric sulcation and fullness of the left middle frontal gyrus that raised concern for FCD versus neoplasm. MRS at TE 35 milliseconds over the lesion (*C*) compared with MRS obtained over the contralateral normal right middle frontal gyrus (*D*) show a reduced NAA/Cr ratio and no elevation in Cho/NAA, findings thought to favor dysplasia instead of neoplasia. The patient became medically refractory during the course of the next 2 years, underwent resection of the left middle frontal gyral lesion, and pathologic examination confirmed a type IIB FCD.

with normal MR imaging volumetric analysis.[14] Cendes and colleagues proposed that MRS may be used in "conventional MR imaging negative" patients to confirm a lesion suggested by EEG.

Part II: how to do MRS: technique.

Major Resonances in Brain ¹H MRS and Their Clinical Relevance

The resonances seen in the brain on MRS are typically low-weight molecules such as NAA,

Cho-containing compounds, Cr/phosphocreatine, lactate, myoinositol (ml), glutamate/glutamine (Glx), and lipids. NAA is predominantly found in neurons and therefore is a marker for neuronal density and viability.[16–19] Cr serves as a marker for energy-dependent systems. Cho concentrations are increased as a result of increased inflammatory/gliotic processes and pathologic changes in membrane turnover.[20,21] Lactate is not normally detected on MRS; however, its presence can be detected after seizures,[22] in cases of

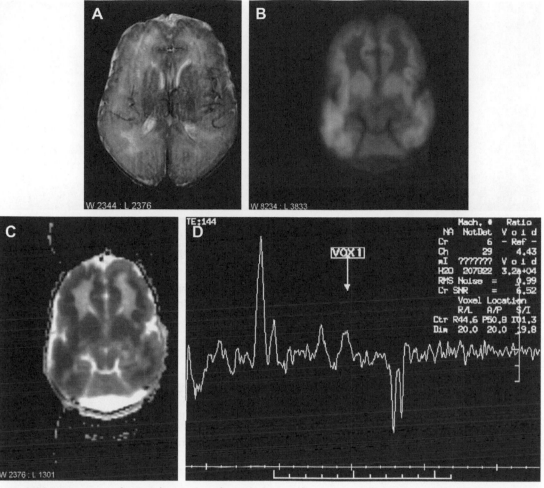

Fig. 4. MRS raises concern for an inborn error of metabolism, sulfite oxidase deficiency, rather than HII in the setting of neonatal encephalopathy. MR imaging and MRS of a 3-day-old term infant who presented with generalized tonic-clonic seizures and hypotonia on the third day of life. Axial T2 (*A*), DWI trace (*B*), and ADC map (*C*) show abnormal high signal on T2 and diminished diffusion that predilects the subcortical white matter and basal ganglia. MRS at TE 144 milliseconds over the involved white matter (*D*) shows prominent peaks at 2 to 2.4 ppm consistent with elevated Glx that may be seen in metabolic disorders (eg, urea cycle disorders),[101] marked decrease in NAA at 2 ppm, and a prominent lactate resonance at 1.3 ppm. The diffuse injury, predilection of the subcortical white matter, marked early reduction in NAA, and prominent peak at 2 to 2.4 ppm raised sufficient concern for an inborn error of metabolism to prompt enzymatic testing that confirmed sulfite oxidase deficiency.

hypoxic-ischemic injury (HII),[23–26] or in mitochondrial disorders[27–29] and in the first hours after birth.[30] Glutamate is the major excitatory neurotransmitter of the brain.[31,32] Excessive stimulation of glutamate can be toxic and can eventually result in neuronal death. mI is an organic osmolite and primarily located in glia, and an increase in mI is commonly thought to be a marker of gliosis.[33]

Acquisition Parameters

As with MR imaging, the choice of echo time (TE) and repetition time (TR) can have a considerable

effect on the appearance of the information obtained in an ^{1}H MRS study.

Spin-lattice TRs

Spin-lattice TRs for selected resonances at 1.5 T vary between 1100 and 1700 milliseconds.[34] Ideally, one has to wait 3 × T1 (3 × 1500 milliseonds = 4500 seconds) to gain approximately 95% of the original magnetization. With longer TRs (>3 seconds), the signal/noise ratio (SNR) and the quantification improve. A long TR, however, results in a long examination time. Therefore, typical TRs for clinical MRS experiments lie between 1 and 3 seconds.

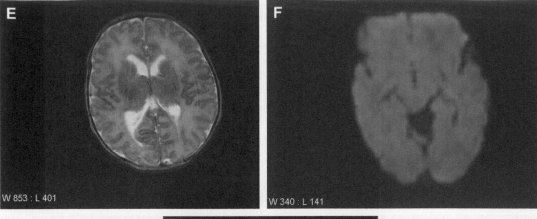

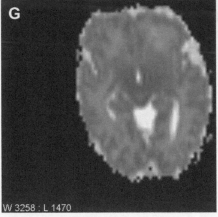

Fig. 4. Axial T2 (*E*), DWI (*F*), and ADC map (*G*) in a developmentally normal 3-day-old infant are provided for comparison.

TEs

MR spectra obtained with shorter TEs (~35 milliseconds) allow the detection of more metabolites, including Glx and mI (see **Fig. 1**A). Specifically, high concentrations of Glx may reflect seizure activity and have been reported in neonates with HII; elevated Glx levels were found to be associated with poor prognosis in HII.[35,36] Furthermore, low levels of mI most likely the result of glial loss were associated with poor outcome.[37]

Spectra obtained with longer TEs (135–144 milliseconds) depict a reduced number of metabolites (**Fig. 6**B). However, spectra are easier to process and analyze because of the relatively flat baseline. In addition, lactate (1.3 ppm) and alanine (1.5 ppm) doublets are inverted, thereby allowing better differentiation between these metabolites and lipids/macromolecules. Spectra obtained at TEs of 270 to 288 milliseconds have the advantage that typically no lipid contamination is present; lactate is once more phased up, but the SNR is considerably decreased because of T2 effects (see **Fig. 6**C).

In our MRS protocol for epilepsy, we suggest initially obtaining short TE MR spectra to detect metabolites such as Glx and mI. In case there is suspicion for the presence of lactate, we suggest repeating the MRS using a longer TE of 144 milliseconds at 1.5 T and 288 milliseconds at 3 T. This technical adjustment at 3 T is necessary, because at higher field strengths, lactate may show reduced or absent signal intensity at a TE of 144 milliseconds.[38]

Editing and 2-Dimensional MRS Techniques

Splitting of resonance lines into multiplets because of J-modulation results in signal loss and cancellation and therefore can make the quantification in an MR spectrum more challenging.[38,39] In addition, in the ^{1}H MR spectrum, many resonances overlap at similar frequencies (eg, the γ-aminobutyric acid [GABA] triplet and the Cr singlet resonate at 3.0 ppm).

In difference editing, a selective and nonselective spin-echo spectrum is acquired, and the difference spectrum contains the contribution of

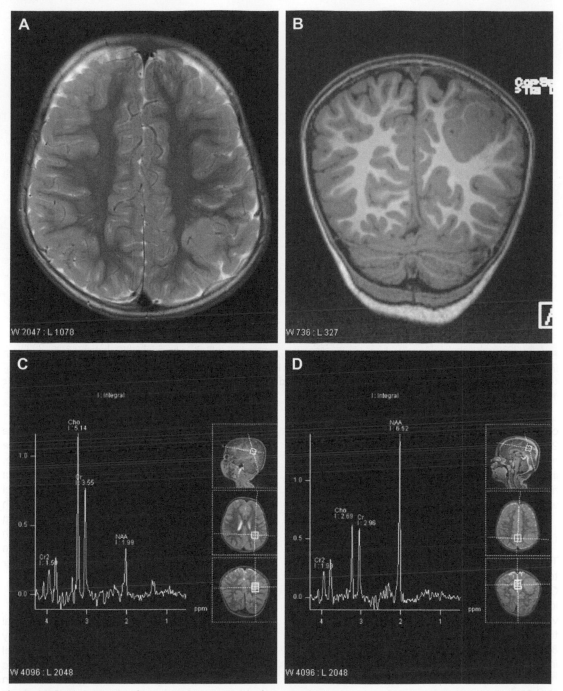

Fig. 5. MRS raises concern for a neoplasm instead of an FCD. MR imaging and MRS in a 7-year-old developmentally normal boy who presents, afebrile, with sudden onset of right face and arm twitching; EEG shows left parietal slowing and spikes. (*A*) An axial T2 and (*B*) a coronal MPRAGE images show a lesion that appears largely isointense to gray matter and that expands the involved left parietal cortex. (*C*) SV MRS performed at TE 288 milliseconds at 3 T shows elevation in Cho and decrease in NAA compared with adjacent normal cortex (*D*), which raised concern for neoplasia; a small lactate peak was also seen over the lesion.

the target metabolite providing the subtraction of all other contributors will null the background.[40,41] For example, the GABA triplet at 3.0 ppm can be detected using this method, canceling

contribution from Cr.[42] Macromolecules, however, are usually edited along with GABA.

An MRS technique called 2-dimensional J-resolved MRS spreads out the resonances that

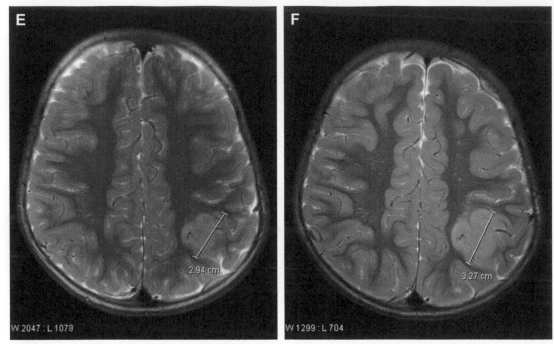

Fig. 5. The lesion was followed closely during a trial of AEDs, and comparison between the presentation MR imaging (*E*) and a follow-up MR imaging several months later (*F*) showed interval increase in size that raised additional suspicion for neoplasm. The lesion was resected and pathologic examination showed an angiocentric astrocytoma.

overlap in conventional 1-dimensional MRS along 2 separate dimensions, improving the definition and specificity of detection of different metabolites.[43] Such metabolite-specific MRS techniques may be useful for the evaluation of GABA levels with antiepileptic treatment.[44–46]

Localization Techniques

To measure MR spectra in vivo, one has to be able to define the spatial origin of the detected signal. Currently, 2 methods exist to obtain the spatially localized metabolic information in vivo: (1) single-voxel spectroscopy (SVS) uses selective excitation pulses to localize a voxel of typically 3 to 8 cm^3 and (2) multivoxel arrays of spectra (MRS imaging) can be obtained in 1, 2, or 3 dimensions resulting in individual voxel sizes of typically 0.5 to 3 cm^3.

SVS

SVS has the advantage of higher SNR and typically shorter acquisition times (~3 minutes) compared with MRS imaging (~8 minutes). In SV MRS, one approach is to survey white matter and deep and cortical gray matter by performing 3 × SV MRS at TE of 35 milliseconds, one each over the centrum semiovale, lentiform nuclei, and midline occipitoparietal cortex. Another approach is to perform one SV MRS over the basal ganglia; in the interest of time, when the conventional/anatomic MR images are negative, we perform one SV MRS over the basal ganglia as a screening technique and reserve the 3-voxel approach for those cases when there is a high clinical suspicion for inborn error of metabolism or when the anatomic MR images raise such concern. To evaluate TLE, 2 single voxels are placed in the left and right temporal lobes over the hippocampi.

MRS imaging or MV MRS

MRS imaging allows one to collect the spectral information from a volume consisting of many voxels. We prefer MRS imaging for clinical studies when it is indicated to obtain metabolic information of a large and heterogeneous lesion (eg, in tumors and in myelin disorders such as adrenoleukodystrophy). In addition, spectral information from control regions may be obtained simultaneously. However, the main limitation of MRS imaging is the lengthy acquisition times, especially with 3-dimensional data acquisition.

Fast MRS imaging techniques Several fast MRS imaging experiments have been presented that promise to reduce data acquisition duration.

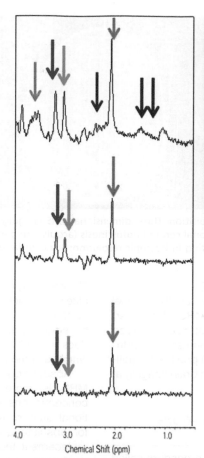
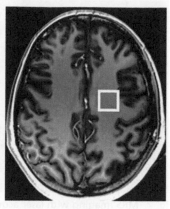

A **Short TE (35 ms)**
MRS spectrum

B **Long TE (144 ms)**
MRS spectrum

C **Very long TE (288 ms)**
MRS spectrum

Myo-inositol

Choline

Creatine

Glutamate/Glutamine

N-acetylaspartate

Lactate and Lipids

4.0   3.0   2.0   1.0
Chemical Shift (ppm)

Fig. 6. MRS of white matter in a normal brain. A typical proton MR spectra from the centrum semiovale acquired at TE of 35, 144, and 288 milliseconds. The 144- to 288- millisecond TE spectra have less baseline distortion and are easy to process and analyze but show fewer metabolites than short TE spectra. Also, the lactate and alanine peaks are inverted at 144 milliseconds, which makes it easier to differentiate them from lipids. Short TE demonstrates peaks attributable to more metabolites, including lipids, Glx, and mI.

Some improvement of sensitivity may be achieved by acquiring data by reduced k-space sampling.[47,48] Fast MRS imaging sequences have evolved from concepts related to spatial encoding using gradient switching during acquisition.[49–53] Spiral trajectories in k-space allow fast encoding of spatial information. A recent study showed that clinical 3-dimensional MRS images can be acquired 4 times faster with spiral protocols than with the elliptical phase encoding protocol at a high spatial resolution of 1 cm^3 in 2.5 minutes.[54]

Chemical Shift Artifact

With increasing field strengths, (1) chemical shift displacement error, (2) spatial nonuniformity of radiofrequency excitation, and (3) contamination with subcutaneous lipid signal from tissues outside the region of interest are becoming increasingly and more severe. To compensate for radiofrequency inhomogeneity, adiabatic pulses can be implemented.[55,56] Recently, a 3-dimensional MRS imaging technique with low-power adiabatic pulses and fast spiral acquisition was implemented,[54] resulting in high-resolution, high-SNR MRS data (**Fig. 7**).

Field strength

MRS has inherently low SNR, resulting in MRS imaging with low spatial resolution or long acquisition times. MRS SNR can be improved significantly by using higher magnetic field strengths, because the SNR is proportional to B0 field strength. Increased chemical shift at 3 and 7 T results in greater separation of the resonance peaks and, as a consequence, allows for better quantification of those metabolites that generally overlap with others, such as Glx[57] and GABA, without using editing techniques.[58]

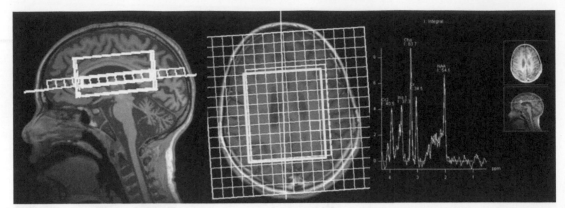

Fig. 7. MRS imaging with laser acquisition. Three-dimensional MRS imaging sequence with laser acquisition and spiral readout of a child with neuronal ceroid lipofuscinosis (acquisition parameters include matrix 16 × 16 × 8 over field of view of 160 mm resulting in isotropic resolution: 1 mL, duration: 6 minutes).

Multichannel array receiver coils

Multichannel receiver coils such as 32-channel brain improves the SNR in MRS. Moreover, a recent study demonstrated that size-optimized multichannel array coils (for neonates, 6-month-olds, and 1-, 4-, and 7-year-olds) provided significant sensitivity gains for pediatric brain imaging at 3 T.[59]

OTHER TECHNICAL CONSIDERATIONS
Shimming

To maximize B0 homogeneity, a procedure called "shimming" must be used at the beginning of every acquisition. Shimming is critical for MRS studies to obtain narrow signals. On most commercial scanners, shimming routines are readily available and are typically performed by generating a B0 field map.[60–63] Rapid imaging techniques such as echo planar or spiral imaging are often used to minimize scan time[64] such as "fastestmap."[65]

Motion Correction

For children between 2 months and 7 years of age, motion artifact and patient cooperation often limit the feasibility of MR imaging and MRS and sedation must often be used. Anesthesia, however, carries risks to patients, so there is a search for motion correction techniques that may allow for the reduction in sedated cases. Using image-based navigators, it is possible to correct motion in structural imaging and SVS prospectively.[66–69]

Quantification

The total area under the metabolite resonance peak is proportional to the concentration of that specific metabolite, and the integration of this area is the primary task needed for quantification.

The easiest quantification method is to use metabolite ratios such as NAA/Cr or Cho/NAA. Ratios reported using Cr as an internal standard are often based on the assumption that the Cr concentration does not change during the disease process, which is sometimes, but not always, true.

"Absolute quantification" of brain metabolites by MRS is more difficult to obtain. Metabolite concentrations are generally expressed in institutional units or units of mmol/kg. Methods used for absolute quantification include (1) phantom replacement techniques,[70–73] (2) water signal as a reference using a second MR spectrum in which the water is unsuppressed,[74,75] and (3) the use of an external reference.[76,77]

Spectral Analysis Methods

To date, automated parametric spectral analysis methods have been implemented that seek to determine the optimum parameters that enable some functions (so-called model functions) to best describe the data. These model functions are based on prior information. Fortunately, considerable information on the observable metabolites and their spectral characteristics are available.[31] Parametric modeling based on a priori spectral information has been made reasonably robust.[78–83] Fitting can be done in the time[84] or frequency[85] domain. Currently, the most commonly used MRS analysis programs are LCModel[78,86,87] and jMRUI.[88–90]

PART III: WHEN DOES MRS HELP? SEMIOLOGIC SPECIFIC EXAMPLES

The International League against Epilepsy has classified epilepsy phenotypes into electroclinical groupings that may serve as a context in which to exemplify when MRS may help in the imaging evaluation of the patient with epilepsy.[91] The following examples are organized by electroclinical grouping and are discussed in the context of the results of the conventional MR images.

Semiology: Focal Epilepsy

Conventional MR imaging: lesional

In this setting, if the seizure semiology and EEG both suggest a focal epilepsy, and conventional MR imaging detects a focal lesion, we have found MRS to be useful in confirming the lesion as a dysplasia (see Fig. 3), in raising concern for alternative interpretations of the lesion as a neoplasm

(see Fig. 5), or, more rarely, as a focal or tumefactive manifestation of a metabolic disorder (Fig. 8). Kaminaga and colleagues[92] studied 15 patients, with conventional MR imaging–defined malformations of cortical development, including 8 cases of focal cortical dysplasia (FCD), by stimulated echo sequence (probe-s) short and long echo MRS on 1.5 T; they found a low NAA to be the only statistically significant difference between the FCD group and the age-matched normal control subjects and did not find a statistically significant difference in Cho levels. Aasly and colleagues[93] performed ex vivo ^{1}H MRS in homogenized brain extracts from 17 patients who underwent surgical resection

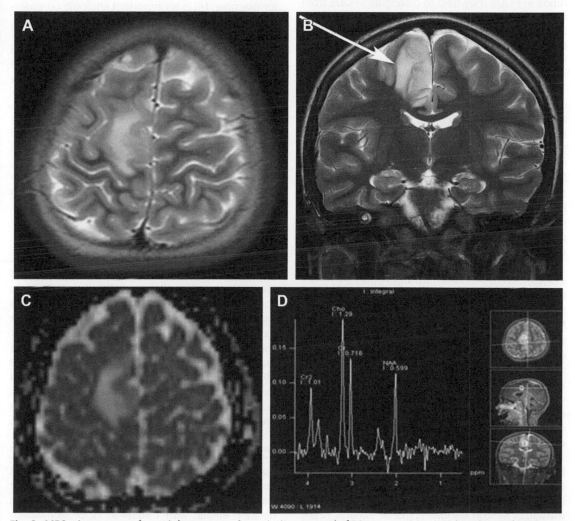

Fig. 8. MRS raises concern for an inborn error of metabolism instead of FCD or neoplasm. MR imaging and MRS were performed on an 8-year-old previously healthy girl brought to the emergency department for severe headache. On arrival to the emergency department, she was afebrile and had generalized tonic-clonic seizures with left focal gaze. (A) Axial and (B) coronal T2-weighted images show a single high signal lesion that involves the cortex and subcortical white matter of the right superior frontal gyrus. (C) The axial ADC map shows increased diffusion. (D) SV MRS at 1.5 T and TE 144 milliseconds shows a small inverted lactate peak at 1.4 ppm and prominent peaks at 2.4 and 3.7 ppm that likely reflect Glx, findings that raised concern for an inborn error of metabolism and seem less consistent with dysplasia or neoplasm. Muscle biopsy and electron transport chain analysis showed a complex I deficiency.

of lesions for medically refractory epilepsy with pathologic correlation; in the 4 cases of FCD from their series, they found statistically significantly lower levels of NAA and higher levels of GABA, alanine, tyrosine, lactate, and inositol, and no statistically significant difference in Cho, compared with age-matched normal control subjects. Elevations in Cho/Cr ratios and decreases in NAA/Cr ratios have been well described in patients with glial neoplasms and in many pediatric patients with brain tumors.[94,95] Although decreased NAA/Cr ratios are thus common findings in both FCDs and some central nervous system neoplasms, the relatively normal Cho/Cr ratios in FCDs may help to distinguish FCDs from neoplasms when the conventional MR imaging findings are equivocal (see **Figs. 3** and **5**). The MRS findings in many inborn errors of metabolism have been presented in the literature.[96] Cackmacki and colleagues,[97] for example, performed ^{1}H MRS on 19 patients with different inborn errors of metabolism and frequently found elevations in lactate or Glx/Cr ratios. The results of ^{1}H MRS of some inborn errors of metabolism, such as elevation in Cho/Cr or decrease in NAA/Cr, may confusingly overlap those of both neoplasia and FCD. Based on published findings, however, in practice, spectroscopic features such as marked elevation in lactate and elevation in Glx/Cr raise enough concern for inborn errors of metabolism as to prompt further serologic or urine metabolic testing that may confirm the diagnosis (see **Fig. 8**).[96,97]

Conventional MR imaging: nonlesional

In the setting of focal epilepsy, if the conventional MR imaging is negative for a lesion, the use of MRS may seem to be less obvious. There is no signal abnormality on the conventional MR images over which to place the voxel. It is important, in this setting, to recall that certain metabolic disorders, such as mitochondrial disorders, can present with a focal epilepsy phenotype and, as discussed earlier, MRS has been shown to evidence mitochondrial dysfunction in some instances when conventional MR imaging may be negative.[5,9]

In TLE, as discussed earlier, MRS can be helpful for lateralization and identification of epileptogenic areas in patients with normal conventional MR imaging.[98] In an attempt to address the issue of the use of MRS in identifying malformations, Krsek and colleagues[99] studied 7 patients with extratemporal epilepsy and conventional MR imaging–negative brains at 1.5 T. They found that in 5 patients that multivoxel MRS findings of decreased NAA/Cho and decreased NAA/Cr overlapped the ictal zone as determined by subdural electrodes and correlated with FCDs on local

resection and that 4 of 5 patients were seizure free or obtained greater than 90% seizure reduction at 12- to 18-month follow-up.[99] Such results raise for consideration that MRS may serve as a localizing technique in extratemporal epilepsy secondary to FCDs that are occult on conventional MR imaging.

Semiology: Generalized Epilepsy

Conventional MR imaging: positive

If the seizure semiology is generalized and the conventional MR imaging findings are positive, MRS may be used to further characterize the abnormal findings. In neonatal encephalopathy, for example, HII is an important etiologic consideration.[100] Certain inborn errors of metabolism, however, can present with neonatal encephalopathy, such as nonketotic hyperglycinemia or sulfite oxidase sufficiency, when MRS may raise concern for an inborn error of metabolism and prompt further testing (see **Fig. 4**).[4]

Conventional MR imaging: negative

If the seizure semiology suggests generalized epilepsy but the conventional MR images reveal no findings specific for a metabolic derangement, we have nevertheless found MRS to be an important tool to screen for inborn errors of metabolism (see **Figs. 1** and **2**).[4,5]

SUMMARY
Part I: Why Do MRS? Indications

During the triage phase of the imaging workup of the patient with epilepsy, MRS is indicated to screen for metabolic derangements such as inborn errors of metabolism. During the presurgical phase of the imaging workup of the patient with epilepsy, MRS is indicated to characterize masses that may be equivocal on conventional MR imaging for dysplasia versus neoplasia and may serve a role for confirmation of EEG-determined lateralization in cases of TLE when the conventional MR image is negative for a lesion.

Part II: How to Do MRS in Epilepsy? Technique

For the patient with epilepsy with conventional MR imaging negative examinations, we recommend at least an SV MRS approach, with the parameters detailed earlier, with 1 voxel at TE of 35 milliseconds placed over the basal ganglia as a screening technique for detection of inborn errors of metabolism. Multivoxel MRS techniques can be considered in conventional MR imaging–negative cases of extratemporal epilepsy.[99]

For patient with epilepsy with pathologic changes detected on conventional MR images

(MR imaging positive), the signal abnormality detected should guide voxel placement. A contralateral voxel should be considered to be used as an internal reference.

For suspected TLE, bilateral rectangular voxels including the hippocampi have been shown in the literature to be useful to demonstrate relatively decreased NAA or increased Cho ratios ipsilateral to the epileptogenic source.[98]

Part III: When to Do MRS? Case Illustrations

If the semiology is focal and the conventional MR imaging shows a focal lesion, ^{1}H MRS may confirm the lesion as a dyplasia or raise concern for a neoplasm or tumefactive manifestation of an inborn error of metabolism. If the conventional MR imaging is negative, ^{1}H MRS is useful to screen for mitochondrial disorders that may exhibit a focal seizure phenotype.

If the semiology is generalized and the conventional MR imaging is positive, as may be seen in neonatal encephalopathy, or if the semiology is generalized and the conventional MR imaging is negative, ^{1}H MRS may help to raise concern for an underlying inborn error of metabolism.

REFERENCES

1. Cendes F, Stanley J, Dubeau F, et al. Proton magnetic resonance spectroscopic Imaging for discrimination of absence and complex partial seizures. Ann Neurol 1997;41:74–81.
2. Parikh S, Cohen BH, Gupta A, et al. Metabolic testing in the pediatric epilepsy unit. Pediatr Neurol 2008;38:191–5.
3. Buist NR, Dulac O, Bottiglieri T, et al. Metabolic evaluation of infantile epilepsy: summary recommendations of the Amalfi Group. J Child Neurol 2002;17(Suppl 3):3S98–102.
4. Wolf N, García-Cazorla A, Hoffmann G. Epilepsy and inborn errors of metabolism in children. J Inherit Metab Dis 2009;32:609–17.
5. Cristina Bianchi M, Tosetti M, Battini R, et al. Proton MR spectroscopy of mitochondrial diseases: analysis of brain metabolic abnormalities and their possible diagnostic relevance. AJNR Am J Neuroradiol 2003;24:1958–66.
6. Newmeyer A, Cecil KM, Schapiro M, et al. Incidence of brain creatine transporter deficiency in males with developmental delay referred for brain magnetic resonance imaging. J Dev Behav Pediatr 2005;26:276–82.
7. Khurana DS, Salganicoff L, Melvin JJ, et al. Epilepsy and respiratory chain defects in children with mitochondrial encephalopathies. Neuropediatrics 2008;39:8–13.
8. Canafoglia L, Franceschetti S, Antozzi C, et al. Epileptic phenotypes associated with mitochondrial disorders. Neurology 2001;56:1340–6.
9. Lee Y, Kang H, Lee J, et al. Mitochondrial respiratory chain defects: underlying etiology in various epileptic conditions. Epilepsia 2008;49:685–90.
10. Nasrallah F, Feki M, Kaabachi N. Creatine and creatine deficiency syndromes: biochemical and clinical aspects. Pediatr Neurol 2010;42:163–71.
11. Stromberger C, Bodamer OA, Stockler-Ipsiroglu S. Clinical characteristics and diagnostic clues in inborn errors of creatine metabolism. J Inherit Metab Dis 2003;26:299–308.
12. Arias A, Corbella M, Fons C, et al. Creatine transporter deficiency: prevalence among patients with mental retardation and pitfalls in metabolite screening. Clin Biochem 2007;40:1328–31.
13. Campos B, Yasuda C, Castellano G, et al. Proton MRS may predict AED response in patients with TLE. Epilepsia 2010;51:783–8.
14. Cendes F, Caramanos Z, Andermann F, et al. Proton magnetic resonance spectroscopic imaging and magnetic resonance imaging volumetry in the lateralization of temporal lobe epilepsy: a series of 100 patients. Ann Neurol 1997;42:737–46.
15. Kuzniecky R, Hugg JW, Hetherington H, et al. Relative utility of 1H spectroscopic imaging and hippocampal volumetry in the lateralization of mesial temporal lobe epilepsy. Neurology 1998;51:66–71.
16. Simmons ML, Frondoza CG, Coyle JT. Immunocytochemical localization of N-acetyl-aspartate with monoclonal antibodies. Neuroscience 1991;45:37–45.
17. Moffett JR, Namboodiri MA, Cangro CB, et al. Immunohistochemical localization of N-acetylaspartate in rat brain. Neuroreport 1991;2:131–4.
18. Urenjak J, Williams SR, Gadian DG, et al. Specific expression of N-acetylaspartate in neurons, oligodendrocyte-type-2 astrocyte progenitors, and immature oligodendrocytes in vitro. J Neurochem 1992;59:55–61.
19. Urenjak J, Williams SR, Gadian DG, et al. Proton nuclear magnetic resonance spectroscopy unambiguously identifies different neural cell types. J Neurosci 1993;13:981–9.
20. Lin A, Bluml S, Mamelak AN. Efficacy of proton magnetic resonance spectroscopy in clinical decision making for patients with suspected malignant brain tumors. J Neurooncol 1999;45:69–81.
21. Bendszus M, Martin-Schrader I, Warmuth-Metz M, et al. MR imaging- and MR spectroscopy-revealed changes in meningiomas for which embolization was performed without subsequent surgery. AJNR Am J Neuroradiol 2000;21:666–9.
22. Breiter SN, Arroyo S, Mathews VP, et al. Proton MR spectroscopy in patients with seizure disorders. AJNR Am J Neuroradiol 1994;15:373–84.

23. Khong PL, Tse C, Wong IY, et al. Diffusion-weighted imaging and proton magnetic resonance spectroscopy in perinatal hypoxic-ischemic encephalopathy: association with neuromotor outcome at 18 months of age. J Child Neurol 2004;19:872–81.

24. Kadri M, Shu S, Holshouser B, et al. Proton magnetic resonance spectroscopy improves outcome prediction in perinatal CNS insults. J Perinatol 2003;23:181–5.

25. da Silva LF, Hoefel Filho JR, Anes M, et al. Prognostic value of 1H-MRS in neonatal encephalopathy. Pediatr Neurol 2006;34:360–6.

26. Zarifi MK, Astrakas LG, Poussaint TY, et al. Prediction of adverse outcome with cerebral lactate level and apparent diffusion coefficient in infants with perinatal asphyxia. Radiology 2002;225:859–70.

27. Cross JH, Gadian DG, Connelly A, et al. Proton magnetic resonance spectroscopy studies in lactic acidosis and mitochondrial disorders. J Inherit Metab Dis 1993;16:800–11.

28. Castillo M, Kwock L, Green C. MELAS syndrome: imaging and proton MR spectroscopic findings. AJNR Am J Neuroradiol 1995;16:233–9.

29. Mathews PM, Andermann F, Silver K, et al. Proton MR spectroscopic characterization of differences in regional brain metabolic abnormalities in mitochondrial encephalomyopathies. Neurology 1993;43:2484–90.

30. Barkovich AJ, Westmark KD, Bedi HS, et al. Proton spectroscopy and diffusion imaging on the first day of life after perinatal asphyxia: preliminary report. AJNR Am J Neuroradiol 2001;22:1786–94.

31. Govindaraju V, Young K, Maudsley AA. Proton NMR chemical shifts and coupling constants for brain metabolites. NMR Biomed 2000;13:129–53.

32. Ross BD. Biochemical considerations in 1H spectroscopy. Glutamate and glutamine; myo-inositol and related metabolites. NMR Biomed 1991;4:59–63.

33. Brand A, Richter-Landsberg C, Leibfritz D. Multinuclear NMR studies on the energy metabolism of glial and neuronal cells. Dev Neurosci 1993;15:289–98.

34. Frahm J, Bruhn H, Gyngell ML, et al. Localized proton NMR spectroscopy in different regions of the human brain in vivo. Relaxation times and concentrations of cerebral metabolites. Magn Reson Med 1989;11:47–63.

35. Groenendaal F, van der Grond J, van Haastert IC, et al. Findings in cerebral proton spin resonance spectroscopy in newborn infants with asphyxia, and psychomotor development. Ned Tijdschr Geneeskd 1996;140:255–9 [in Dutch].

36. Zhu W, Zhong W, Qi J, et al. Proton magnetic resonance spectroscopy in neonates with hypoxic-ischemic injury and its prognostic value. Transl Res 2008;152:225–32.

37. Ancora G, Soffritti S, Lodi R, et al. A combined a-EEG and MR spectroscopy study in term newborns with hypoxic-ischemic encephalopathy. Brain Dev 2010;32:835–42.

38. Lange T, Dydak U, Roberts TP, et al. Pitfalls in lactate measurements at 3T. AJNR Am J Neuroradiol 2006;27:895–901.

39. Thrippleton MJ, Edden RA, Keeler J. Suppression of strong coupling artefacts in J-spectra. J Magn Reson 2005;174:97–109.

40. De Graaf RA. In vivo NMR spectroscopy: principles and techniques. Chichester (UK): John Wiley & Sons; 1998.

41. Campbell ID, Dobson CM. The application of high resolution nuclear magnetic resonance to biological systems. Methods Biochem Anal 1979;25:1–133.

42. Mescher M, Merkle H, Kirsch J, et al. Simultaneous in vivo spectral editing and water suppression. NMR Biomed 1998;11:266–72.

43. Ludwig C, Viant MR. Two-dimensional J-resolved NMR spectroscopy: review of a key methodology in the metabolomics toolbox. Phytochem Anal 2010;21:22–32.

44. Ke Y, Cohen BM, Bang JY, et al. Assessment of GABA concentration in human brain using two-dimensional proton magnetic resonance spectroscopy. Psychiatry Res 2000;100:169–78.

45. Levy LM, Degnan AJ. GABA-based evaluation of neurologic conditions: MR spectroscopy. AJNR Am J Neuroradiol 2012. [Epub ahead of print].

46. Puts NA, Edden RA. In vivo magnetic resonance spectroscopy of GABA: a methodological review. Prog Nucl Magn Reson Spectrosc 2012;60:29–41.

47. Maudsley AA, Matson GB, Hugg JW, et al. Reduced phase encoding in spectroscopic imaging. Magn Reson Med 1994;31:645–51.

48. Kuehn B. Fast proton spectroscopic imaging employing k-space weighing achieved by variable repetition times. Magn Reson Med 1996;35:457–64.

49. Mansfield P. Spatial mapping of the chemical shift in NMR. Magn Reson Med 1984;1:370–86.

50. Guilfoyle DN, Blamire A, Chapman B, et al. PEEP: a rapid chemical-shift imaging method. Magn Reson Med 1989;10:282–7.

51. Webb P, Spielman D, Macovski A. A fast spectroscopic imaging method using a blipped phase encode gradient. Magn Reson Med 1989;12:306–15.

52. Twieg DB. Multiple-output chemical shift imaging (MOCSI): a practical technique for rapid spectroscopic imaging. Magn Reson Med 1989;12:64–73.

53. Posse S, Tedeschi G, Risinger R, et al. High speed 1H spectroscopic imaging in human brain by echo planar spatial-spectral encoding. Magn Reson Med 1995;33:34–40.

54. Andronesi OC, Gagoski BA, Sorensen AG. Neurologic 3D MR spectroscopic imaging with low-power adiabatic pulses and fast spiral acquisition. Radiology 2012;262:647–61.

55. Garwood M, Uğurbil K, Rath AR, et al. Magnetic resonance imaging with adiabatic pulses using a single surface coil for RF transmission and signal detection. Magn Reson Med 1989;9:25–34.

56. Andronesi OC, Ramadan S, Ratai EM, et al. Spectroscopic imaging with improved gradient modulated constant adiabaticity pulses on high-field clinical scanners. J Magn Reson 2010;203:283–93.

57. Tkac I, Andersen P, Adriany G, et al. In vivo 1H NMR spectroscopy of the human brain at 7 T. Magn Reson Med 2001;46:451–6.

58. Wijtenburg SA, Rowland LM, Spieker IA, et al. Reproducibility of anterior cingulate 1H MRS data at 7T. In: Proc Intl Soc Mag Reson Med. Melbourne (Australia): 2012. p. 4391.

59. Keil B, Alagappan V, Mareyam A, et al. Size-optimized 32-channel brain arrays for 3 T pediatric imaging. Magn Reson Med 2012;66:1777–87.

60. Webb P, Macovski A. Rapid, fully automatic, arbitrary-volume in vivo shimming. Magn Reson Med 1991;20:113–22.

61. Schneider E, Glover G. Rapid in vivo proton shimming. Magn Reson Med 1991;18:335–47.

62. Kanayama S, Kuhara S, Satoh K. In vivo rapid magnetic field measurement and shimming using single scan differential phase mapping. Magn Reson Med 1996;36:637–42.

63. Hetherington HP, Chu WJ, Gonen O, et al. Robust fully automated shimming of the human brain for high-field 1H spectroscopic imaging. Magn Reson Med 2006;56:26–33.

64. Reese TG, Davis TL, Weisskoff RM. Automated shimming at 1.5 T using echo-planar image frequency maps. J Magn Reson Imaging 1995;5:739–45.

65. Gruetter R, Tkac I. Field mapping without reference scan using asymmetric echo-planar techniques. Magn Reson Med 2000;43:319–23.

66. Hess AT, Tisdall MD, Andronesi OC, et al. Real-time motion and B0 corrected single voxel spectroscopy using volumetric navigators. Magn Reson Med 2011;66:314–23.

67. Tisdall MD, Hess AT, Reuter M, et al. Volumetric navigators for prospective motion correction and selective reacquisition in neuroanatomical MRI. Magn Reson Med 2011;68(2):389–99.

68. Kuperman JM, Brown TT, Ahmadi ME, et al. Prospective motion correction improves diagnostic utility of pediatric MRI scans. Pediatr Radiol 2011;41:1578–82.

69. Brown TT, Kuperman JM, Erhart M, et al. Prospective motion correction of high-resolution magnetic resonance imaging data in children. Neuroimage 2010;53:139–45.

70. Jacobs MA, Horska A, van Zijl PC, et al. Quantitative proton MR spectroscopic imaging of normal human cerebellum and brain stem. Magn Reson Med 2001;46:699–705.

71. Soher BJ, van Zijl PC, Duyn JH, et al. Quantitative proton MR spectroscopic imaging of the human brain. Magn Reson Med 1996;35:356–63.

72. Alger JR, Symko SC, Bizzi A, et al. Absolute quantitation of short TE brain 1H-MR spectra and spectroscopic imaging data. J Comput Assist Tomogr 1993;17:191–9.

73. Michaelis T, Merboldt KD, Bruhn H, et al. Absolute concentrations of metabolites in the adult human brain in vivo: quantification of localized proton MR spectra. Radiology 1993;187:219–27.

74. Barker PB, Soher BJ, Blackband SJ, et al. Quantitation of proton NMR spectra of the human brain using tissue water as an internal concentration reference. NMR Biomed 1993;6:89–94.

75. Christiansen P, Henriksen O, Stubgaard M, et al. In vivo quantification of brain metabolites by 1H-MRS using water as an internal standard. Magn Reson Imaging 1993;11:107–18.

76. Hennig J, Pfister H, Ernst T, et al. Direct absolute quantification of metabolites in the human brain with in vivo localized proton spectroscopy. NMR Biomed 1992;5:193–9.

77. Tofts PS, Wray S. A critical assessment of methods of measuring metabolite concentrations by NMR spectroscopy. NMR Biomed 1988;1:1–10.

78. Provencher SW. Estimation of metabolite concentrations from localized in vivo proton NMR spectra. Magn Reson Med 1993;30:672–9.

79. Stanley JA, Drost DJ, Williamson PC, et al. The use of a priori knowledge to quantify short echo in vivo 1H MR spectra. Magn Reson Med 1995;34:17–24.

80. Soher BJ, Young K, Govindaraju V, et al. Automated spectral analysis III: application to in vivo proton MR spectroscopy and spectroscopic imaging. Magn Reson Med 1998;40:822–31.

81. Young K, Govindaraju V, Soher BJ, et al. Automated spectral analysis I: formation of a priori information by spectral simulation. Magn Reson Med 1998;40:812–5.

82. Young K, Soher BJ, Maudsley AA. Automated spectral analysis II: application of wavelet shrinkage for characterization of non-parameterized signals. Magn Reson Med 1998;40:816–21.

83. Slotboom J, Boesch C, Kreis R. Versatile frequency domain fitting using time domain models and prior knowledge. Magn Reson Med 1998;39:899–911.

84. Vanhamme L, Sundin T, Hecke PV, et al. MR spectroscopy quantitation: a review of time-domain methods. NMR Biomed 2001;14:233–46.

85. Mierisova S, Ala-Korpela M. MR spectroscopy quantitation: a review of frequency domain methods. NMR Biomed 2001;14:247–59.

86. Provencher SW. Automatic quantitation of localized in vivo 1H spectra with LCModel. NMR Biomed 2001;14:260–4.

87. Pfeuffer J, Tkac I, Provencher SW, et al. Toward an in vivo neurochemical profile: quantification of 18 metabolites in short-echo-time (1)H NMR spectra of the rat brain. J Magn Reson 1999; 141:104–20.

88. van den Boogaart A, Van Hecke P, Van Huffel S, et al. MRUI: a graphical user interface for accurate routine MRS data analysis. In: Proceedings of the ESMRMB, 13th Annual Meeting. Prague: 1996. p. 318.

89. Naressi A, Couturier C, Castang I, et al. Java-based graphical user interface for MRUI, a software package for quantitation of in vivo/medical magnetic resonance spectroscopy signals. Comput Biol Med 2001;31:269–86.

90. Naressi A, Couturier C, Devos JM, et al. Java-based graphical user interface for the MRUI quantitation package. MAGMA 2001;12:141–52.

91. Berg AT, Berkovic SF, Brodie MJ, et al. Revised terminology and concepts for organization of seizures and epilepsies: report of the ILAE Commission on Classification and Terminology, 2005-2009. Epilepsia 2010;51:676–85.

92. Kaminaga T, Kobayashi M, Abe T. Proton magnetic resonance spectroscopy in disturbances of cortical development. Neuroradiology 2001;43:575–80.

93. Aasly J, Silfvenius H, Aas TC, et al. Proton magnetic resonance spectroscopy of brain biopsies from patients with intractable epilepsy. Epilepsy Res 1999;35:211–7.

94. Negendank WG, Sauter R, Brown TR, et al. Proton magnetic resonance spectroscopy in patients with glial tumors: a multicenter study. J Neurosurg 1996; 84:449–58.

95. Panigrahy A, Krieger MD, Gonzalez-Gomez I, et al. Quantitative short echo time 1H-MR spectroscopy of untreated pediatric brain tumors: preoperative diagnosis and characterization. AJNR Am J Neuroradiol 2006;27:560–72.

96. Cecil KM. MR spectroscopy of metabolic disorders. Neuroimaging Clin N Am 2006;16:87–116, viii.

97. Cakmakci H, Pekcevik Y, Yis U, et al. Diagnostic value of proton MR spectroscopy and diffusion-weighted MR imaging in childhood inherited neurometabolic brain diseases and review of the literature. Eur J Radiol 2010;74:e161–71.

98. Chernov MF, Ochiai T, Ono Y, et al. Role of proton magnetic resonance spectroscopy in preoperative evaluation of patients with mesial temporal lobe epilepsy. J Neurol Sci 2009;285:212–9.

99. Krsek P, Hajek M, Dezortova M, et al. (1)H MR spectroscopic imaging in patients with MRI-negative extratemporal epilepsy: correlation with ictal onset zone and histopathology. Eur Radiol 2007;17:2126–35.

100. Blair E, Stanley FJ. Intrapartum asphyxia: a rare cause of cerebral palsy. J Pediatr 1988;112:515–9.

101. Gropman AL, Fricke ST, Seltzer RR, et al. 1H MRS identifies symptomatic and asymptomatic subjects with partial ornithine transcarbamylase deficiency. Mol Genet Metab 2008;95:21–30.

Magnetic Resonance Spectroscopy in Metabolic Disorders

Andrea Rossi, MD[a],*, Roberta Biancheri, MD, PhD[b]

KEYWORDS

- Hypomyelination • Leukodystrophy • Leukoencephalopathy • Metabolic diseases
- MR spectroscopy • White matter

KEY POINTS

- Proton magnetic resonance spectroscopy (MRS) is an important adjunct to conventional MRI in the diagnosis of metabolic disorders.
- Some metabolic diseases are associated with entirely specific characteristic MRS findings, consisting of either abnormal elevation or reduction of a single normal peak or detection of abnormal metabolites.
- Specific MRS patterns are mainly found in Canavan disease (elevated NAA), creatine deficiency (reduced Cr), nonketotic hyperglycinemia (presence of glycine), and maple syrup urine disease (detection of branched-chain amino acids).
- In most the inherited metabolic disorders, MRS findings are abnormal but not specific for a single disease or syndrome.
- Nonspecific MRS patterns are either unremarkable (ie, similar to normal age-matched controls) or consisting of a variable degree of modification of the ratios between the various normal metabolites in the MR spectra, possibly associated with presence of lactate.

INTRODUCTION

Metabolic diseases comprise a large host of inherited disorders that may predominantly involve the cerebral gray matter, white matter, or both. The underlying, causative enzyme defects have been elucidated in several of these conditions, and research constantly adds new information to this already relevant body of knowledge; however, a significant proportion of metabolic diseases remain without a specific etiology despite extensive clinical, imaging, and laboratory investigations.[1,2] Magnetic resonance imaging (MRI) plays a pivotal role in the diagnostic evaluation of patients suspected of harboring metabolic disease.[1] The specificity of MRI findings increases significantly when a pattern recognition approach is used,[3] but may remain unsatisfactory, because different metabolic disorders may result in similar signal intensity changes on conventional magnetic resonance (MR) images. Magnetic resonance spectroscopy (MRS) plays an important supportive role to conventional MRI in the diagnosis of metabolic disorders, based on its capability to detect and quantify in vivo both normal and abnormal metabolites in the brain.[4,5]

The technical basis of MRS is related to the identification of metabolites based on their differences in resonance frequencies, which is translated into a graph in which the various peaks correspond to individual compounds. Thus, when used in association, MRI and MRS enable one to correlate

[a] Pediatric Neuroradiology Unit, Istituto Giannina Gaslini, 5 Via Gerolamo Gaslini, Genoa 16147, Italy;
[b] Infantile Neuropsychiatry Unit, Istituto Giannina Gaslini, 5 Via Gerolamo Gaslini, Genoa 16147, Italy
* Corresponding author. Department of Pediatric Neuroradiology, Istituto Giannina Gaslini, Largo G. Gaslini 5, Genoa 16147, Italy.
E-mail address: andrearossi@ospedale-gaslini.ge.it

Neuroimag Clin N Am 23 (2013) 425–448
http://dx.doi.org/10.1016/j.nic.2012.12.013
1052-5149/13/$ – see front matter © 2013 Elsevier Inc. All rights reserved.

neuroimaging.theclinics.com

anatomic and physiopathological characteristics within preselected areas of the brain. MRS can be performed based on signal generated by hydrogen protons (^{1}H), carbon (^{13}C), or phosphorus (^{31}P) atoms. Unlike ^{13}C or ^{31}P MRS, however, ^{1}H-MRS has become widely available in a routine clinical setting. In fact, hydrogen is the most abundant atom in the human body and its nucleus emits a strong radiofrequency signal, which generates a sufficient signal-to-noise ratio at 1.5 T to become detectable with a sufficient resolution. At higher magnetic field strength (ie, 3 T) the resolution of ^{1}H spectra improves, providing better resolution of the individual compounds. On the other hand, also at 3 T, the number of metabolites that can be detected is necessarily limited by the narrow chemical shift range, which unfavorably influences their identification and quantification.

TECHNICAL ASPECTS

The most commonly used techniques of ^{1}H-MRS are single-voxel and multivoxel (ie, chemical-shift imaging) techniques. Single-voxel MRS provides spectral information on predetermined selected brain volumes (usually at least 2 × 2 × 2 cm) in a reasonable amount of time (usually less than 5 minutes) (Fig. 1). Multivoxel MRS, although usually longer in terms of acquisition time, provides spectra from multiple, small, and contiguous volumes on a particular region of interest that may involve both the gray and white matter, which enables one to map metabolic tissue distributions, usually at higher spatial resolution than single-voxel ^{1}H-MRS (Fig. 2). On both single-voxel and multivoxel MRS, the possibility to detect the various metabolites, and their relative orientation with respect to the baseline,

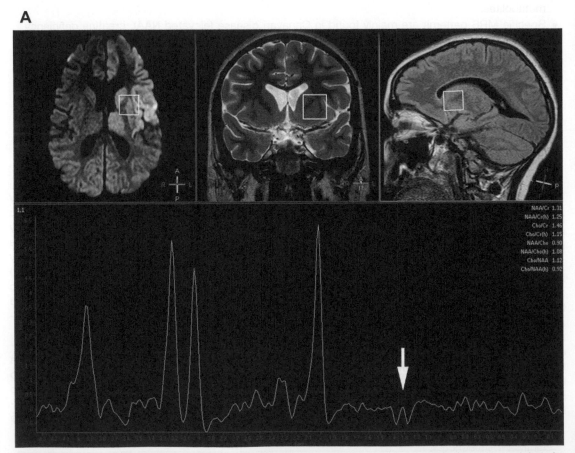

Fig. 1. (A) MRI and single-voxel ^{1}H-MRS at TE 144 ms in a 10-year-old girl with an unclassified peroxisomal disorder. *Upper row:* Axial DWI (*left*) shows restricted diffusion involving the left fronto-insular cortex and the homolateral striate and thalamus, whereas axial T2-weighted (*center*) and FLAIR (*right*) images are normal. A single MRS sampling voxel is depicted on the left basal ganglia region. *Lower row:* Intermediate-TE (144 ms) water-suppressed ^{1}H-MRS spectrum shows reduced NAA and a lactate doublet (*arrow*). (B) Intermediate-TE (144 ms) water-suppressed ^{1}H-MRS spectrum centered on the lateral ventricles shows huge lactate doublet, which correlated with laboratory findings of CSF lactic acidosis in this case. Cho, choline; Cr, creatine; NAA, N-acetylaspartate.

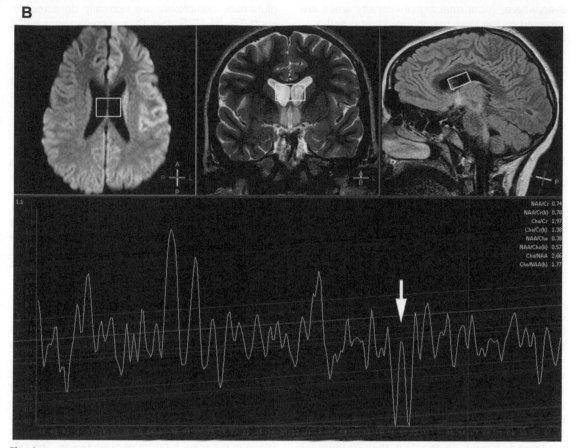

NAA/Cr 0.74
NAA/Cr(h) 0.78
Cho/Cr 1.97
Cho/Cr(h) 1.38
NAA/Cho 0.38
NAA/Cho(h) 0.57
Cho/NAA 2.66
Cho/NAA(h) 1.77

Fig. 1.

depends on several variables. Among these, the choice of the echo-time (TE) is of critical importance. MRS can be performed at short (20–35 ms), intermediate (135–144 ms), and long (270–288 ms) TE, with different results regarding number, sharpness, and orientation of metabolite peaks, as well as the amount of background noise. At short TE, a larger number of metabolites are detected but peak superimposition may occur, rendering interpretation more problematic. On the other hand, the number of detected metabolites is lower at longer TE, but the peaks are typically better defined. At intermediate TE, lactate is typically inverted below the baseline because of the J-coupling phenomenon (see **Fig. 1**B).

Obtaining more than one spectrum at different TEs or in different brain locations obviously has a significant influence over scan duration and must be evaluated carefully in each individual case, depending on the clinical suspicion and the findings on conventional MRI. Although, in theory, in many metabolic conditions the sampling voxel may be placed anywhere in the brain, as abnormal metabolites are presumably present diffusely

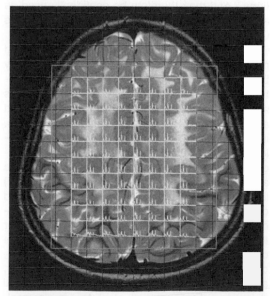

Fig. 2. Multivoxel ^{1}H-MRS (chemical shift imaging) at TE 144 ms in a 10-year-old boy with Alexander disease highlights regional differences in the spectral pattern among different gray and white matter areas.

everywhere,[1] abnormal signal intensity areas are sampled in the vast majority of clinical settings. In this case, care should be used to avoid necrotic, hemorrhagic, or calcified regions in which tissue samples may no longer be representative of the metabolic status of the rest of the brain or in which the presence of magnetic field inhomogeneity may result in excessively noisy or uninterpretable spectra.[1]

SIGNIFICANCE OF THE INDIVIDUAL PEAKS

Regardless of the TE or other technical aspects, under normal conditions ¹H-MRS consistently detects 3 main peaks: N-acetylaspartate (NAA), a marker of the neuronal population and viability; choline (Cho), a membrane marker; and creatine (Cr), representing energy storage compounds. Other normal peaks that are detected only at short TE include myo-inositol (mI), a glial function marker. The absolute and relative concentrations of these metabolites vary normally with age.[6,7] In the neonate, Cho and, at short TE, mI are the prominent peaks, whereas NAA is low; by 4 months, NAA becomes more prominent, whereas Cho and mI decrease; an adult appearance is reached by 6 months of age.[1] In most clinical instances, absolute metabolite quantitation is not routinely obtained; instead, relative concentrations to Cr (the so-called ratios) are usually measured, based on the fact that Cr remains stable throughout life, reflecting the stability of energy storage in the brain under normal conditions,[6] and may therefore be confidently used as a control value in relation to other metabolites under most circumstances.

Under abnormal conditions, including inherited metabolic disorders, other metabolites may become detectable on ¹H-MRS. The most important of these is lactate, whose presence indicates anaerobic metabolism and must be considered abnormal, with the sole exception of newborns, in which mild amounts of lactate may be physiologic. MRS detection of lactate in the brain parenchyma is a more precise indicator of cerebral lactic acidosis than blood and cerebrospinal fluid (CSF) lactate levels.[8] Lactate is particularly elevated during phases of metabolic unbalance in mitochondrial diseases, and may be used to monitor the response to therapy.[9] Lactate can also be demonstrated in a wide variety of metabolic disorders causing secondary lactic acidosis, however, and is therefore not specific for mitochondrial diseases. Evidence of lactate in normal-appearing brain areas on conventional MRI is an important indicator of an underlying generalized metabolic impairment (see **Fig. 1**).[8] Glutamine/

glutamate complexes are normally detected on short-TE ¹H-MRS, but their increase in several metabolic diseases is a sign of excitotoxicity,[10,11] which may portend neuronal death. Other metabolites only show up in specific conditions, such as glycine in nonketotic hyperglycinemia, and may therefore significantly assist in a specific diagnosis.

SPECIFIC MRS PATTERNS

Only a small number of entities are associated with entirely specific and characteristic findings on ¹H-MRS. In these conditions, spectral abnormalities may result from either abnormal elevation or reduction of a single normal peak or from the appearance of abnormal metabolites that are specifically associated with a given metabolic condition. Only the most relevant entities are discussed here.

Canavan Disease

Canavan disease is an autosomal recessive disease caused by mutation of the ASPA gene on chromosome 17 encoding for aspartoacylase, an enzyme metabolizing NAA into acetate and aspartate. This results in brain accumulation of NAA, a neuron-specific marker that is present in neuron bodies and axons and indicates their density and viability.[1] Production of NAA takes place in the mitochondria of brain tissue. The role of NAA is still incompletely elucidated; it is proposed that it regulates the molecular efflux water pump system that accounts for fluid balance between intracellular and extracellular spaces within the myelinated white matter. Thus, excessive NAA would lead to water accumulation in white matter with resulting intramyelinic edema, spongy degeneration, demyelination, and glial cell loss.[12] Canavan disease occurs in 3 clinical variants: neonatal, infantile, and juvenile, of which the infantile (presenting by age 3–6 months) is the most common. Patients are affected with macrocrania, hypotonia, lethargy, seizures, spasticity, optic atrophy, and developmental delay, with variably severe phenotypes depending on the degree of residual enzyme activity.

MRI shows a diffuse leukoencephalopathy with swelling of the white matter, involving both the supratentorial and the infratentorial compartments with relative sparing of the internal capsules and corpus callosum.[13] The affected white matter appears hypointense on T1-weighted images, hyperintense on T2-weighted images, and shows restricted diffusivity on diffusion-weighted images (DWI) owing to intramyelin edema.[14] The gray matter of the thalami and globi pallidi is also involved, whereas the caudate nuclei, putamina, and claustra are spared.[13] Canavan disease has a pathognomonic appearance on ^{1}H-MRS, characterized by marked, isolated increase of the NAA peak (**Fig. 3**)[15]; other nonspecific features include decrease of Cho and Cr, increase of ml, and the frequent presence of lactate.[1]

Creatine Deficiency

Creatine phosphate is required for adenosine triphosphate synthesis during energy use, and is obtained through phosphorylation of creatine. Creatine deficiency may result from defective primary synthesis because of deficiency of 1 of 2 enzymes, guanidinoacetate-methyltransferase or arginine: glycine amidinotransferase,[16] or from an X-linked defect of the creatine transport mechanism that

delivers creatine to the brain.[17] The latter is the most common form of creatine deficiency, and occurs in males with global developmental delay with a prevailing impairment of language.

Conventional MRI is typically unremarkable. On the other hand, MRS is highly specific, showing profound reduction or even absence of the Cr peak regardless of sampling voxel positioning in the brain (**Fig. 4**).[18] MRS is also useful to monitor therapy, which consists of oral creatine monohydrate administration and is typically efficacious in synthetic defects, but not in transport abnormalities.

Nonketotic Hyperglycinemia

Glycine is a neurotransmitter with inhibitory functions at level of the spinal cord and brainstem,

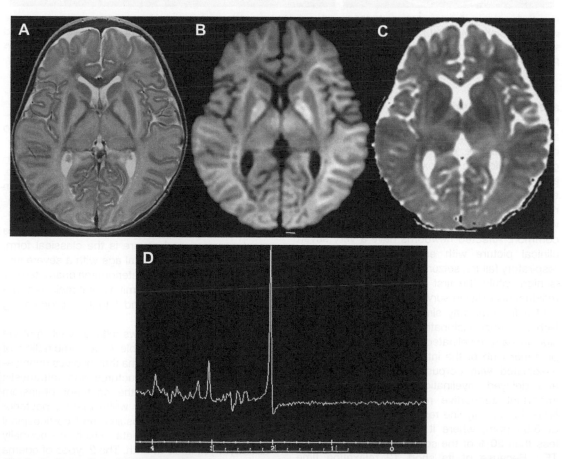

Fig. 3. Canavan disease: MRI and MRS in a 1.5-year-old boy. (*A*) Axial T2-weighted image shows diffuse abnormality of the supratentorial white matter with involvement of subcortical fibers and sparing of the corpus callosum and internal capsule. There is swelling and abnormal signal intensity of the thalami and globi pallidi with sparing of the striatum and claustrum bilaterally. (*B*) Diffusion-weighted image and (*C*) ADC map show restricted diffusion throughout the involved white matter, consistent with intramyelin edema, as well as in both thalami and globi pallidi. (*D*) Intermediate TE (144 ms) water-suppressed ^{1}H-MRS spectrum shows pathognomonic increase of the NAA peak. (*Courtesy of* C. Hoffmann, MD, Tel Aviv, Israel.)

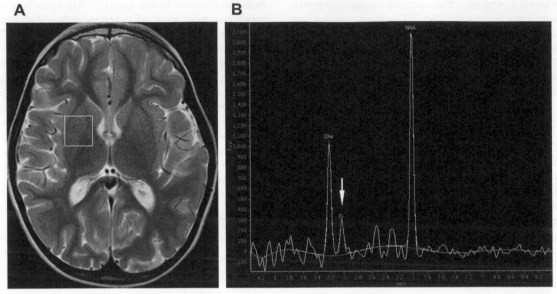

Fig. 4. Creatine deficiency: MRI and MRS in a 5-year-old boy with psychomotor delay and prevailing language skill compromise. (*A*) Axial T2-weighted image is unremarkable except for a mild prominence of the subarachnoid spaces. The MRS sampling voxel is shown. (*B*) Intermediate TE (144 ms) water-suppressed ^{1}H-MRS spectrum shows pathognomonic decrease of the Cr peak (*arrow*). Cho, choline; Cr, creatine; NAA, N-acetylaspartate.

and playing an excitatory role in the forebrain. Nonketotic hyperglycinemia (NKH), also known as glycine encephalopathy, is caused by defective glycine cleavage enzyme. As a consequence, glycine builds up to toxic levels in body fluids and in the brain, where it causes glutaminergic excitotoxicity.[19] NKH presents with 4 variants: neonatal, infantile, late onset, and transient, of which the neonatal or classical form is the most common. Affected newborns have a very severe clinical picture with encephalopathy, lethargy, respiratory failure, seizures, and hiccups; mortality is high within the first year of life, with severe residual disability in survivors.[20]

MRI findings may simulate those of hypoxic-ischemic encephalopathy, with restricted diffusion in early myelinated pathways, such as the posterior limb of the internal capsule,[21] possibly associated with corpus callosum abnormalities and delayed myelination.[22] ^{1}H-MRS plays an important supportive role in the diagnosis of NKH. In fact, glycine resonates together with ml at 3.56 ppm, where it normally contributes to less than 20% of the so-called ml peak at short TE.[1] Because of its short T2 relaxation time, however, ml is not normally detected on intermediate or long TE MRS. Therefore, persistence of a conspicuous "ml" peak at intermediate and long TEs indicates elevated glycine, thus supporting the diagnosis of NKH in a concordant clinical setting (**Fig. 5**).

Maple Syrup Urine Disease

Maple syrup urine disease (MSUD) is related to deficiency of branched-chain α-keto acid dehydrogenase enzyme, leading to increased concentrations of branched-chain amino acids (leucine, valine, and isoleucine) and their derivatives in blood, urine, and CSF. There are 4 clinical phenotypes of MSUD: classical, intermediate, intermittent, and thiamine responsive forms, of which the most common and severe is the classical form, which presents in neonatal age with a severe and progressive neurologic deterioration characterized by feeding problems, vomiting, ketoacidosis, hypoglycemia, seizures, and lethargia progressing to coma.[23]

Conventional MRI shows diffuse swelling of the brain, which is attributable to a combination of extensive vasogenic edema that involves nonmyelinated white matter structures and intramyelin edema at the level of the posterior brainstem tracts, central cerebellar white matter, posterior limbs of the internal capsules, and corticospinal tracts in the corona radiata, which are normally already myelinated at birth. The 2 types of edema can be confidently differentiated from one another on DWI, resulting in a pathognomonic appearance of restricted diffusion in the myelinated areas at birth.[14,23]

In MSUD, especially during stages of metabolic decompensation, elevations in the branched-chain

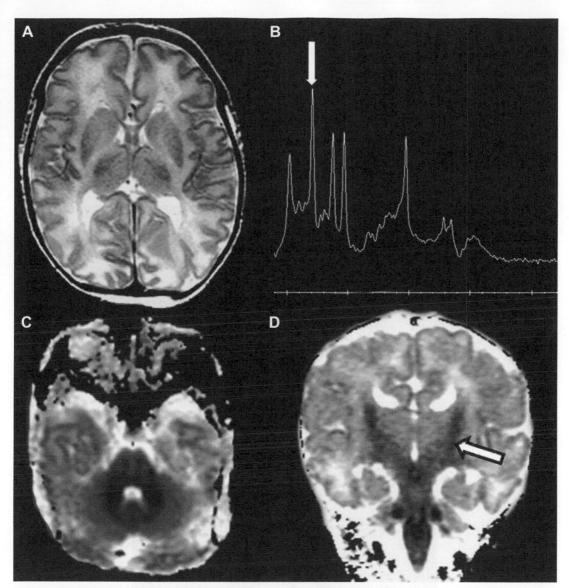

Fig. 5. Nonketotic hyperglycinemia: MRI and MRS in a 5-day newborn. (*A*) Axial T2-weighted image reveals white matter swelling. (*B*) Short TE (32 ms) water-suppressed ^{1}H-MRS spectra from basal ganglia shows an elevated peak (*arrow*) at 3.55 ppm, which was attributed to glycine based on its persistence at longer TE (not shown). (*C*) Axial ADC map shows diffuse cerebellar and brainstem diffusion restriction. (*D*) Coronal ADC map demonstrates involvement in the corticospinal tracts (*arrow*). The "bull's head" appearance of the ventricular system suggests agenesis or severe hypogenesis of the corpus callosum. (*Courtesy of* A. Poretti and T.A. Huisman, Baltimore, MD.)

amino acids leucine, isoleucine, and valine and their ketoacids can be detected on ^{1}H-MRS as a peak at 0.9 ppm. This peak is present on both short-TE and long-TE spectra and may be associated with evidence of lactate and/or reduction of the NAA peak (**Fig. 6**).[24,25]

NONSPECIFIC MRS PATTERNS

In most inherited metabolic disorders, findings on ^{1}H-MRS are abnormal but not specific for a single

disease or syndrome. This nonspecific appearance may either be unremarkable (ie, similar to normal age-matched controls) or entail a variable degree of modification of the ratios between the various normal metabolites in the MR spectra, in which (1) the NAA peak is variably decreased owing to depletion of the neuronal population with loss of neuroaxonal integrity; (2) Cho may be variably increased or decreased in function of the degree of membrane turnover, demyelination, and gliosis; (3) Cr is usually stable in most

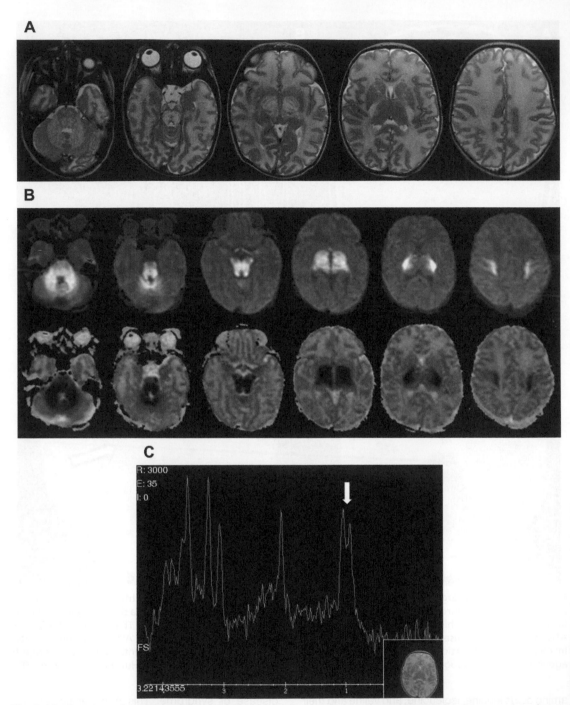

Fig. 6. Maple syrup urine disease: MRI and MRS in a 10-day newborn. (*A*) Axial T2-weighted images show hyperintense signal and swelling of the cerebellar white matter, dorsal pons, corticospinal tracts in the basis pontis, midbrain, posterior limb of the internal capsule, thalami, and central corona radiata. (*B*) DWI images (*top row*) and ADC maps (*bottom row*) show hyperintense signal on DWI and hypointensity on ADC maps representing restricted diffusion in the cerebellar white matter, dorsal pons, corticospinal tracts in the basis pontis, midbrain, posterior limb of the internal capsule, thalami, and central corona radiata. (*C*) Short-TE (35 ms) water-suppressed ¹H-MRS spectrum from the posterior limb of the internal capsule demonstrates an abnormal wide peak at 0.9 ppm representing branched-chain amino acids and ketoacids (*arrow*). (*Courtesy of* A. Poretti and T.A. Huisman, Baltimore, MD.)

instances; (4) elevation of the mI peak, probably as a result of gliosis, may be seen at short-TE; and (5) lactate may also show up as an indicator of anaerobic glycolysis owing to defective energy metabolism. MRS findings may vary with time in function of the disease stage (active metabolic stress vs burnt-out), and also regionally in the brain depending on the degree of involvement of individual structures. MR spectra may be abnormal also in areas that appear unaffected on conventional MR images, as a result of widespread metabolic derangement. Sampling of the CSF in the ventricular cavities is also possible and may provide a gross appraisal of CSF lactic acidosis, which may be relevant in cases in which CSF examination is not available (see **Fig. 1**).

Despite the nonspecific appearance in terms of identification of a definite diagnosis of a specific disease entity, studies have shown that quantitative MRS can assist in discriminating between different types of white matter disorders and classifying white matter lesions of unknown origin with respect to underlying pathologic conditions.[2,26]

The following section deals with some of the most prominent metabolic diseases characterized by an aspecifically pathologic spectrum, aiming to identify a role for ^{1}H-MRS in the neuroimaging diagnostic process.

Pelizaeus-Merzbacher Disease

The Pelizaeus-Merzbacher disease (PMD) is the prototype of the large, heterogeneous group of hypomyelinating disorders.[27] PMD is caused by various types of mutations of the X-linked proteolipid protein 1 gene (PLP1), located on Xp22 and encoding for the proteolipid protein (PLP), which contributes to 50% of all central nervous system (CNS) myelin protein. These mutations include copy number changes (most commonly duplications), point mutations, and insertions or deletions of a few bases, corresponding to a wide clinical spectrum that ranges from the most severe connatal PMD to the classic infantile PMD, the PLP1 null syndrome, and the least severe spastic paraplegia 2 (SPG2).[28] Affected patients are invariably males,

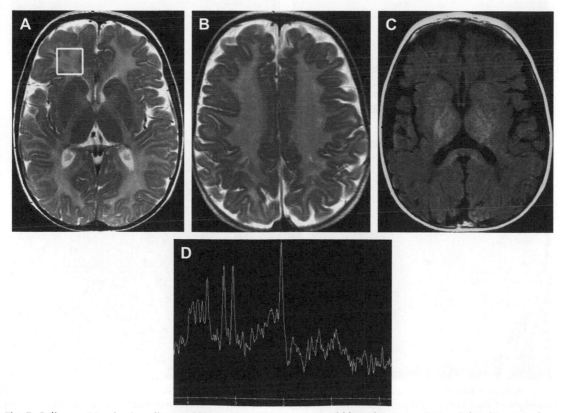

Fig. 7. Pelizaeus-Merzbacher disease: MRI and MRS in a 9-month-old boy. (*A, B*) Axial T2-weighted images show diffuse hypomyelination involving the supratentorial white matter. An MRS sampling voxel is shown in the right frontal white matter. (*C*) Axial T1-weighted image confirms lack of myelination with a diffusely hypointense white matter. Traces of myelin are found at the thalamus bilaterally. (*D*) Short TE (32 ms) water-suppressed ^{1}H-MRS spectrum centered at the right frontal white matter shows an essentially normal spectrum.

and present variably depending on their clinical form, ranging from severe failure to thrive to variably severe developmental delay, seizures, spasticity, and, characteristically for the classical PMD form, nystagmus. A more recently described entity within the PMD disease group is PMD-like disease 1 (PMLD1). This particular entity is caused by mutations of the GJC2 gene on chromosome 1q41-q42.[28] Affected patients have a similar clinical picture as classic PMD, but with higher cognitive and intellectual function, greater levels of motor performance, earlier onset, and more rapid neurologic deterioration.

In both PMD and PMLD1, conventional MRI shows a diffuse pattern of hypomyelination of the white matter, with increased signal intensity on T2-weighted or fluid-attenuated inversion recovery (FLAIR) images and isointensity to mild hypointensity on T1-weighted images.[1] Affected white matter regions include the cerebral hemispheres,

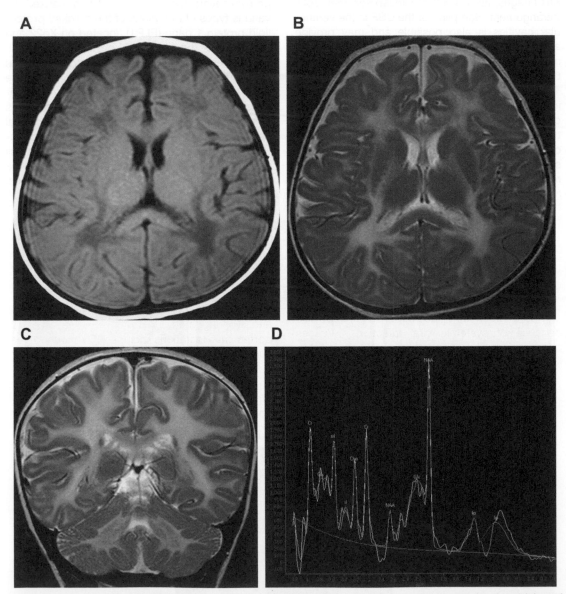

Fig. 8. Pelizaeus-Merzbacher-like disease: MRI and MRS in a 6-month-old boy. (*A*) Axial T1-weighted and (*B*) axial T2-weighted images show diffusely abnormal signal consistent with hypomyelination of the supratentorial white matter; the splenium of the corpus callosum is relatively spared. (*C*) Coronal T2-weighted image shows abnormal signal consistent with hypomyelination also involving the cerebellar white matter. (*D*) Short TE (23 ms) water-suppressed ¹H-MRS spectrum sampling of the right parietal white matter shows mildly reduced Cho; NAA is within normal range. Cho, choline; Cr, creatine; Glx, glutamine-glutamate complex; Lip, lipids; mI, myo-inositol; NAA, N-acetylaspartate; sI, scyllo-inositol.

cerebellum, and brainstem in the connatal and classical forms of PMD as well as in PMLD1, whereas hypomyelination is patchy in SPG2.[28] Findings on ^{1}H-MRS are nonspecific, and often not profoundly dissimilar to those of age-matched controls (Figs. 7 and 8). In PMD, Cho has been described to be variably reduced (reflecting hypomyelination) or increased (reflecting on-going demyelination in the early stages), whereas NAA may range from mildly to moderately reduced.[28] In general, MRS findings may vary depending on clinical phenotypes, genotypes, or stages of disease progression.[29]

Hypomyelination and Congenital Cataract

Hypomyelination and congenital cataract (HCC), also known as hypomyelinating leukodystrophy 5 (HLD5), is a recently described[30] hypomyelinating disorder caused by deficiency of FAM126, a gene located on chromosome 7 and encoding hyccin,[30] a neuronal protein that is presumed to be involved in neuron-to-glia signaling to initiate or maintain myelination.[31] Affected patients present with congenital cataract, variably severe psychomotor delay and neurologic impairment, and, in the vast majority of cases, peripheral

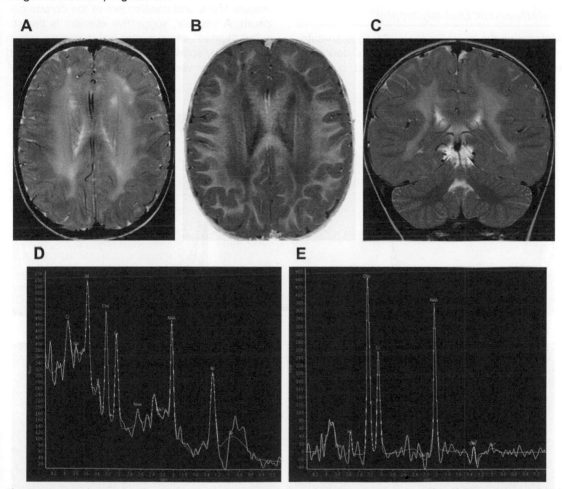

Fig. 9. Hypomyelination and congenital cataract (HCC): MRI and MRS in a 20-month-old boy. (A) Axial T2-weighted and (B) axial IR image show abnormal signal of the supratentorial white matter consistent with hypomyelination that involves prevailingly the periventricular and deep white matter with some degree of sparing of the subcortical fibers. Increased T2 signal with corresponding hypointensity in the IR image in the deep frontal white matter is consistent with increased white matter water content, a typical feature of HCC that becomes more prominent as the disease progresses. (C) Coronal T2-weighted image shows spared cerebellar white matter in this particular case. Notice that T2 signal of the deep supratentorial white matter is intermediate between those of CSF and gray matter, a typical finding in hypomyelinating disorders. (D) Short TE (23 ms) water-suppressed ^{1}H-MRS spectrum sampling of the right parietal white matter shows increased mI, slightly increased Cho, and reduced NAA peaks, and an abnormally high lipid peak. (E) Intermediate TE (144 ms) water-suppressed ^{1}H-MRS spectrum sampling of the same region as D shows increased Cho, mildly reduced NAA, and a mild amount of lactate. Cho, choline; Cr, creatine; Glx, glutamine-glutamate complex; Lip, lipids; mI, myo-inositol; NAA, N-acetylaspartate; sI, scyllo-inositol.

neuropathy.[32,33] MRI shows hypomyelination of the supratentorial white matter and, often, the cerebellum; areas of increased white matter water content are typically found in the periventricular white matter, especially around the frontal horns.[34] ¹H-MRS shows variable findings depending on the stage of the disease. MR spectra in patients studied early during the course of their disease show elevated mI/Cr and Cho/Cr ratios with normal to reduced NAA, whereas Cho decreases in older patients.[34] Lactate and lipid peaks may be found (**Fig. 9**).[34]

Metachromatic Leukodystrophy

Metachromatic leukodystrophy (MLD) is an autosomal recessive disorder caused by deficiency of arylsulfatase A, an enzyme that catalyzes degradation of sulfatides, or by deficiency in the sphingolipid activator protein, saposin B. In both cases, accumulation of sulphatides and reduction of cerebrosides in the myelin sheath lead to myelin instability and demyelination.[35] Three subtypes of MLD exist: the late infantile, the juvenile, and the adult type, of which the late infantile variant is the most common. Affected patients present after the first year of life with gait abnormalities, ataxia, hypotonia, and peripheral neuropathy, progressing to spasticity and mental regression.

MRI shows symmetric periventricular white matter abnormalities with early sparing of the arcuate fibers and involvement of the corpus callosum. A peculiar, suggestive element is the so-called "tigroid" white matter lesion pattern, which is caused by sparing of perivascular myelin around the medullary vessels in the centrum semiovale.

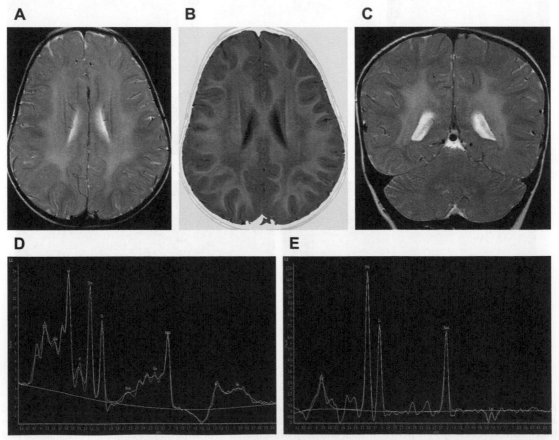

Fig. 10. Metachromatic leukodystrophy: MRI and MRS in a 2-year-old girl. (*A*) Axial T2-weighted and (*B*) axial IR images show abnormal signal intensity involving the periventricular and deep white matter, with sparing of the subcortical fibers. There is not a typical tigroid pattern in this case, although white matter signal abnormalities are somewhat heterogeneous. (*C*) Coronal T2-weighted image shows mild hyperintensity of the cerebellar white matter, resulting in a blurred appearance. (*D*) Short TE (31 ms) water-suppressed ¹H-MRS spectrum sampling of the right centrum semiovale shows significant increase of mI; Cho is also mildly increased, and NAA reduced. (*E*) Intermediate TE (144 ms) water-suppressed ¹H-MRS spectrum sampling of the same region as *D* shows increased Cho, mildly reduced NAA, and a mild amount of lactate. Cho, choline; Cr, creatine; Glx, glutamine-glutamate complex; Lip, lipids; mI, myo-inositol; NAA, N-acetylaspartate; sI, scyllo-inositol.

Progression of white matter involvement is centrifugal, leading to brain atrophy in the advanced stages of disease.[36] In the affected white matter, the ¹H-MRS pattern at intermediate to long TE is entirely aspecific, with elevated Cho, decreased NAA, and elevated lactate peaks. At short TE, elevated ml appears to be a distinctive feature among other leukodystrophies,[37] and probably results from glial abnormalities and membrane instability (**Fig. 10**).[8]

Globoid Cell Leukodystrophy (Krabbe Disease)

Globoid cell leukodystrophy (GCLD) is a lysosomal disease caused by deficiency of galactocerebroside-β-galactosidase, an enzyme catalyzing cerebroside into galactose and ceramide. Cerebroside is almost exclusively found in oligodendrocytes, Schwann cells, and myelin sheaths, and its metabolism is related to the metabolism of myelin. Accumulation of cerebroside into phagocytic cells is responsible for transformation of these cells into globoid cells. The deacylated form of cerebroside, psychosine, is a cytotoxic substance that accumulates within oligodendrocytes, causing their death and therefore demyelination.[35] There are infantile, juvenile, and adult variants of GCLD. In the classic early infantile form, patients present before 6 months of age with irritability followed by rigidity and tonic spasms, whereas in the late-infantile form, symptoms appear between 6 months and 3 years of life with ataxia, weakness, spasticity, and dysarthria.

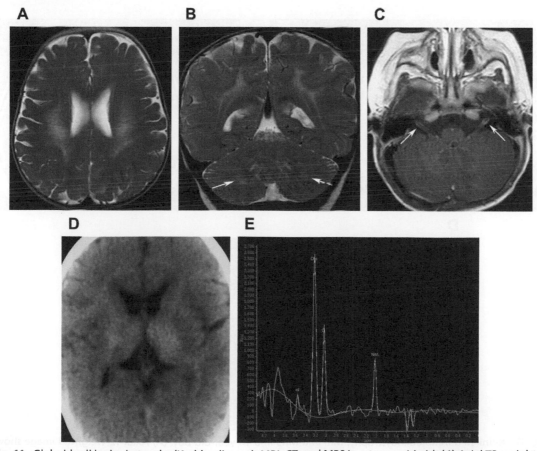

Fig. 11. Globoid cell leukodystrophy (Krabbe disease): MRI, CT, and MRS in a 1-year-old girl. (A) Axial T2-weighted image shows abnormally hyperintense deep white matter with a posterior-to anterior gradient of involvement, with spared subcortical regions. Notice a typical striated, "tigroid" pattern that results from relative sparing of perivenular myelin. (B) Coronal T2-weighted image, slightly affected by motion artifacts, shows patchy involvement of the deep cerebellar white matter bilaterally (*arrows*). (C) Contrast-enhanced axial T1-weighted image shows enhancement of cranial nerves VII and VIII bilaterally (*arrows*). There also was enhancement of cranial nerves III and V, as well as the nerve roots of the cauda equina (not shown). (D) Unenhanced axial CT scan shows mildly hyperdense thalami. (E) Intermediate TE (144 ms) water-suppressed ¹H-MRS spectrum sampling of the deep white matter of the left parietal lobe shows significantly increased Cho, reduced NAA, and presence of lactate, resulting in an aspecifically pathologic spectrum. Cho, choline; Cr, creatine; Lac, lactate; ml, myo-inositol; NAA, N-acetylaspartate.

Conventional MRI shows demyelination of the deep white matter, progressing from the posterior to the anterior regions and initially sparing the subcortical white matter. A "tigroid" pattern can be identified also in GCLD.[1] The cerebellum, pyramidal tracts in the brainstem, and spinal cord are often involved, and the optic chiasm is frequently thickened. One hallmark of GCLD is calcifications within the thalami, basal ganglia, and corona radiata, which are better shown by computed tomography (CT) scan. Postcontrast imaging shows enhancement of the cranial nerves and caudal nerve roots, a finding in common with MLD.[38] In the involved white matter areas, ^{1}H-MRS shows a similar pattern as in MLD: an aspecific appearance with increased Cho, reduced NAA, and an usually prominent lactate peak (**Fig. 11**).[39]

X-linked Adrenoleukodystrophy

X-linked adrenoleukodystrophy (X-ALD) is a peroxisomal disease caused by mutations of ABCD1, a gene encoding ALDP, a peroxisome membrane protein required for the peroxisomal localization of very long-chain fatty acids (VLCFA). As a consequence of this defect, VLCFA cannot be metabolized into shorter-chain fatty acids and becomes incorporated within myelin, resulting in destabilization of the myelin sheath.[35] An important pathophysiologic component is the presence of microglial inflammatory response, which is a unique phenomenon among inherited white matter diseases and contributes to the peculiar MRI picture, characterized by positive contrast enhancement. X-ALD has several clinical phenotypes, of which the childhood

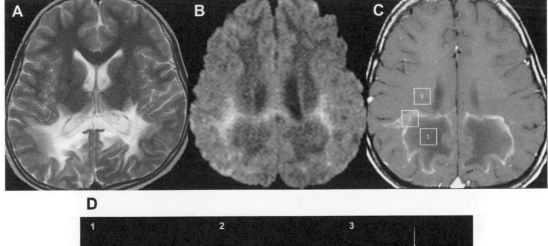

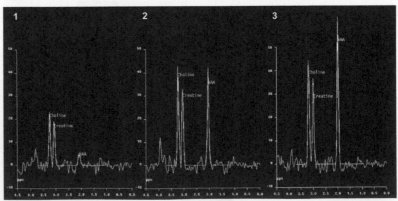

Fig. 12. X-linked adrenoleukodystrophy: MRI and MRS in a 14-year-old boy. (*A*) Axial T2-weighted image shows symmetric bilateral white matter lesions involving the parieto-occipital regions; the posterior parts of internal, external, and extreme capsules; and the splenium of corpus callosum. (*B*) Axial DWI (b = 1000 s) shows the central zones of the parieto-occipital lesions are markedly hypointense, the intermediate zone is markedly hyperintense, and the peripheral zone is faintly hyperintense, corresponding to a concentric pattern of gliosis, inflammation, and demyelination. (*C*) Postcontrast axial T1-weighted image shows the intermediate inflammatory zone enhances. It also shows placement of MRS sampling voxels in the gliotic (1), inflammatory/demyelinating (2), and normal-appearing (3) zones. (*D*) Intermediate TE (144 ms) water-suppressed ^{1}H-MRS spectrum sampling shows significant decrease of all normal brain metabolites and abnormal lactate in the gliotic zone (1); decreased NAA, slightly decreased Cr, increased Cho, and a small lactate peak in the inflammatory/demyelinating zone; and slightly increased Cho in the normal-appearing white matter (3). (*Courtesy of* Z. Patay, Memphis, TN.)

cerebral form is the most common and presents between 4 and 8 years with subtle cognitive decline followed by spasticity, pseudobulbar signs, dementia, and impaired vision and hearing, associated with adrenocortical impairment.

Conventional MRI shows a pathognomonic appearance of extensive white matter lesions in the parieto-occipital regions with involvement of the splenium of the corpus callosum and sparing of the subcortical fibers; early involvement of the pyramidal and occipito-parieto-temporo-pontine tracts is also seen.[40] A more rare variant prevails in the frontal lobes. The involved deep white matter shows a characteristic appearance of concentric zones, of which the central portion corresponds to the fully demyelinated, gliotic component; the intermediate region corresponds to inflammatory phenomena (characterized by restricted diffusion and contrast enhancement); and the peripheral region shows active demyelination.[1,14] ^{1}H-MRS shows an aspecifically pathologic appearance with increased Cho, reduced NAA, and presence of lactate in the initial stages of the disease,[41,42] whereas global metabolite reduction, with the exception of mI, occurs in later stages. There are regional differences depending on the sampling region (ie, burnt-out zone, active inflammation-demyelination, and apparently normal tissue).[43] In the fully demyelinated, burnt-out zone, NAA is severely reduced because of neuroaxonal degeneration. In the inflammatory and demyelinating zones, Cho is increased because of myelin breakdown, and NAA is reduced because of loss of neuroaxonal integrity; mI is normal or slightly increased, whereas lactate is present wherever in the affected white matter. Increased Cho within apparently normal white matter on conventional MRI indicates increased myelin turnover or mild demyelination,

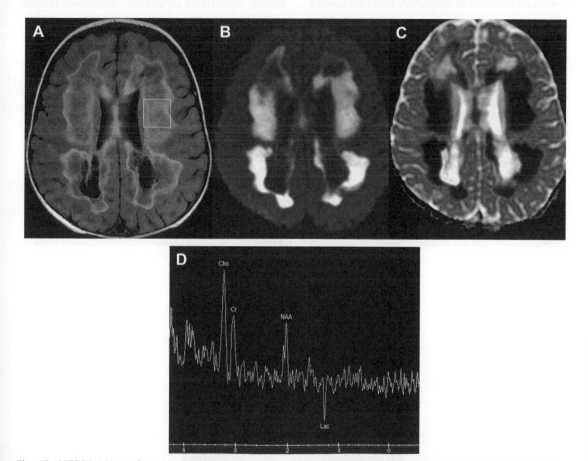

Fig. 13. MERRF: MRI and MRS in an 18-month-old boy. (A) Axial FLAIR image shows a concentric pattern of leukoencephalopathy with central cavitations, intermediate isointensity, and an outer hyperintense rim. The subcortical white matter is spared. (B) Axial diffusion-weighted image and (C) corresponding ADC map show extensive restriction of diffusivity in the abnormal white matter with increased diffusivity in the central cavitations. (D) Intermediate TE (144 ms) water-suppressed ^{1}H-MRS spectrum sampling of the abnormal white matter of the left frontal lobe shows increased choline, reduced NAA, and presence of lactate at 1.44 ppm. Cho, choline; Cr, creatine; Lac, lactate; NAA, N-acetylaspartate.

and suggests progression of the disease to those areas (**Fig. 12**).[41–43]

Mitochondrial Disorders

Mitochondrial diseases (MCD) are a heterogeneous group of disorders caused by a large number of mutations in the mitochondrial DNA (mtDNA) or nuclear DNA (nDNA), which cause impaired function of the respiratory chain, oxydative phosphorylation, pyruvate dehydrogenase (PDH) complex, or beta-oxidation. The CNS is prominently involved in MCD, together with the muscles (mitochondrial encephalomyopathies) and/or other organs in the human body. Muscle biopsy plays a crucial role in the diagnostic process, showing ragged-red muscle fibers, reduced cytochrome-C activity, increased succinate dehydrogenasis activity, or abnormal mitochondria. Biochemical confirmation of reduced activities of respiratory chain complexes

or the PDH complex, and eventual genetic verification of mtDNA or nDNA mutations, complete the diagnostic evaluation of patients suspected of harboring MCD. The clinical phenotypes are variable, and classifications are complex and challenging. Several syndromic entities are recognized in the spectrum of MCD, prominently including Leigh syndrome, Kearns-Sayre syndrome, mitochondrial encephalomyopathy with lactacidosis and strokelike episodes (MELAS), myoclonic epilepsy with ragged red fibers (MERRF), and many others.[44]

Conventional MRI findings in MCD are extremely variegated, and lack specificity.[45,46] Focal or widespread white matter lesions, showing up as high signal on T2-weighted or FLAIR images, are a frequent finding in MCDs, sometimes characterized by restricted diffusion on DWI, consistent with myelin edema, and associated with central cavitations (**Fig. 13**).[47] Strokelike lesions,

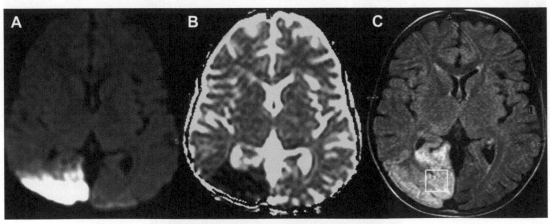

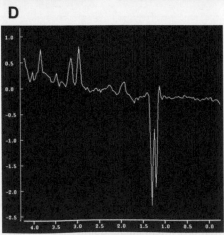

Fig. 14. MELAS: MRI and MRS in a 10-year-old girl presenting with seizures, left hemianopia, hypertrophic cardiomyopathy, and gastrointestinal symptoms. (*A*) Axial DWI and (*B*) corresponding ADC map show profoundly restricted diffusion in the right occipital lobe. (*C*) Axial FLAIR image shows positioning of the MRS voxel. (*D*) Intermediate TE (144 ms) water-suppressed ¹H-MRS spectrum shows huge inverted lactate doublet associated with marked reduction of the other metabolites. (*Courtesy of* T. Krings, MD, PhD, University of Toronto, Canada.)

typically found in MELAS, comprise cortico-subcortical areas of abnormal signal intensity, hyperintense on T2-weighted and FLAIR images, and variably described as restricted or increased diffusion on DWI, which do not conform to a specific vascular territory (**Fig. 14**).[48] Focal, bilateral, symmetric brain lesions involving the basal ganglia, periaqueductal gray matter, and brainstem nuclei and tracts are frequent in MCDs, typically in the context of Leigh syndrome (**Fig. 15**); involvement of specific nuclei may sometimes suggest a specific diagnosis, such as in the case of the subthalamic nuclei in cytochrome-C oxidase deficiency (**Fig. 16**).[49]

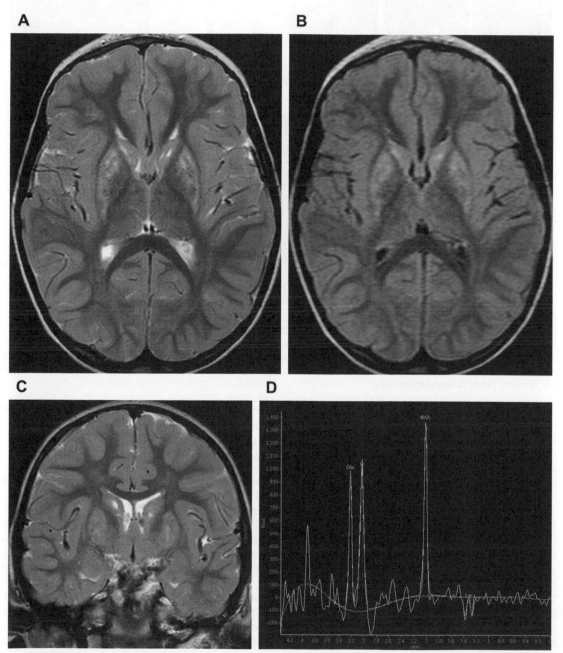

Fig. 15. Leigh syndrome: MRI and MRS in a 5-year-old girl. (*A*) Axial T2-weighted and (*B*) axial FLAIR images show somewhat heterogeneously hyperintense striatum bilaterally. (*C*) Coronal T2-weighted image confirms heterogeneously hyperintense striatum bilaterally. (*D*) Intermediate TE (144 ms) water-suppressed ¹H-MRS spectrum centered on the right putamen shows presence of lactate. Cho, choline; Cr, creatine; Lac, lactate; NAA, N-acetylaspartate.

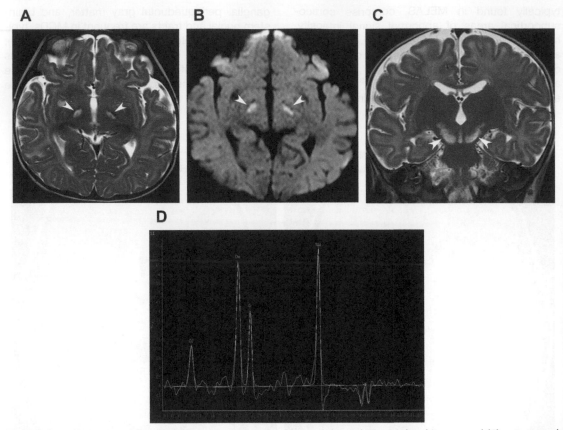

Fig. 16. Cytochrome-c oxidase deficiency in a 6-month-old boy. (*A*) Axial T2-weighted image and (*B*) corresponding DWI show abnormal hyperintensity of the subthalamic nuclei with restricted diffusion (*arrowheads*). (*C*) Coronal T2-weighted image confirms focal involvement of the thalamic nuclei (*arrowheads*). (*D*) Intermediate TE (144 ms) water-suppressed ¹H-MRS spectrum centered on a 20 × 20 × 20-mm region of interest including the right subthalamic nucleus shows mild Cho elevation and presence of lactate. Cho, choline; Cr, creatine; Lac, lactate; NAA, N-acetylaspartate.

¹H-MRS plays an important role in the diagnostic workup of patients with suspected MCD, because it allows the noninvasive determination of cerebral lactate, which may be elevated in the absence of peripheral lactic acidemia. MRS evidence of lactate elevation is a consistent feature in Leigh syndrome, especially in patients with respiratory chain complex deficiencies (see **Figs. 15** and **16**).[50] Lactate elevations are also common in MELAS, both in macroscopically involved areas (see **Fig. 14**) and in normal-appearing brain tissues,[51] and may be an earlier indicator of nervous tissue dysfunction than DWI.[52] Modifications of lactate levels can be measured by ¹H-MRS as a result of disease exacerbation or remission.[53] Elevations of lactate may be dramatic in MELAS, whereas the other peaks are significantly reduced (see **Fig. 14**); in general, NAA is often decreased in lesion areas owing to neuroaxonal compromise, whereas Cho may be elevated, yielding an aspecifically pathologic spectrum that highlights the importance of

correlating the MRS findings with the clinical picture and conventional MRI.

Alexander Disease

Alexander disease (AD) is caused by deficiency of GFAP, a gene located on chromosome 17 and encoding for the glial fibrillary acidic protein (GFAP), an astrocytic protein. This results in fibrinoid white matter degeneration with accumulation of Rosenthal fibers, the histopathologic hallmark of AD, which are astrocytic inclusions containing GFAP in association with small heat-shock proteins.[35] There are 4 clinical variants of AD (ie, neonatal, infantile, juvenile, and adult), of which the infantile form is the most common. In this variant, patients present at approximately 6 months of age with macrocrania, developmental delay, seizures, and progressive spasticity.

In the infantile variant of AD, conventional MRI shows hyperintensity of the supratentorial white matter on T2-weighted and FLAIR images that prevails in the frontal regions and in the deep white matter, but tends to extend both posteriorly and superficially toward the subcortical region, according to an anteroposterior, centrifugal gradient of white matter involvement. Contrast enhancement is often visible along the ependymal margins of the lateral ventricles and in the deep gray matter nuclei.[54] ^{1}H-MRS shows regional variation depending on where the sampling voxel is placed. The abnormal white matter regions in the frontal lobes show decrease of NAA and presence of lactate (**Fig. 17**). In relatively preserved white matter regions in the posterior part of the brain, mild decrease of the NAA peak without associated lactate is found.[55] In the context of a virtually pathognomonic conventional MRI picture, MRS does not add significant value to the diagnosis of AD, but may assist in determining the extent and severity of the anteroposterior gradient of white matter involvement.[1]

Megalencephalic Leukoencephalopathy with Subcortical Cysts

Megalencephalic leukoencephalopathy with subcortical cysts (MLC), also known as van der Knaap disease, is a recently described leukodystrophy, caused in most cases by homozygous or compound heterozygous mutations in the MLC1 gene on chromosome 22. MLC is characterized by extensive white matter changes associated with a discrepantly mild clinical course. Patients present during the first year of life with macrocephaly and an initially normal or slightly delayed motor and mental development; the clinical course is slowly progressive with development of ataxia, spasticity, gait disturbances, and, in later stages of the disease, mental deterioration and seizures.[56,57]

MRI shows a characteristic pattern of involvement of the white matter in a context of severe

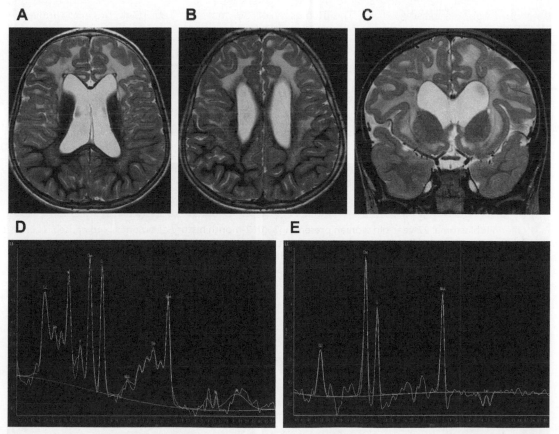

Fig. 17. Alexander disease: MRI and MRS in a 10-year-old boy. (*A, B*) Axial modulus IR images show abnormal hyperintensity of the white matter of the frontal lobes with an anterior-to-posterior gradient of severity. Notice striated, "tigroid" pattern in the posterior periventricular white matter. (*C*) Coronal T2-weighted image shows partial preservation of the temporal white matter. (*D*) Short TE (32 ms) water-suppressed ^{1}H-MRS spectrum centered on the right frontal white matter shows slightly reduced NAA. (*E*) Intermediate TE (144 ms) water-suppressed ^{1}H-MRS spectrum centered at the same level as D shows mild Cho increase, which was not readily evident on the short TE spectrum. Also notice reduced NAA and evidence of lactate. Cho, choline; Cr, creatine; Glx, glutamine/glutamate complex; Lac, lactate; Lip, lipids; mI, myo-inositol; NAA, N-acetylaspartate; sI, scyllo-inositol.

macrocephaly. The hemispheric white matter is markedly swollen and abnormally hyperintense on T2-weighted images, with relative sparing of the corpus callosum, internal capsule, and brainstem. The subcortical white matter in the anterior temporal, and often fronto-parietal, region shows characteristic cystic formations that are isointense with CSF. The cerebellar white matter usually is only mildly abnormal and is not swollen. ^{1}H-MRS shows an aspecific pattern with increased Cho and reduced NAA in the affected white matter; no abnormal metabolites, including lactate, are found. The spectra from the basal ganglia are normal (**Fig. 18**).[58]

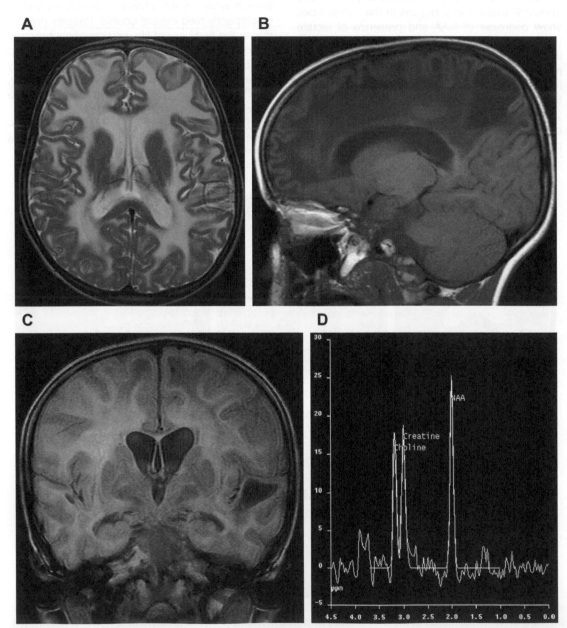

Fig. 18. Megalencephalic leukoencephalopathy with subcortical cysts: MRI and MRS in a 3-year-old boy. (*A*) Axial T2-weighted image shows diffuse involvement of the supratentorial white matter with relative sparing of the corpus callosum and posterior limb of the internal capsule bilaterally. (*B*) Sagittal and (*C*) coronal T1-weighted images show subcortical cysts in the left parietal and temporal regions. (*D*) Intermediate TE (144 ms) water-suppressed ^{1}H-MRS spectrum sampling of the right basal ganglia does not show significant abnormalities other than a mildly reduced NAA peak. (*Courtesy of* Z. Patay, Memphis, TN.)

Vanishing White Matter Disease

Vanishing white matter disease (VWMD), also referred to as childhood ataxia with central hypomyelination or CACH, is a recently identified inherited white matter disorder caused by mutations of any of the 5 genes encoding the 5 subunits of the so-called eukaryotic translation initiation factor (eIF2B), and enzyme implicated in the final step of protein production under circumstances of mild stress.[59] Clinically, after an initially normal or mildly delayed psychomotor development, patients show slowly progressive neurologic deterioration that may be transiently precipitated by episodes of stress, including minor infection or head trauma, leading to lethargy or coma. Cerebellar ataxia and spasticity are the main neurologic signs, and optic atrophy and seizures may occur.[35]

Conventional MRI shows swelling of the brain with broadened gyri; the white matter shows central areas of cavitation, with signal properties paralleling those of CSF, which may, however, be absent during the early stage of the disease. There is a diffuse background of hypomyelination. The central white matter of the posterior limbs of the internal capsules, the external, and extreme capsules is involved, whereas the anterior limbs of the internal capsules are spared. The corpus callosum is also involved, except for its outer rim, whereas the cerebellar white matter is also abnormal, including the hili of the dentate nuclei. The gray matter structures, including the cerebral

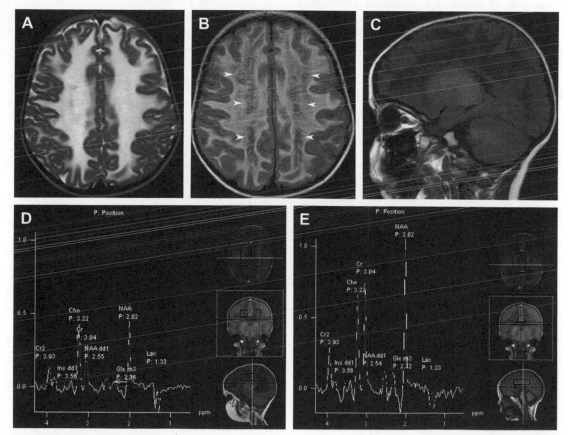

Fig. 19. Vanishing white matter disease: MRI and MRS in 2 different patients. (A) Axial T2-weighted image in a 3-year-old boy shows swollen, diffusely hyperintense white matter. (B) Axial FLAIR image reveals central hypointense areas within the abnormal white matter, consistent with vacuolization (*arrows*). (C) Sagittal T1-weighted image shows a relatively macrocephalic head and diffuse hypointensity of the supratentorial white matter. (D, E) ¹H-MRS spectrum obtained from the pathologic white matter in a 19-month-old boy (CSI performed at repetition time [TR]/TE = 1500/135 ms) shows reduced levels of inositol, choline, creatine, glutamate, and N-acetylaspartate. There is evidence of lactate and α-glucose multiplet peaks around 3.8 ppm. (E) Spectrum obtained from the unaffected gray matter (CSI performed at TR/TE = 1500/135 ms) in the same patient as D shows normal findings. Cho, choline; Cr, creatine; Glx, glutamine/glutamate complex; Lac, lactate; Lip, lipids; Ins, inositol; NAA, N-acetylaspartate; sl, scyllo-inositol. ([C] *Courtesy of* A. Nastro, Naples, Italy; and [D, E] L. Meiners and P. Sjiens, Groningen, the Netherlands.)

cortex and basal ganglia, appear to be normal.[1] ^{1}H-MRS has shown severely reduced Cho, Cr, and NAA in the affected white matter, with appearance of glucose and lactate signals, consistent with neuroaxonal damage (**Fig. 19**).[60]

SUMMARY

^{1}H-MRS proves useful as a complementary method to conventional brain MRI in the diagnostic evaluation of patients suspected of harboring metabolic diseases, and is also useful to monitor treatment response; it can be applied in a routine clinical setting, and provides detailed information about the neurochemical properties of affected brain areas noninvasively. Although the MRI findings may remain aspecific in a large proportion of cases, the additional information provided by ^{1}H-MRS may prove significant to restrict the scope of the differential diagnosis and, in some cases, to indicate a specific diagnosis.

REFERENCES

1. Patay Z. Metabolic disorders. In: Tortori-Donati P, Rossi A, editors. Pediatric neuroradiology. Berlin: Springer; 2005. p. 543–722.

2. Bizzi A, Castelli G, Bugiani M, et al. Classification of childhood white matter disorders using proton MR spectroscopic imaging. AJNR Am J Neuroradiol 2008;29:1270–5.

3. van der Knaap MS, Breiter SN, Naidu S, et al. Defining and categorizing leukoencephalopathies of unknown origin: MR imaging approach. Radiology 1999;213:121–33.

4. Tzika AA, Ball WS Jr, Vigneron DB, et al. Clinical proton MR spectroscopy of neurodegenerative disease in childhood. AJNR Am J Neuroradiol 1993;14:1267–81.

5. Vion-Dury J, Meyerhoff DJ, Cozzone PJ, et al. What might be the impact on neurology of the analysis of brain metabolism by in vivo magnetic resonance spectroscopy. J Neurol 1994;241:354–71.

6. van der Knaap MS, van der Grond J, van Rijen PC, et al. Age-dependent changes in localized proton and phosphorus MR spectroscopy of the brain. Radiology 1990;176:509–15.

7. Lam WW, Wang ZJ, Zhao H, et al. 1H MR spectroscopy of the basal ganglia in childhood: a semiquantitative analysis. Neuroradiology 1998;40:315–23.

8. Takahashi S, Oki J, Miyamoto A, et al. Proton magnetic resonance spectroscopy to study the metabolic changes in the brain of a patient with Leigh syndrome. Brain Dev 1999;21:200–4.

9. Detre JA, Wang ZY, Bogdan AR, et al. Regional variation in brain lactate in Leigh syndrome by localized 1H magnetic resonance spectroscopy. Ann Neurol 1991;29:218–21.

10. Connelly A, Cross JH, Gadian G, et al. Magnetic resonance spectroscopy shows increased brain glutamine in ornithine carbamoyl transferase deficiency. Pediatr Res 1993;33:77–81.

11. Bergman AJ, van der Knaap MS, Smeitink JA, et al. Magnetic resonance imaging and spectroscopy of the brain in propionic acidemia: clinical and biochemical considerations. Pediatr Res 1996;40:404–9.

12. Moffett JR, Ross B, Arun P, et al. N-Acetylaspartate in the CNS: from neurodiagnostics to neurobiology. Prog Neurobiol 2007;81:89–131.

13. McAdams HP, Geyer CA, Done SL, et al. CT and MR imaging of Canavan disease. AJNR Am J Neuroradiol 1990;11:397–9.

14. Patay Z. Diffusion-weighted MR imaging in leukodystrophies. Eur Radiol 2005;15:2284–303.

15. Janson CG, McPhee SW, Francis J, et al. Natural history of Canavan disease revealed by proton magnetic resonance spectroscopy (1H-MRS) and diffusion-weighted MRI. Neuropediatrics 2006;37:209–21.

16. Battini R, Leuzzi V, Carducci C, et al. Creatine depletion in a new case with AGAT deficiency: clinical and genetic study in a large pedigree. Mol Genet Metab 2002;77:326–31.

17. Cecil KM, Salomons GS, Ball WS Jr, et al. Irreversible brain creatine deficiency with elevated serum and urine creatine: a creatine transporter defect? Ann Neurol 2001;49:401–4.

18. Stöckler S, Holzbach U, Hanefeld F, et al. Creatine deficiency in the brain: a new, treatable inborn error of metabolism. Pediatr Res 1994;36:409–13.

19. Tada K, Kure S. Non-ketotic hyperglycinemia: molecular lesion, diagnosis and pathophysiology. J Inherit Metab Dis 1993;16:691–703.

20. Lu FL, Wang PJ, Hwu WL, et al. Neonatal type of nonketotic hyperglycinemia. Pediatr Neurol 1999; 20:295–300.

21. Mourmans J, Majoie CB, Barth PG, et al. Sequential MR imaging changes in nonketotic hyperglycinemia. AJNR Am J Neuroradiol 2006;27:208–11.

22. Press GA, Barshop BA, Haas RH, et al. Abnormalities of the brain in nonketotic hyperglycinemia: MR manifestations. AJNR Am J Neuroradiol 1989;10:315–21.

23. Poretti A, Blaser SI, Lequin MH, et al. Neonatal neuroimaging findings in inborn errors of metabolism. J Magn Reson Imaging 2013;37:294–312.

24. Jan W, Zimmerman RA, Wang ZJ, et al. MR diffusion imaging and MR spectroscopy of maple syrup urine disease during acute metabolic decompensation. Neuroradiology 2003;45:393–9.

25. Felber SR, Sperl W, Chemelli A, et al. Maple syrup urine disease: metabolic decompensation monitored by proton magnetic resonance imaging and spectroscopy. Ann Neurol 1993;33:396–401.

26. van der Voorn JP, Pouwels PJ, Hart AA, et al. Childhood white matter disorders: quantitative MR imaging and spectroscopy. Radiology 2006;241: 510–7.

27. Steenweg ME, Vanderver A, Blaser S, et al. Magnetic resonance imaging pattern recognition in hypomyelinating disorders. Brain 2010;133:2971–82.

28. Hobson GM, Garbern JY. Pelizaeus-Merzbacher disease, Pelizaeus-Merzbacher-like disease 1, and related hypomyelinating disorders. Semin Neurol 2012;32:62–7.

29. Pizzini F, Fatemi AS, Barker PB, et al. Proton MR spectroscopic imaging in Pelizaeus-Merzbacher disease. AJNR Am J Neuroradiol 2003;24:1683–9.

30. Zara F, Biancheri R, Bruno C, et al. Deficiency of hyccin, a newly identified membrane protein, causes hypomyelination and congenital cataract. Nat Genet 2006;38:1111–3.

31. Gazzerro E, Baldassari S, Giacomini C, et al. Hyccin, the molecule mutated in the leukodystrophy hypomyelination and congenital cataract (HCC), is a neuronal protein. PLoS One 2012;7:e32180.

32. Biancheri R, Zara F, Bruno C, et al. Phenotypic characterization of hypomyelination and congenital cataract. Ann Neurol 2007;62:121–7.

33. Biancheri R, Zara F, Rossi A, et al. Hypomyelination and congenital cataract: broadening the clinical phenotype. Arch Neurol 2011;68:1191–4.

34. Rossi A, Biancheri R, Zara F, et al. Hypomyelination and congenital cataract: neuroimaging features of a novel inherited white matter disorder. AJNR Am J Neuroradiol 2008;29:301–5.

35. Di Rocco M, Biancheri R, Rossi A, et al. Genetic disorders affecting white matter in the pediatric age. Am J Med Genet B Neuropsychiatr Genet 2004;129B:85–93.

36. Kim TS, Kim IO, Kim WS, et al. MR of childhood metachromatic leukodystrophy. AJNR Am J Neuroradiol 1997;18:733–8.

37. Kruse B, Hanefeld F, Christen HJ, et al. Alterations of brain metabolites in metachromatic leukodystrophy as detected by localized proton magnetic resonance spectroscopy in vivo. J Neurol 1993; 241:68–74.

38. Morana G, Biancheri R, Dirocco M, et al. Enhancing cranial nerves and cauda equina: an emerging magnetic resonance imaging pattern in metachromatic leukodystrophy and Krabbe disease. Neuropediatrics 2009;40:291–4.

39. Zarifi MK, Tzika AA, Astrakas LG, et al. Magnetic resonance spectroscopy and magnetic resonance imaging findings in Krabbe's disease. J Child Neurol 2001;16:522–6.

40. Kim JH, Kim HJ. Childhood X-linked adrenoleukodystrophy: clinical-pathologic overview and MR imaging manifestations at initial evaluation and follow-up. Radiographics 2005;25:619–31.

41. Confort-Gouny S, Vion-Dury J, Chabrol B, et al. Localised proton magnetic resonance spectroscopy in X-linked adrenoleukodystrophy. Neuroradiology 1995;37:568–75.

42. Tzika AA, Ball WS Jr, Vigneron DB, et al. Childhood adrenoleukodystrophy: assessment with proton MR spectroscopy. Radiology 1993;189:467–80.

43. Kruse B, Barker PB, van Zijl PC, et al. Multislice proton magnetic resonance spectroscopic imaging in X-linked adrenoleukodystrophy. Ann Neurol 1994;36:595–608.

44. Mitochondrial Medicine Society's Committee on Diagnosis, Haas RH, Parikh S, Falk MJ, et al. The in-depth evaluation of suspected mitochondrial disease. Mol Genet Metab 2008;94:16–37.

45. Friedman SD, Shaw DW, Ishak G, et al. The use of neuroimaging in the diagnosis of mitochondrial disease. Dev Disabil Res Rev 2010;16:129–35.

46. Finsterer J. Central nervous system imaging in mitochondrial disorders. Can J Neurol Sci 2009;36: 143–53.

47. Biancheri R, Rossi D, Cassandrini D, et al. Cavitating leukoencephalopathy in a child carrying the mitochondrial A8344G mutation. AJNR Am J Neuroradiol 2010;31:E78–9.

48. Sue CM, Crimmins DS, Soo YS, et al. Neuroradiological features of six kindreds with MELAS tRNA Leu A3243G point mutation: implications for pathogenesis. J Neurol Neurosurg Psychiatry 1998;65: 233–40.

49. Rossi A, Biancheri R, Bruno C, et al. Leigh syndrome with COX deficiency and SURF1 gene mutations: MR imaging findings. AJNR Am J Neuroradiol 2003;24:1188–91.

50. Dinopoulos A, Cecil KM, Schapiro MB, et al. Brain MRI and proton MRS findings in infants and children with respiratory chain defects. Neuropediatrics 2005;36:290–301.

51. Castillo M, Kwock L, Green C. MELAS syndrome: imaging and proton MR spectroscopic findings. AJNR Am J Neuroradiol 1995;16:233–9.

52. Abe K, Yoshimura H, Tanaka H, et al. Comparison of conventional and diffusion-weighted MRI and proton MR spectroscopy in patients with mitochondrial encephalomyopathy, lactic acidosis, and stroke-like events. Neuroradiology 2004;46:113–7.

53. Bianchi MC, Sgandurra G, Tosetti M, et al. Brain magnetic resonance in the diagnostic evaluation of mitochondrial encephalopathies. Biosci Rep 2007; 27:69–85.

54. van der Knaap MS, Naidu S, Breiter SN, et al. Alexander disease: diagnosis with MR imaging. AJNR Am J Neuroradiol 2001;22:541–52.

55. Grodd W, Krageloh-Mann I, Klose U, et al. Metabolic and destructive brain disorders in children: findings with localized proton MR spectroscopy. Radiology 1991;181:173–81.

56. van der Knaap MS, Scheper GC. Megalencephalic leukoencephalopathy with subcortical cysts [Internet]. In: Pagon RA, Bird TD, Dolan CR, et al, editors. Genereviews™. Seattle (WA): University of Washington, Seattle; 1993 - 2003 Aug 11 [updated 2011 Nov 03].

57. van der Knaap MS, Barth PG, Stroink H, et al. Leukoencephalopathy with swelling and a discrepantly mild clinical course in eight children. Ann Neurol 1995;37:324–34.

58. Brockmann K, Finsterbusch J, Terwey B, et al. Megalencephalic leukoencephalopathy with subcortical cysts in an adult. quantitative proton MR spectroscopy and diffusion tensor MRI. Neuroradiology 2003;45:137–42.

59. Leegwater PA, Vermeulen G, Konst AA, et al. Subunits of the translation initiation factor eIF2B are mutant in leukoencephalopathy with vanishing white matter. Nat Genet 2001;29:383–8.

60. Sijens PE, Boon M, Meiners LC, et al. 1H chemical shift imaging, MRI, and diffusion-weighted imaging in vanishing white matter disease. Eur Radiol 2005; 15:2377–9.

Hypoxic-Ischemic Injuries
The Role of Magnetic Resonance Spectroscopy

Lara A. Brandão, MD[a,b,*], Cristiana Caires, MD[a]

KEYWORDS

- MR • MR spectroscopy • Hypoxia • Lactate • NAA • Prognosis

KEY POINTS

- Magnetic resonance spectroscopy (MRS) is perhaps more sensitive to injury and more indicative of the severity of injury in the first 24 hours after a hypoxic-ischemic episode, when conventional magnetic resonance imaging and diffusion-weighted imaging may yield false-negative findings or lead to significant underestimation of the extent of injury.
- Neonates with asphyxia have statistically significant correlations between proton MRS results and both neurologic and cognitive status by 12 months of age.
- The optimal regions for determining the abnormalities associated with hypoxic injury include the occipital cortex, the basal ganglia, and watershed zones.
- Lactate is an early observation within the first 12 to 24 hours after insult, and is the best prognostic indicator in the early stage.
- In the late stage, *N*-acetyl-aspartate is the preferred prognostic indicator.
- Proton MRS should be performed as early as possible, preferably in the first week of life, so that abnormalities caused by hypoxia can be identified.

INTRODUCTION

Several conditions may result in hypoxic encephalopathy (HE):

- Low Apgar score at birth
- Neonatal asphyxia/hypoxemia
- Severe asthma
- Drowning
- Congestive heart failure
- Extensive myocardial infarction
- Congenital cardiopathy
- Bronchoaspiration
- Head injury
- Respiratory failure

Although computed tomography and magnetic resonance imaging (MRI) are useful for assessing hypoxic injury, changes in images often do not occur immediately.[1,2] In addition, the lack of myelination in the neonatal brain can obscure white matter hypoxic ischemic changes on T2-weighted images (**Fig. 1**).[3]

Distinct patterns of brain injury are observed and result from various combinations of 3 primary factors: the level of brain maturation at the time of the insult and the severity and duration of the hypoperfusion event. The vascular supply to the brain changes with brain maturation. In the immature brain, ventriculopetal penetrating arteries extend

Funding Sources: None.
Conflict of Interest: None.
[a] Clínica Felippe Mattoso, Av. Das Américas 700, sala 320, Barra da Tijuca, Rio de Janeiro 22640-100, Brazil;
[b] Clínica IRM - Resonancia Magnetica, Rua Capitão Salomão 44-Humaitá, Rio De Janeiro 22271040, Brazil
* Corresponding author. Clínica Felippe Mattoso, Av. Das Américas 700, sala 320, Barra da Tijuca, Rio de Janeiro 22640-100.
E-mail address: larabrandao.rad@terra.com.br

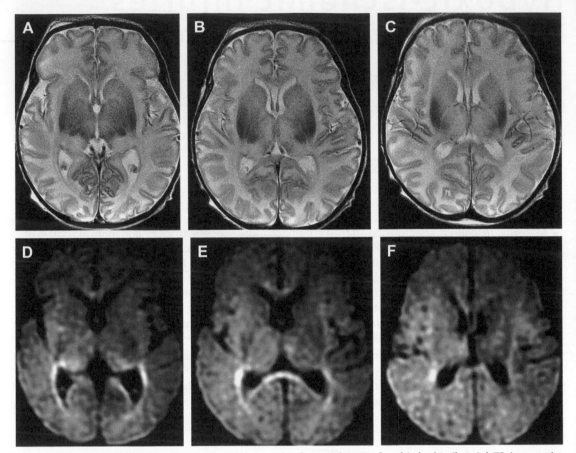

Fig. 1. Term baby, Apgar score 2/5, and seizures in the first 24 hours after birth. (*A–C*) Axial T2 is negative, whereas the diffusion-weighted images (*D–F*) readily demonstrate injury to the occipital watershed zones bilaterally.

inward from the surface of the brain to supply the periventricular regions; hence, periventricular leukomalacia is the most common pathologic finding in hypoperfusion injury. With maturation of the brain (36 weeks' gestation), vessels extend into the brain from the lateral ventricles, and the intervascular border zone moves peripherally to a parasagittal location (**Fig. 2**).

A hypoxic-anoxic event lasting more than 10 minutes is required to induce parenchymal changes, and the extent of injury increases with prolonged duration of the insult.[4]

PROTON MAGNETIC RESONANCE SPECTROSCOPY: CLINICAL APPLICATIONS

Proton magnetic resonance spectroscopy (MRS) has proven very useful in the assessment of patients with HE.[5–8]

MRS and diffusion-weighted imaging (DWI) are the most sensitive imaging modalities for detecting hypoxic ischemic encephalopathy (HIE) in the acute period.

MRS is perhaps more sensitive to injury and more indicative of the severity of injury in the first 24 hours after a hypoxic-ischemic episode, when conventional MRI and DWI may yield false-negative findings or lead to significant underestimation of the extent of injury.[9–12]

Proton MRS may show abnormalities earlier than conventional MRI,[1] documenting the severity of the encephalopathy[13,14] and predicting the neuropsychological and motor development of patients. Neonates with asphyxia show statistically significant correlations between proton MRS results and both neurologic and cognitive status by 12 months of age.[13] Nevertheless, it is important to correlate the MRS findings with MRI findings to interpret the spectra properly.

Clinical progression can be followed by serial spectroscopy.[15,16]

VOXEL POSITIONING

Because HE is a global event, single voxel spectroscopy can be used to assess it.[16] The optimal

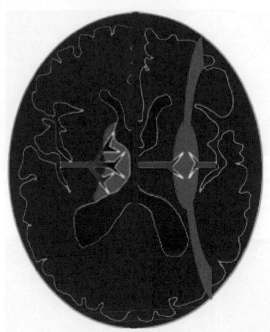

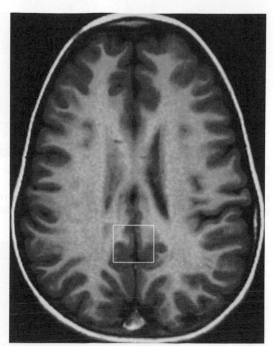

Fig. 2. Patterns of brain injury in mild to moderate hypoperfusion. The premature neonatal brain (*left*) has a ventriculopetal vascular pattern, and hypoperfusion results in a periventricular border zone (*red shaded area*) of white matter injury. In the term infant (*right*), a ventriculofugal vascular pattern develops as the brain matures, and the border zone during hypoperfusion is more peripheral (*red shaded area*) with subcortical white matter and parasagittal cortical injury. (*From* Chao CP, Zaleski CG, Patton AC. Neonatal hypoxic-ischemic encephalopathy: multimodality imaging findings. Radiographics 2006;26:S159–72; with permission.)

regions for determining the abnormalities associated with hypoxic injury include the occipital cortex (**Fig. 3**), basal ganglia (**Fig. 4**A), and watershed or border zones (see **Fig. 4**B).[13]

HE abnormalities are generally more severe in the cortex than in white matter,[9] and the occipital cortex is severely affected in cases of neonatal hypoxia.

The basal ganglia are very vulnerable to asphyxia.[17–19] Pavlakis and colleagues[17] demonstrated that the 1-minute Apgar score is more directly related to N-acetyl-aspartate (NAA)/choline (Cho) and NAA/Cho plus creatine (Cr) ratios in basal ganglia than in watershed zones.

MAIN SPECTRAL FINDINGS
NAA, NAA/Cr

Reduction of the NAA and NAA/Cr ratio is significant in severe injury, particularly in the subacute and chronic settings.[1,7,14,20]

Fig. 3. Voxel positioning within the occipital cortex.

Cr, Cho, myo-inositol

Cr, Cho, and myo-inositol peaks may be normal in early-stage hypoxia.

Significant abnormalities in the Cho level are not observed in early and subacute HE, meaning that an increase in the Cho/Cr ratio should indicate reduction of Cr and, thus, a poor prognosis.[14] Cho elevations may be seen weeks and months after insult.

Glutamate and Glutamine

A glutamine/glutamate (Glx) peak may also be detected at 2.3 parts per million, probably reflecting the release of glutamate that occurs in HIE.[6,9]

Lactate

In early-stage hypoxia, as early as 2 to 8 hours after insult,[6,12] lactate can be the only metabolic abnormality, typically more exuberant on the site affected by the hypoxia (**Figs. 5** and **6**).[13]

Lipids

Lipids represent one of the metabolic markers of neonatal hypoxia. The increase in lipids is a response to cerebral injuries that is more common in infants than in toddlers and adults.[14] However, a small amount of lipids can normally be detected in infants.

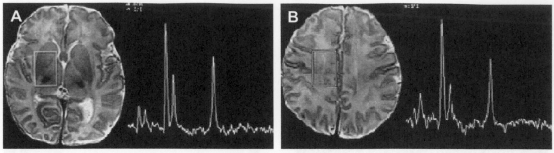

Fig. 4. Neonate. (A) Normal proton MRS in right basal ganglia. Echo time (TE) of 288 ms. (B) Normal proton MRS in watershed zone. TE of 288 ms. (From Barkovich AJ, Baranski K, Vigneron D, et al. Proton MR spectroscopy for the evaluation of brain injury in asphyxiated, term neonates. AJNR Am J Neuroradiol 1999;20:1399–405; with permission. Copyright © 1999, American Society of Radiology.)

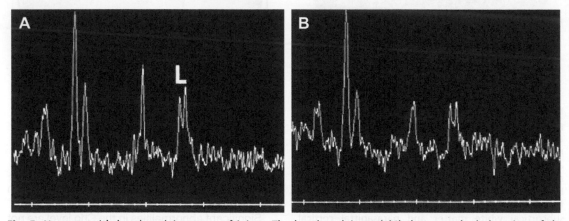

Fig. 5. Neonate with basal nuclei pattern of injury. The basal nuclei voxel (A) shows marked elevation of the lactate peak (L). The watershed voxel (B) shows less elevated lactate. In this acute phase, NAA, Cho, and Cr peaks are normal. (From Barkovich AJ, Baranski K, Vigneron D, et al. Proton MR spectroscopy for the evaluation of brain injury in asphyxiated, term neonates. AJNR Am J Neuroradiol 1999;20:1399–405; with permission. Copyright © 1999, American Society of Radiology.)

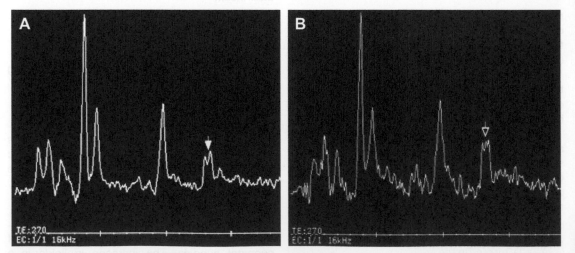

Fig. 6. Neonate with watershed pattern of injury. The spectrum from the basal nuclei voxel (A) shows a smaller elevation of lactate (arrow) than the spectrum from the watershed voxel (arrow) (B). (From Barkovich AJ, Baranski K, Vigneron D, et al. Proton MR spectroscopy for the evaluation of brain injury in asphyxiated, term neonates. AJNR Am J Neuroradiol 1999;20:1399–405; with permission. Copyright © 1999, American Society of Radiology.)

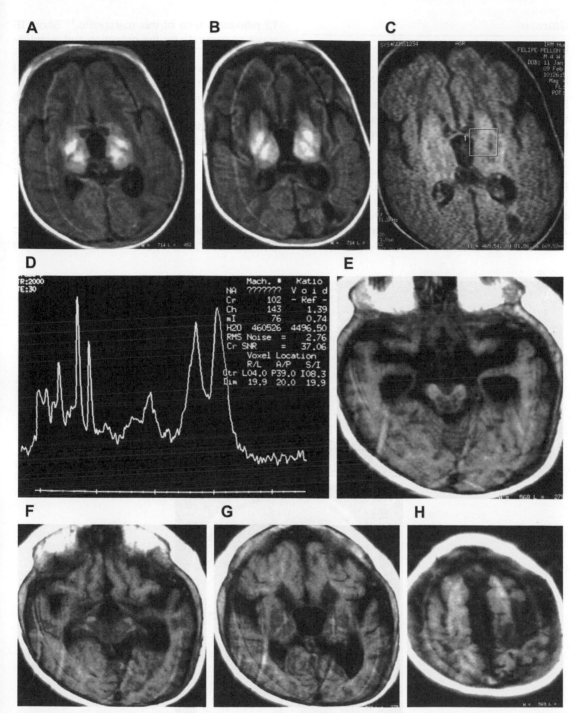

Fig. 7. Neonate, born term after prolonged delivery, presenting with severe asphyxia. MR performed at the age of 1 month. Axial T1 image (*A, B*) shows extensive hypoxic ischemic injury to the basal ganglia and thalami bilaterally. A huge lipid-lactate peak and severe reduction of the NAA peak are demonstrated, indicating poor prognosis (*C, D*). Note also elevation of the Cho peak and Cho/Cr ratio. A follow-up MR was performed 3 years later (*E, F*). At that time, the child presented with microcephaly and was completely dependent on oxygen. Some areas of malacia are seen in the brainstem (*E, F*), the basal ganglia and thalami have shrunk (*G*) and there is also malacia in the perirolandic regions bilaterally (*H*).

Glucose

Glucose may be present.

FINDINGS PREDICTIVE OF PROGNOSIS

Some metabolic abnormalities are directly related to poor prognosis, indicating a possible progression to death or persistent vegetative state.[13,14]

Lactate

Lactate is related to poor outcome.[2,6,13,21,22] An increase in lactate is the abnormality most consistently detected in proton MRS of neonates with asphyxia. It is better detected and quantitated on long echo time (TE) spectra because of the long T2 relaxation time of this metabolite.[13] Short TE is not as accurate for the detection and quantitation of lactate,[13] because of overlap with lipid signals. Lactate is an early observation within the first 12 to 24 hours after insult, and is the best prognostic indicator in the early stage (see **Figs. 5** and **6**).[13]

Several studies have shown a correlation between high lactate level and severity of progression (**Fig. 7**).[7,8,13]

Two lactate elevations are believed to occur during the acute to subacute period of HIE.[9] In animal models, lactate levels increase almost immediately after a hypoxic-ischemic insult, probably as a result of hypoxemia and ensuing anaerobic glycolysis, only to decrease nearly to baseline

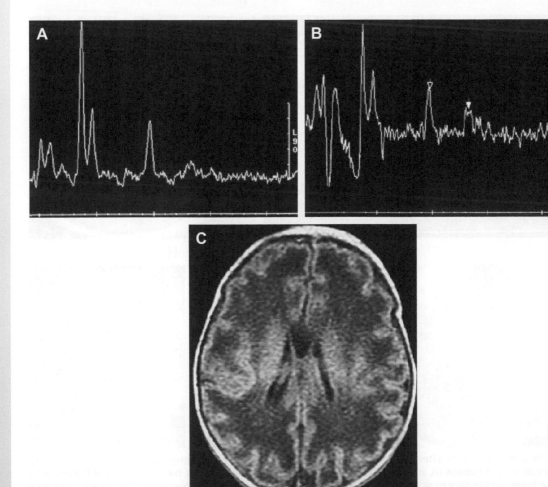

Fig. 8. Premature neonate, 36-week gestational age, 2 days after birth. (*A*) Basal ganglia spectroscopy shows reduced NAA levels, indicating an immature brain. (*B*) Spectrum from the less-mature watershed zone reveals a greater drop in NAA levels (*open arrow*) and a discrete lactate peak (*solid arrow*). (*C*) Axial T1 image indicates an immature gyrus pattern, confirming brain immaturity. (*From* Barkovich AJ, Baranski K, Vigneron D, et al. Proton MR spectroscopy for the evaluation of brain injury in asphyxiated, term neonates. AJNR Am J Neuroradiol 1999;20:1399–405; with permission. Copyright © 1999, American Society of Radiology.)

over the next few hours as a result of restored perfusion. Over the following 24 to 48 hours, a second increase occurs that is thought to be the result of a process known as "secondary energy failure," in which neurons that survived the initial insult develop delayed energy depletion, probably as a result of mitochondrial failure. This process probably partly explains why initial DWI leads to underestimation of injury in the acute setting, as mentioned earlier. Injury because of secondary energy failure will result in elevated cerebral lactate after 24 hours on MRS, and carries a grave prognosis.[8,9] In general, the finding of elevated lactate in the first few days of life portends a poor neurologic outcome.

However, it is important to remember that a small amount of lactate can be observed in the watershed regions of neonatal brain, especially in preterm infants, which is not solely evidence of cerebral injury (**Fig. 8**).[13]

NAA

A significant reduction of NAA level and NAA/Cr ratio is considered by some authors as the single most significant piece of information to determine prognosis.[14]

However, reduction of NAA is not significant in the first 3 days of insult[13]; thus, at an early stage, lactate is the best prognostic indicator. Zarifi and colleagues[23] showed that a lactate-choline ratio of 1 indicates a greater than 95% probability of adverse neurodevelopmental outcome, whereas the absence of lactate predicts a normal outcome.

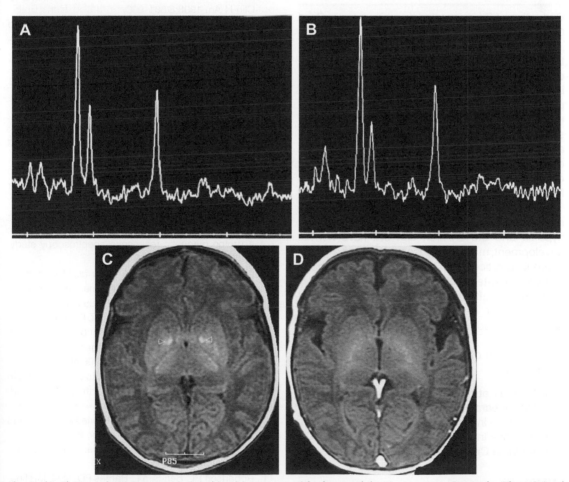

Fig. 9. (A, B) Normal spectroscopy in a 2-day-old neonate with abnormal development at 12 months. The minimal lactate peak observed in the spectrum from the basal nuclei voxel (A) is normal. The spectrum from the watershed zones (B) is also normal. (C) Axial T1 image shows globular hyperintensity (*arrows*) in the lentiform nuclei, indicative of an injury that is more than 1 week old. (D) Axial T1 image in a child with a normal neonatal course and normal postnatal development shows the normal appearance of the neonatal basal nuclei. (*From* Barkovich AJ, Baranski K, Vigneron D, et al. Proton MR spectroscopy for the evaluation of brain injury in asphyxiated, term neonates. AJNR Am J Neuroradiol 1999;20:1399–405; with permission. Copyright © 1999, American Society of Radiology.)

In the late stage, when lactate may not be detected, NAA is the preferred indicator.

A reduction of NAA levels is a normal finding in the brain of preterm children (see **Fig. 8**).

Glx

An increase of glutamine and glutamate should not be an isolated criterion of poor prognosis because it may merely reflect seizure activity.

Lipids

The presence of lipids, associated with the previously listed abnormalities, also indicates poor prognosis. However, when lipids are the single abnormality, prognosis is still good.

Cr

Reduction of Cr, suggested by an increase in Cho/Cr ratio, is another poor prognosis factor.

Barkovich and colleagues,[13] after assessing 31 term newborns who had experienced hypoxia, observed that an increase in lactate and reduction in NAA are the main spectral findings related to the presence of neurologic and developmental abnormalities at the age of 12 months. Proton MRS should be performed as early as possible, preferably in the first week of life, so that abnormalities caused by hypoxia can be identified. If the injury occurred during the intrauterine period, proton MRS may be normal (**Fig. 9**).[13]

Conventional MRI and proton MRS can show abnormalities in the watershed zone in neonates with hypoxia and the children can still have normal development, mainly because this area has a higher neuronal plasticity than the basal ganglia. In these children, long-term follow-up is necessary.[13]

In severely affected patients, who experienced acute oxygen deprivation, a predominance of lactate and reduction of all normal metabolites are seen.

In the stage of hypoxia recovery, the following can be found:

- Normalization of NAA and Glx
- Disappearance of lipids and lactate
- Increase in Cho and Cho/Cr
- Increase in myo-inositol and myo-inositol/Cr
- Variable Cr levels

SUMMARY

Proton MRS has proven very useful in the assessment of patients with HE.

Barkovich and colleagues[24] found that MRS performed in the first 24 hours after birth is more sensitive to the severity of hypoxic-ischemic brain injury than diffusion-weighted MRI, which can demonstrate the injury but underestimates its extent.

Proton MRS may show abnormalities earlier than conventional MRI, documenting the severity of the encephalopathy[13,14] and predicting the neuropsychological and motor development of patients.

With the voxel positioned in the basal ganglia and watershed zones, spectral abnormalities related to HE can be demonstrated.

The severity of the HE and the prognosis can also be estimated.

REFERENCES

1. Ricci PE. Proton MR spectroscopy in ischemic stroke and other vascular disorders. Neuroimaging Clin N Am 1998;8:881–900.
2. Barkovich AJ. MR and CT evaluation of profound neonatal and infantile asphyxia. AJNR Am J Neuroradiol 1992;13:959–72.
3. Barkovich AJ. Destructive brain disorders of childhood. In: Barkovich AJ, editor. Pediatric neuroimaging. 2nd edition. Philadelphia: Lippincott Raven; 1996. p. 107–75.
4. Chao CP, Zaleski CG, Patton AC. Neonatal hypoxic-ischemic encephalopathy: multimodality imaging findings. Radiographics 2006;26:S159–72.
5. Shu SK, Ashwal S, Holshouser BA, et al. Prognostic value of 1-H ERM in perinatal CNS insults. Pediatr Neurol 1997;17:309–18.
6. Hanrahan JD, Sargentoni J, Azzopardi D, et al. Cerebral metabolism within 18 hours of birth asphyxia: a proton magnetic resonance spectroscopy study. Pediatr Res 1996;39:584–90.
7. Leth H, Toft PB, Pettersen B, et al. Use of brain lactate levels to predict outcome after perinatal asphyxia. Acta Paediatr 1996;85:859–64.
8. Penrice J, Cady EB, Lorek A, et al. Proton magnetic resonance spectroscopy of the brain in normal preterm infants, and early changes after perinatal hypoxia-ischemia. Pediatr Res 1996;40:6–14.
9. Huang BY, Castillo M. Hypoxic-ischemic brain injury:imaging findings from birth to adulthood. Radiographics 2008;28:417–39.
10. Barkovich AJ. Brain and spine injuries in infancy and childhood. In: Barkovich AJ, editor. Pediatric neuroimaging. 4th edition. Philadelphia: Lippincott Williams & Wilkins; 2005. p. 190–290.
11. Robertson RL, Ben-Sira L, Barnes PD, et al. MR line-scan diffusion-weighted imaging of term neonates with perinatal brain ischemia. AJNR Am J Neuroradiol 1999;20:1658–60.
12. Barkovich AJ, Westmark K, Partridge C, et al. Perinatal asphyxia: MR findings in the first 10 days. AJNR Am J Neuroradiol 1995;16:427–38.

13. Barkovich AJ, Baranski K, Vigneron D, et al. Proton MR spectroscopy for the evaluation of brain injury in asphyxiated, term neonates. AJNR Am J Neuroradiol 1999;20:1399–405.

14. Danielsen ER, Ross B. Magnetic resonance spectroscopy diagnosis of neurological diseases. Marcel Dekker Incorporated; 1999. p. 147–85.

15. Patel J, Edwards AD. Prediction of outcome after perinatal asphyxia. Curr Opin Pediatr 1997;9:128–32.

16. Auld KZ, Ashwal S, Holshouser BA, et al. Proton magnetic resonance spectroscopy in children with acute central nervous system injury. Pediatr Neurol 1995;12:323–34.

17. Pavlakis SG, Kingsley PB, Harper R, et al. Correlation of basal ganglia magnetic resonance spectroscopy with Apgar score in perinatal asphyxia. Arch Neurol 1999;56(12):1476–81.

18. Roland EH, Poskitt K, Rodriguez E, et al. Perinatal hypoxic-ischemic thalamic injury: clinical features and neuroimaging. Ann Neurol 1998;44:161–6.

19. Johnston MV. Selective vulnerability in the neonatal brain. Ann Neurol 1998;44:155–6.

20. Ross BD, Ernest T, Kries R. Proton magnetic resonance spectroscopy in hypoxic–ischemic disorders. In: Bax M, Faerber EN, editors. MRI of the central nervous system in infants and children. London: MacKeith Press; 1995. p. 279–306.

21. Groenendaal F, Veenhoven RH, van der Grond J, et al. Cerebral lactate and N-acetyl-aspartate/choline ratios in asphyxiated full-term neonates demonstrated in vivo using proton magnetic resonance spectroscopy. Pediatr Res 1994;35:148–51.

22. Passe TJ, Charles HC, Rajagopalan P, et al. Nuclear magnetic resonance spectroscopy: a review of neuropsychiatric applications. Prog Neuropsychopharmacol and Biol Psychiat 1995;19:541–63.

23. Zarifi MK, Astrakas LG, Poussaint TY, et al. Prediction of adverse outcome with cerebral lactate level and apparent diffusion coefficient in infants with perinatal asphyxia. Radiology 2002;225:859–70.

24. Barkovich AJ, Westmark KD, Bedi HS, et al. Proton spectroscopy and diffusion imaging on the first day of life after perinatal asphyxia: preliminary report. AJNR ãAm J Neuroradiol 2001;22:1786–94.

^{1}H Magnetic Resonance Spectroscopy in Multiple Sclerosis and Related Disorders

Àlex Rovira, MD*, Juli Alonso, PhD

KEYWORDS

• Multiple sclerosis • Diagnosis • Magnetic resonance spectroscopy • Brain • Spinal cord

KEY POINTS

- Proton magnetic resonance spectroscopy (^{1}H-MRS) is a useful technique to understand the pathophysiological changes, namely neurodegeneration and demyelination, which occur both in lesions and in normal-appearing tissue in multiple sclerosis.
- ^{1}H-MRS could provide useful diagnostic information to MR imaging for distinguishing pseudotumoral demyelinating lesions from tumors.
- N-acetylaspartate is the metabolite that most consistently correlates with irreversible disability in patients with multiple sclerosis, supporting its use as a surrogate marker of neuroaxonal dysfunction in research studies.
- The available evidence does not support the use of ^{1}H-MRS as a marker of disease severity or progression in clinical practice.

INTRODUCTION

Multiple sclerosis (MS) is a chronic, persistent inflammatory-demyelinating disease of the central nervous system (CNS), characterized pathologically by areas of inflammation, demyelination, axonal loss, and gliosis scattered throughout the CNS with a predilection for the optic nerves, brainstem, spinal cord, and cerebellum, as well as the cerebral periventricular white matter, although cortical and subcortical gray matter damage is also prominent.[1,2] Conventional magnetic resonance (cMR) imaging techniques, such as T2-weighted sequences and gadolinium-enhanced T1-weighted sequences, are highly sensitive for detecting MS plaques and can provide quantitative assessment of inflammatory activity and lesion load. These conventional MR imaging–derived metrics have become established as the most important paraclinical tool in the diagnosis of MS,[3–5] and contribute to understanding the natural history of the disease and monitoring the efficacy of disease-modifying treatments.[6] However, the correlation between the extent of lesions observed on cMR imaging and the clinical manifestations of the disease is weak and underlines the fact that these techniques do not suffice to explain the entire spectrum of the disease process.[7] This clinical-radiological paradox may be partially explained by several limitations of cMR imaging: (1) limited specificity for the various pathologic substrates of MS, which contribute differently to the development of permanent disability; (2) inability to quantify the extent of damage in normal-appearing white matter; (3) inability to detect and quantify the extent of gray matter damage; (4) variability in the clinical expression of MS plaques in different anatomic locations (eg, the spinal cord and optic nerve); and (5) inability to assess the effectiveness of reparative mechanisms in MS, such as cortical adaptive reorganization.

Department of Radiology, Magnetic Resonance Unit (IDI), Vall d'Hebron Research Institute, Vall d'Hebron University Hospital, Pg. Vall d'Hebron 119-129, Barcelona 08035, Spain
* Corresponding author.
E-mail address: alex.rovira@idi-cat.org

Neuroimag Clin N Am 23 (2013) 459–474
http://dx.doi.org/10.1016/j.nic.2013.03.005
1052-5149/13/$ – see front matter © 2013 Elsevier Inc. All rights reserved.

Over the past years, the MR research community has dedicated enormous effort to overcoming these limitations by applying new techniques, such as quantitative analysis of brain volume (global and regional), magnetization transfer ratio, diffusion-tensor imaging, proton MR spectroscopy, and functional MR imaging, which can reveal the underlying substrate of intrinsic pathology, monitor the neurodegenerative and reparative mechanisms of the disease, and assess the effects of experimental treatments.

Proton MR spectroscopy (^{1}H-MRS) is the first nonconventional MR technique used in MS and has proved to be particularly informative by revealing metabolic abnormalities related to the 2 primary pathologic processes of the disease. These are active inflammatory demyelination and neuronal/axonal injury in both T2-visible lesions and in brain regions that are not associated with evident structural abnormalities on cMR imaging, the so-called normal-appearing brain tissue (NABT).[8] However, the high technical demands of ^{1}H-MRS have generally limited its use in research studies, and currently available data do not suffice to support its use as a biomarker of the neurodegenerative process of MS in clinical practice.

The aim of this article is to review the main brain and spinal cord ^{1}H-MRS features in MS and other idiopathic inflammatory-demyelinating diseases, the potential diagnostic value of this technique in specific situations, and its use as a biomarker of the neurodegenerative component of these diseases.

TECHNICAL ASPECTS OF ^{1}H-MRS IN MS

The first 2 articles of this issue are devoted to technical aspects of ^{1}H-MRS that should be considered for clinical use of this technique in various CNS disorders. Here, we present some additional data about technical aspects related to specific use of this method in patients with MS.

In MS, most ^{1}H-MRS examinations use the standard acquisition techniques provided by the manufacturers; that is, localized spin-echo or stimulated-echo pulse sequences with single-voxel or multivoxel mode. These standard pulse sequences provide metabolic information on predefined regions, and although they are useful for assessing metabolic changes in T2-visible lesions or specific NABT regions, they cannot provide overall metabolic information within the brain. To overcome this limitation, one proposal is to obtain localized spectra from a large volume of interest centered on the corpus callosum, including the superior lateral ventricular regions where axonal

projections converge after traversing large volumes of white matter. The rationale of this approach is based on the concept that damaged axons undergo anterograde shrinkage and Wallerian degeneration; hence, decreases in the amino acid N-acetylaspartate (NAA), considered a marker of neuronal/axonal function and density, should reflect brain damage inside and outside this volume of interest.[9,10] Studies using this approach have demonstrated that the metabolite ratios obtained from this volume are equivalent to and highly correlate with those obtained from a whole supratentorial volume.[11] Another approach proposes the use of a nonlocalized pulse sequence to allow acquisition of a spectrum to study changes in the whole-brain NAA.[12] Although whole-brain NAA seems a more sensitive indicator of disease progression than lesion load or atrophy, and it could be an optimal surrogate marker for the overall load of neuronal and axonal dysfunction and damage in the disease, some unresolved technical issues have prevented its use in clinical MR scanners.

^{1}H-MRS has an important limitation in terms of acquisition time and size of the volume of interest because of the low sensitivity of the technique. To obtain a useful spectrum in a reasonable time, the minimum volume of interest is typically about 1 cm,[3] but most MS lesions are smaller, and this can lead to partial volume effects that should be taken into account when interpreting the results.

Absolute quantitation is highly desirable but not easy; therefore, relative quantitation is generally used in clinical practice. The most common relative method is the use of ratios between metabolites, with NAA usually expressed relative to creatine-phosphocreatine (Cr), assuming that this metabolite is kept constant. Although this approach may be dubious in MS, where the Cr concentration may not be unaffected by MS pathology, NAA/Cr ratio is a practical compromise to acquiring surrogate measures of neuroaxonal integrity.[13]

^{1}H-MRS OF THE BRAIN IN MS

MS is one of the neurologic diseases in which ^{1}H-MRS has been most widely used. The first studies appeared in the early phases of clinical application of this technique at the beginning of the 1990s.[14,15] MS is a diffuse, dynamic disease that evolves over time. Thus, to summarize the ^{1}H-MRS features of the brain in this condition, it is useful to divide the metabolic patterns into 2 groups: those observed in T2-visible lesions, including both active and chronic lesions, and those in NABT, which is known to be affected in MS. ^{1}H-MRS is particularly useful to provide evidence of neurodegeneration even from the earliest stages of the disease based on the resonance intensity of NAA, a marker of neuronal integrity, and other metabolites, such as choline-containing compounds (Cho) and myo-inositol (mIns), which are affected by damage and repair of non-neuronal brain cells.

^{1}H-MRS in Focal Brain Lesions: Acute and Chronic

The presence of CNS lesions disseminated in space and time is one of the main features of MS, and the aim of the first ^{1}H-MRS studies was characterization of MS lesions in their different stages (Table 1). In general, acute inflammatory-demyelinating lesions, which usually enhance with contrast on T1-weighted images, show increases in Cho and lactate (Lac) resonances during the first 6 to 10 weeks following lesion development. Changes in the resonance intensity of Cho can be interpreted as a measure of membrane phospholipids released during active myelin breakdown, whereas Lac increases mainly seem to reflect the metabolism of inflammatory cells or neuronal mitochondrial dysfunction. The NAA pattern in the acute phase of lesion development is highly variable, ranging from almost no change with respect to normal brain tissue to significant decreases. Because NAA is detected almost exclusively in neurons in the healthy adult brain, decreases in this metabolite are interpreted as a measure of neuronal/axonal dysfunction or loss.[16,17] This initial NAA decrease may persist over time, indicating irreversible neuroaxonal injury, or show partial recovery starting a few weeks after the onset of lesion development and continuing for several months.[18,19] Few studies have focused on the changes occurring in other metabolites in the proton spectrum, and the results are sometimes contradictory. Of particular relevance in MS plaques is the behavior of Cr, a metabolite present in both neurons and glial cells, with higher concentrations in glia than neurons.[20] Cr, which commonly remains stable, can show significant increases in some plaques,[21] or decreases.[22,23] These changes may be related to varying amounts of neuroaxonal loss, oligodendroglial loss, and astrocytic proliferation.

Short echo time spectra provide evidence of transient increases in visible lipids in some lesions, probably released during myelin breakdown.[24] These lipid peaks have been identified in prelesional areas (areas of normal-appearing white matter [NAWM] that subsequently developed a plaque visible on MR imaging). A localized increase in Cho has also been described in areas of NAWM months before subsequent development of a plaque visible on MR imaging,[24,25] consistent with focal prelesional myelin membrane disease. These observations suggest that demyelination can occur months before acute inflammatory changes become evident. Other nonconventional MR techniques, such as magnetization transfer imaging, diffusion, and dynamic susceptibility weighted sequences have also shown abnormalities in this prelesional stage, further supporting the presence of subtle progressive alterations in tissue integrity before focal leakage of the blood-brain barrier as part of plaque formation in MS.[26–30] Increases have been reported in mIns, a proposed glial marker likely related to microglial proliferation,[21,22,31,32] and in glutamate,[21] which is consistent with active inflammatory infiltrates (large quantities of glutamate are produced and released by activated leucocytes, macrophages, and microglial cells).[33] In addition, application of metabolite-nulling techniques that differentiate between macromolecular

Table 1
Summary of the changes in the main metabolites of the proton magnetic resonance spectrum that may be present in multiple sclerosis brain lesions

Metabolite	Acute Stage	Evolution	Chronic
Macromolecules	↑	Tendency to ↓	Not present
Lipid	↑	Tendency to ↓	↓ or not present
Lactate	↑	Tendency to ↓	Not present
N-acetylaspartate	↓	Further ↓ partial ↑	↓
Glutamic/glutamine	↑	Tendency to ↓	
Creatine/phosphocreatine	↓, stable or ↑	Further ↑ partial ↓	↑
Choline compounds	↑	Further ↑ partial ↓	↑
Myo-inositol	↑	Remain or further ↑	↑

resonances and metabolites have shown elevated macromolecule resonances in the range of 0.9 to 1.3 ppm in acute lesions, whereas in chronic lesions, the values are similar to those of healthy controls. These macromolecules do not fit the spectral pattern of lipids, and may be interpreted as markers of myelin fragments (**Figs. 1** and **2**).[34]

Acute MS plaques usually evolve to chronic irreversible plaques (with varying degrees of neuronal/axonal loss) as inflammatory activity abates, edema resolves, and reparative mechanisms, such as remyelination, become active. These pathologic changes are reflected on cMR imaging, which usually shows cessation of contrast uptake after several weeks, associated with a T2 lesion size decrease. A percentage of active lesions become irreversibly hypointense on T1-weighted imaging (chronic black holes), which correlates pathologically with permanent demyelination and severe axonal loss. These pathologic changes also can be assessed using ^{1}H-MRS as changes in the spectral pattern of the lesions.[18,23,35–37] Among the more generally recognized changes, there is a progressive return of Lac to normal levels within weeks, whereas Cho and lipids decrease for some months, but do not always return to normal values (see **Fig. 2**). A moderate increase in Cr may also be detected, likely resulting from gliosis and remyelination.[36] NAA may further decrease, indicating progressive neuronal/axonal damage, or show partial recovery over several months without reaching normality. This recovery cannot be explained simply by resolution of edema and inflammation; other processes, such as increases in the diameter of previously shrunken axons secondary to remyelination, and reversible metabolic changes in neuronal mitochondria, also seem to have an important role (see **Table 1**).[16,17]

^{1}H-MRS of NABT: White and Gray Matter

In addition to focal demyelinated plaques, diffuse global injury outside the focal MS lesions (in NABT) is also found in the brains of patients with MS. These abnormalities include diffuse astrocytic hyperplasia, patchy edema, and perivascular cellular infiltration, as well as axonal damage myelin loss and microscopic focal lesions. In vivo demonstration of this widespread abnormality has been achieved by several nonconventional MR techniques, such as magnetization transfer imaging (reduced magnetization transfer ratio), diffusion-weighted sequences (increased diffusivity and decreased fractional anisotropy), and ^{1}H-MRS, which reveals several abnormalities that are more pronounced in the progressive forms of the disease, but also can be detected in patients with clinically isolated syndromes, the earliest stage of possible MS.

The most consistent change reported is a decrease in NAA or in the NAA/Cr ratio within the NAWM, suggesting diffuse axonal loss or dysfunction.[38–41] At least in the early phases of the relapsing forms of MS, when the inflammatory component of the disease predominates over the neurodegenerative component, this NAA decrease of 7% to 9% relative to healthy controls tends to recover from baseline, indicating that the neuronal/axonal injury is partially reversible.[42] Increases in mIns, Cr, Cho, and glutamate (Glu) levels have been demonstrated within the NAWM of patients with MS, likely indicating gliosis and inflammation.[21,32,43–45]

NAA decreases have also been demonstrated in the NAWM of the primary progressive form of MS (PPMS) and have been proposed as a marker of disease progression in this MS phenotype. Nonetheless, in a study performed in 40 patients with PPMS, Narayana and colleagues[46] found no

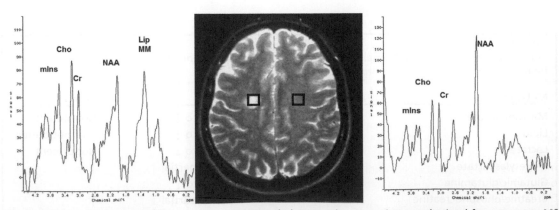

Fig. 1. Stimulated echo acquisition mode spectra recorded at an echo time of 20 ms obtained from an acute MS lesion (*left*) and the contralateral NAWM (*right*). The lesion spectrum shows a moderate decrease in NAA, and an increase in Cho and mIns. There is also elevation of the lipid peak (Lip) and macromolecules (MM).

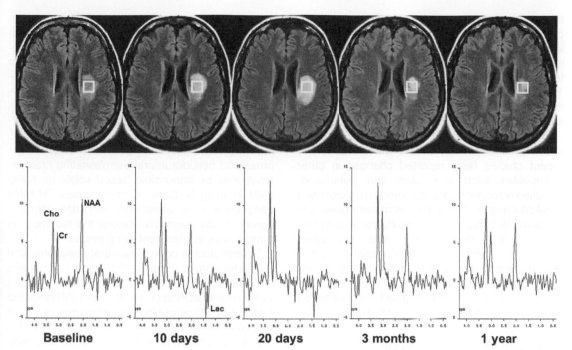

Fig. 2. Serial MRI and spin-echo spectra recorded at an echo time of 135 ms from an acute multiple sclerosis plaque. FLAIR images show an initial progressive lesion size increase followed by decrease over 1 year of follow-up. ¹H-MRS during the acute stage shows the presence of lactate, a slight decrease in NAA, and an increase in Cho. The longitudinal study demonstrates lactate disappearance at 3 months, persistent low levels of NAA, a progressive Cho increase during the first weeks followed by partial recovery, and relatively stable Cr at all time points.

significant differences in NAA levels between T2 lesions and NAWM. Lipid peaks in NAWM were identified in most patients with PPMS in that study. Last, in patients with clinically isolated syndromes, several studies have shown a decrease in NAA, with normal or elevated mIns and Cho levels, indicating that axonal damage occurs during the first demyelinating episode, but absent or only minimal increase of the activity of glial cells.[47–49]

Gustafsson and colleagues[50] performed ¹H-MRS in a group of patients with a clinical diagnosis of MS in whom brain MR imaging was normal. This group, which accounts for approximately 3% of all patients with MS, showed a significant decrease in NAA, indicating diffuse neuronal/axonal damage. However, in contrast to studies in patients with MS with brain T2 lesions, a decrease in Cho and Cr was detected, a finding that could reflect an increase in protective or healing abilities in this particular and unusual group of patients with MS.

Although MS is considered a disease of the white matter, demyelination can also be found in the deep cerebral nuclei, cerebral cortex, and gray matter of the spinal cord and brainstem. Cerebral cortex involvement may contribute to neurologic and cognitive impairment, particularly in advanced disease stages, as a result of axon and dendrite

transection, synapse loss, and neuron apoptosis. Unfortunately, currently available MR imaging techniques are not optimal for detecting cortical lesions because of poor contrast resolution between normal-appearing gray matter (NAGM) and the plaques in question, and because of the partial volume effects of the subarachnoid spaces and cerebrospinal fluid surrounding the cortex. New MR techniques, such as double inversion recovery (DIR) sequences, which selectively suppress the white matter signal and cerebrospinal fluid and phase-sensitive inversion recovery sequences, which generate a high signal-to-noise ratio image, significantly increase the sensitivity for detecting cortical MS lesions, although most purely intracortical lesions remain invisible. ¹H-MRS offers detection of diffuse gray matter involvement, and several studies have demonstrated an NAA decrease in the cortical and subcortical NAGM of patients with MS.[51–61] In addition, significantly lower Cr[53,59,62] and glutamine-glutamate (Glx)[52,57] values have been described, which could be interpreted as an indirect expression of metabolic dysfunction. Lipid resonances consistent with an active process of demyelination/remyelination can also be present.[63] There are reports showing either an increase or decrease in mIns, which is thought to be the result of gliosis[58] or a possible combination of reduced neuronal cellularity and a lack of gliosis.[51] Similarly, there are reports of increases in the Cho resonance, likely attributable to microscopic lesions that are not visible on T2-weighted imaging,[56,60] as well as decreases in this metabolite, which could indicate reduced cellular density and metabolic activity (**Table 2**).[52,59]

In addition to detection of changes in levels of the above-mentioned metabolites within the NABT, recent studies have reported changes in other metabolites, such as citrulline and glutathione. Citrulline resonances are more frequently identified in NAWM and in chronic lesions of early-onset patients with MS than in healthy subjects, suggesting an association between increased citrullination of myelin proteins and demyelinating disease.[64] Furthermore, a decrease in glutathione has been reported in NAWM, NAGM, and T2 lesions of patients with MS.[65,66] This metabolite is considered a biomarker of oxidative stress in the cell.

^{1}H-MRS IN THE DIAGNOSIS OF PSEUDOTUMORAL IDIOPATHIC INFLAMMATORY-DEMYELINATING LESIONS

Idiopathic inflammatory demyelinating diseases can present as single or multiple focal brain lesions that may be clinically and radiographically indistinguishable from tumors. This situation is a diagnostic challenge and reasonably calls for biopsy despite clinical suspicion of demyelination.[67–71] However, even the biopsy specimen may resemble a brain tumor because of the hypercellular nature of the lesions, which are often associated with large protoplasmatic glial cells with fragmented chromatin and abnormal mitosis (Creutzfeldt cells).[72] On MR imaging, these pseudotumoral lesions usually present as large, single or multiple focal lesions

---

Table 2
Summary of the changes in the main metabolites of the proton magnetic resonance spectrum that may be present in normal appearing white matter (NAWM) and normal appearing gray matter (NAGM)

Metabolite	NAWM	NAGM
Lipids	↑	↑
N-acetylaspartate	↓	↓
Glutamic/glutamine	↑	↓
Creatine/phosphocreatine	↑ or ↓	↓
Choline compounds	↑ or ↓	↑ or ↓
Myo-inositol	↑	↑ or ↓

Up arrows, increase; Down arrows, decrease.

---

located in the brain hemispheres.[73] Clues that can help to differentiate these lesions from a brain tumor include a relatively minor mass effect or vasogenic edema, incomplete ring-enhancement on T1-weighted gadolinium-enhanced images sometimes associated with a rim of peripheral hypointensity on T2-weighted sequences, and an internal pattern of alternating bands on T2-weighted images (Balo-like pattern). Nonetheless, the differential diagnosis between malignant gliomas and pseudotumoral demyelinating brain lesions may be impossible based solely on these cMR imaging features. In these cases, ^{1}H-MRS can provide useful additional information, although reports on the diagnostic value of this technique in tumors have yielded conflicting results.

Several studies have shown that pseudotumoral demyelinating lesions and glial tumors can present with similar spectral patterns.[74–78] Others suggest that the combination of ^{1}H-MRS and cMR imaging features can facilitate the correct diagnosis,[79] and that an increase in Glx should suggest a pseudotumoral demyelinating lesion.[80–82] More sophisticated methods rely on statistical analysis of the spectrum using pattern recognition techniques or combining results obtained from spectra acquired at short and long echo times. Pattern recognition techniques applied to ^{1}H-MRS data obtained from acute large solitary demyelinating lesions and astrocytic tumors (low-grade, anaplastic astrocytomas and glioblastoma multiforme) can correctly classify the lesions, based on the leave-one-out technique. However, classification of chronic lesions with this approach is limited because the metabolic patterns of low-grade astrocytomas can overlap those of chronic lesions.[83] Hourani and colleagues[84] studied 36 brain tumors and 33 non-neoplastic pseudotumoral lesions (10 demyelinating) using a discriminant function analysis that correctly classified 84% of the cases. More recently, Majós and colleagues[85] analyzed the spectra of different focal noncystic and nonnecrotic brain lesions (68 glial tumors World Health Organization grade II and III, and 16 pseudotumoral lesions), and found differences in NAA, Glx, Cho, and mIns. This study proposed a classifier based on the mIns/NAA and Cho/NAA ratios obtained at short and at long echo times, tested with a test-set group of 28 cases. Accuracy was about 80%, and the confidence of neuroradiologists in establishing a correct differential diagnosis between tumoral and nontumoral lesions improved in 5% to 27% of cases (**Figs. 3** and **4**). A different and probably more challenging situation is when acute pseudotumoral demyelinating lesions present with a ring-enhancement pattern of contrast uptake (cystic/necrotic appearance) on

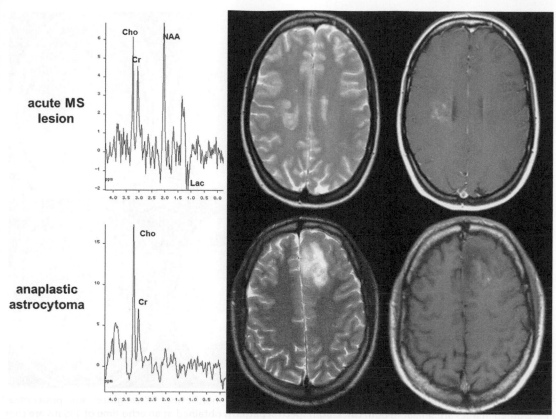

Fig. 3. Comparison of 2 tumefactive lesions. An acute MS lesion and an anaplastic astrocytoma. T2-weighted and post-contrast T1-weighted images are similar in the 2 cases. Spectra recorded at an echo time of 135 ms. The spectral pattern of the pseudotumoral MS lesion is characterized by the presence of lactate, a moderate decrease in NAA, and a slight increase in Cho relative to Cr, whereas in anaplastic astrocytoma there is a marked increase in Cho relative to Cr, and NAA is absent.

cMR imaging, mimicking high-grade primary tumors or metastasis. The [1]H-MR spectra of these lesions are characterized by the presence of Lac, macromolecules/lipids, and Cho with a marked decrease in NAA. On follow-up, these lesions show rapid disappearance of the Lac and macromolecule/lipid signal, whereas NAA shows progressive and partial recovery,[86] associated with a decrease in lesion size and cessation of contrast uptake. These findings suggest the existence of an inflammatory process that produces an accumulation of edema in the extracellular space with an almost complete absence of cells. With elimination of the inflammation, there is a reduction in the edema and almost complete normalization of the spectral pattern, indicating that cell destruction is less important than was initially expected (**Fig. 5**).

In summary, although some conventional MR imaging features (Balo-like pattern and open-ring enhancement) can help differentiate tumoral from pseudotumoral lesions, in some situations these features do not suffice to suggest a precise diagnosis. In these cases, ^{1}H-MRS obtained at different echo times can provide useful additional diagnostic information by assessing the relative concentrations of NAA, Cho, mIns, and Glx, which can, sometimes, help distinguishing between tumoral and pseudotumoral lesions, avoiding unnecessary aggressive diagnostic or therapeutic procedures.

^{1}H-MRS FEATURES OF THE SPINAL CORD IN MS

Spinal cord damage significantly contributes to the degree of disability in patients with MS. ^{1}H-MRS has rarely been applied to assess neuronal/axonal spinal cord damage, however, because of technical challenges, including the small size of the cord, susceptibility differences between the vertebral bodies, intervertebral discs and surrounding tissue leading to strong magnetic field inhomogeneities, and the pulsatile flow of cerebrospinal fluid induced by cardiac and respiratory motion, which causes phase fluctuations, water suppression failure, and spinal cord movement. Because of these

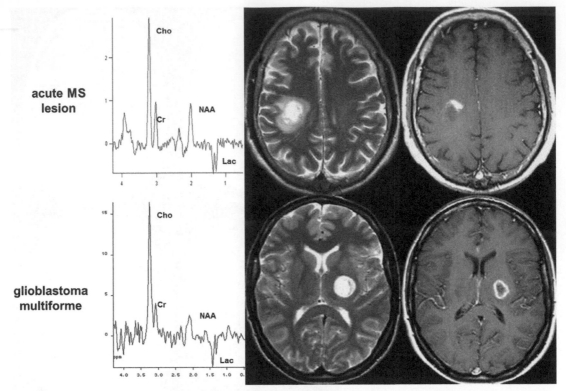

Fig. 4. Comparison of an acute MS lesion and a glioblastoma multiforme. T2-weighted and postcontrast T1-weighted images are similar in both cases. Both spectral patterns obtained at an echo time of 135 ms are characterized by increased Cho and the presence of lactate. The glioblastoma shows a more important decrease in NAA (or other N-acetylated compounds) and increase in Cho relative to Cr than the acute MS lesion.

circumstances, few spinal cord ^{1}H-MRS studies have been undertaken in patients with MS and most are restricted to the uppermost segment of the cervical spine. Recent technical improvements, such as a combination of electrocardiogram triggering, inner-volume saturation, highly selective pulses and localized shimming, minimize the technical limitations of ^{1}H-MRS and extend the applicability of spectroscopy to the entire length of the spinal cord.[87] A recent ^{1}H-MRS study of spinal cord lesions has shown decreases in NAA/Cr and NAA/Cho ratios, whereas Cho/Cr and mIns/Cr ratios were increased.[88] These results partially agree with a previous study that reported a decrease in NAA, which correlates with the 9-hole peg test, whereas mIns, Cr, and Cho correlate with disability.[89] In addition, some studies have shown an NAA decrease in the normal-appearing spinal cord.[90,91]

^{1}H-MRS AND CLINICAL CORRELATIONS

Several studies examining NABT or T2 lesions in patients with MS have reported significant, although moderate, correlations of ^{1}H-MRS findings with clinical disability. NAA is the metabolite that most consistently correlates with disability measured with the Kurtzke Expanded Disability Scale Score (EDSS), supporting the notion that neuronal dysfunction is a mechanism of disability.[22,39,50,62,92–95] Patients with relapsing-remitting multiple sclerosis (RRMS) and advanced clinical disability, those with secondary progressive multiple sclerosis (SPMS), and those with long disease duration generally show the most severe NAA loss. However, correlations between the NAA/Cr ratio and disability are stronger in patients with mild disability (EDSS <5) than in patients with severe disability (EDSS ≥5). When a similar analysis was performed in patients grouped by disease duration, the subgroup with short duration (<5 years) showed a significant correlation between the NAA/Cr ratio and EDSS, which was not seen in patients with long disease duration.[96] Furthermore, a correlation of NAA/Cr with disability has been found in RRMS but not SPMS patients.[97] A study in RRMS and SPMS showed a correlation between the cortical gray matter NAA/Cr ratio and EDSS only when data from both groups were combined.[61] All these findings support the

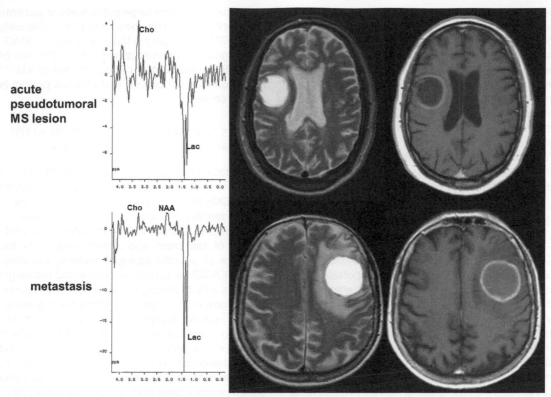

acute pseudotumoral MS lesion

metastasis

Fig. 5. Comparison of an acute pseudotumoral cystlike demyelinating lesion and a metastatic lesion. T2-weighted and postcontrast T1-weighted images are similar in both cases. Spectral patterns obtained at an echo time of 135 ms are characterized by the presence of lactate. Residual Cho is present in both cases and NAA (probably due to other N-acetylated compounds) is more clearly seen In the metastasis.

concept that axonal damage is the primary determinant of disability from the early stages of the disease.

Studies in NAWM have shown that in addition to NAA, mIns and Glx also correlate with disability.[50,57,98] Correlations of the Multiple Sclerosis Functional Composite (MSFC) score were found with cortical NAGM Cr and Glx, and with NAWM mIns, but not with NAA in patients with early RRMS, whereas EDSS correlated only with cortical NAGM Glx.[52] However, other studies based on spectra analysis in different NAGM[53,58] and NAWM regions,[48,99] in large volumes[46,100,101] and in whole brain studies[102,103] did not find correlations between NAA or other metabolites and disability.

As well as disability, NAA has been correlated with fatigue and cognitive dysfunction in patients with MS. Téllez and colleagues[104] reported a significant decrease in NAA/Cr in the lentiform nucleus in patients with fatigue, supporting the idea that specific dysfunction or involvement of the basal ganglia might contribute to the development of this common MS-related symptom. ^{1}H-MRS has a good sensitivity for determining the cognitive status of patients with MS, mainly by measuring NAA in the NABT, and can differentiate patients with MS with and without cognitive impairment (Fig. 6). Some studies have shown correlations between specific cognitive deficits and NAA levels assessed in particular brain structures. In a study performed in early-stage MS, Gadea and colleagues[105] reported NAA decreases in the right

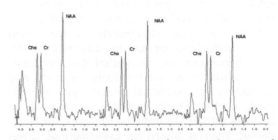

Fig. 6. Proton spectra obtained at an echo time of 135 ms from the frontal region in a control subject (*left*), a cognitively unimpaired patient (*center*), and a cognitively impaired patient (*right*). There is a reduction in NAA relative to Cr in the cognitively impaired patient compared with the control and the unimpaired patient with MS.

locus ceruleus in the pons that correlated to selective attention deficit, measured by a dichotic listening paradigm. More recently, Pfueller and colleagues[106] described a correlation between retinal nerve fiber layer and visual cortex NAA, but not with normal-appearing white matter NAA that was connected with the patients' history of a previous optic neuritis. These data suggest the existence of functional pathway-specific damage patterns exceeding global neurodegeneration. Taken together, these ^{1}H-MRS studies demonstrate that metabolic changes in specific brain areas correlate with specific cognitive deficits.

^{1}H-MRS AS A MARKER OF TREATMENT RESPONSE IN MS

Conventional MR imaging techniques have become established as the most important paraclinical tool for monitoring the efficacy of disease-modifying treatments with a predominant anti-inflammatory effect. Clinical trials assessing the efficacy of glatiramer acetate (GA), interferon (IFN)-β, and natalizumab in relapsing forms of MS have all shown a significant decrease in cMR imaging measures of disease activity. Going further, there is now growing interest in developing neuroprotective agents in MS and this demands new imaging strategies to more specifically monitor the neurodegenerative, irreversible component of the disease. Although NAA has been proposed as a marker for this purpose, it is rarely used as an outcome measure of therapeutic response in clinical trials. The technical demands of ^{1}H-MRS and its low reproducibility across centers have limited its use to single-center trials, and usually in small patient cohorts.

Studies analyzing the effect of interferon in small cohorts of relapsing patients with MS have shown conflicting results that range from improvement or stabilization to little effect on NAA.[107–110] In a pilot study in patients with RRMS, Khan and colleagues[111] reported that NAA/Cr increased significantly in the group treated with glatiramer acetate compared with untreated patients, and suggested that this treatment leads to axonal metabolic recovery and protection from sublethal axonal injury. In contrast, another study, including a subgroup of patients with PPMS from the PROspective Multicenter Imaging Study for Evaluation of Chest Pain (PROMISE) trial[112] found no changes in metabolite ratios between the placebo group and glatiramer acetate–treated group.[113]

The data from these studies does not suffice to establish the sensitivity of ^{1}H-MRS in therapeutic interventions, although the feasibility of using this technique to monitor large subcohorts of patients in multicenter trials has been reported.[46] Recently the MAGNetic Imaging in Multiple Sclerosis (MAGNIMS) group proposed guidelines for the use of ^{1}H-MRS in multicenter, clinical studies of MS[114] to standardize acquisition and analysis protocols across centers.

^{1}H-MRS FEATURES OF THE BRAIN IN ACUTE DISSEMINATED ENCEPHALOMYELITIS

Acute disseminated encephalomyelitis (ADEM) is a severe, immune-mediated inflammatory disorder of the CNS that is usually triggered by an inflammatory response to viral or bacterial infections or vaccinations, and predominantly affects the white matter of the brain and spinal cord.[115] In the absence of specific biologic markers, the diagnosis of ADEM is based on clinical and radiologic features. ADEM usually has a monophasic course, but recurrent or multiphasic forms have been reported, raising diagnostic difficulties in distinguishing these cases from MS. Unlike lesions in MS, ADEM lesions are often large, patchy, and poorly marginated on MR imaging. There is usually asymmetrical involvement of the subcortical and central white matter and cortical gray-white junction of the cerebral hemispheres, cerebellum, brainstem, and spinal cord. The gray matter of the thalami and basal ganglia is often affected, particularly in children and typically in a symmetric pattern. Lesions confined to the periventricular white matter and corpus callosum are less common than in MS.[116]

Advanced MR techniques, including ^{1}H-MRS, have been proposed to differentiate ADEM lesions from others having a similar appearance on MR imaging, such as tumors, acute MS lesions, and infections, but few studies in small patient samples have analyzed the ^{1}H-MRS characteristics in ADEM. In the acute phase, ADEM lesions show a decreased NAA/Cr ratio and increased Cho/Cr ratio, along with increased lipid peaks,[117–121] following the same pattern described in acute MS plaques. The presence of lactate, which normalized within days, was reported in one study,[122] whereas another described decreased NAA in an ADEM lesion during relapse that normalized in tandem with MR imaging abnormalities.[117] These abnormalities have been described together in other studies in addition to new findings, such as the presence of macromolecules/lipids and Cho.[118,120] In a study of 8 patients with ADEM, focusing on characterization of the metabolic pattern of NAWM and lesions in the acute and subacute stages, Cho/Cr and NAA/Cho ratios in the subacute stage were higher and lower, respectively, than in the acute stage or in NAWM.[123] Another study involving 7 patients longitudinally evaluated ^{1}H-MRS changes and reported partial recovery of the Cho/Cr ratio between the acute and chronic phases. Major lipid elevations and decreases in the mIns/Cr ratio were detected in all patients during the acute phase, followed by a reduction in the lipid peak and a mIns/Cr ratio elevation above normal during the chronic phase. The investigators concluded that an mIns/Cr decrease may help to differentiate ADEM from other demyelinating diseases.[121]

^{1}H-MRS FEATURES OF THE BRAIN IN NEUROMYELITIS OPTICA (DEVIC DISEASE)

Devic neuromyelitis optica (NMO) is an uncommon and topographically restricted form of idiopathic inflammatory demyelinating disease that is considered a distinct disease rather than a variant of MS. NMO is characterized by severe unilateral or bilateral optic neuritis and complete transverse myelitis, which occur simultaneously or sequentially within a varying period of time (weeks or years), without clinical involvement of other CNS regions. Initially it was thought that brain MRI might not show white matter lesions, at least in the first stages of the disease; however, about 60% of patients present large confluent and diencephalic lesions (not typically seen in MS) that are related to the presence of aquaporin-4 channel sites.[124]

Few studies have analyzed the metabolic pattern of focal brain lesions in NMO using ^{1}H-MRS. Matsushita and colleagues[125] studied focal brain lesions in 5 antiaquaporin-4 antibody-positive patients and demonstrated increased Cho/Cr and decreased NAA/Cr ratios, as well as the presence of lactate, data consistent with acute inflammation. These findings have been described in other acute inflammatory demyelinating disorders. Of greater interest are the studies analyzing the metabolic pattern in NABT of patients with NMO, in which no differences were found in the pattern of NAWM or NAGM between patients with NMO and healthy subjects, or between patients with normal or abnormal brain MR imaging findings. This contrasts with what has been described in patients with MS, in whom axonal metabolic changes and damage may be found even in early phases of the disease. These data reinforce the concept that axonal damage does not diffusely affect the brain tissue in Devic disease,[126–128] and are consistent with the relapsing-remitting nature of NMO, which rarely has a progressive course, a feature that distinguishes this disease from MS.

SUMMARY

In summary, the results obtained from ^{1}H-MRS studies have not established a specific spectral pattern in MS lesions or NABT because of the highly variable changes documented in the metabolites studied. The same heterogeneity of results is found when examining the relationship between brain metabolites and disability. This can partially be attributed to technical considerations, including differences in acquisition conditions, postprocessing routines, quantification methods, and regions studied. Other factors may come from the complexity of an illness that displays several clinical forms evolving over time and involves various physiopathological processes. Nonetheless, ^{1}H-MRS can provide more detailed information about the physiopathological processes occurring during the disease course as a complement to cMR imaging. Regarding the use of ^{1}H-MRS information to aid in the differential diagnosis of pseudotumoral demyelinating lesions and tumors, the results to date indicate that the need for a biopsy cannot be completely eliminated, but the combination of ^{1}H-MRS and cMR imaging findings can increase the physician's confidence in the diagnosis. Last, despite the efforts made in the past years, the available evidence does not support the use of ^{1}H-MRS as a marker of disease severity and progression in MS, or as a surrogate marker of neuronal/axonal loss and neuronal protection in clinical trials. New studies applying recent technical developments in ^{1}H-MRS data acquisition and postprocessing are required to further investigate the value of this technique in determining the accumulated irreversible disability, and in monitoring the potential neuroprotective effects of new experimental treatments.

REFERENCES

1. Confavreux C, Vukusic S, Moreau T, et al. Relapses and progression of disability in multiple sclerosis. N Engl J Med 2000;343:1430–8.

2. Pirko I, Lucchinetti CF, Sriram S, et al. Gray matter involvement in multiple sclerosis. Neurology 2007; 68:634–42.

3. Barkhof F, Filippi M, Miller DH, et al. Comparison of MRI criteria at first presentation to predict conversion to clinically definite multiple sclerosis. Brain 1997;120:2059–69.

4. Tintoré M, Rovira A, Martínez MJ, et al. Isolated demyelinating syndromes: comparison of different MR imaging criteria to predict conversion to clinically definite multiple sclerosis. AJNR Am J Neuroradiol 2000;21:702–6.

5. Polman CH, Reingold SC, Banwell B, et al. Diagnostic criteria for multiple sclerosis: 2010 revisions to the McDonald criteria. Ann Neurol 2011;69: 292–302.

6. Filippi M, Grossman RI. MRI techniques to monitor MS evolution: the present and the future. Neurology 2002;58:1147–53.

7. Barkhof F. The clinico-radiological paradox in multiple sclerosis revisited. Curr Opin Neurol 2002; 15:239–45.

8. De Stefano N, Bartolozzi ML, Guidi L, et al. Magnetic resonance spectroscopy as a measure of brain damage in multiple sclerosis. J Neurol Sci 2005;233:203–8.

9. Arnold DL, Riess GT, Matthews PM, et al. Use of proton magnetic resonance spectroscopy for monitoring disease progression in multiple sclerosis. Ann Neurol 1994;36:76–82.

10. Matthews PM, Pioro E, Narayanan S, et al. Assessment of lesion pathology in multiple sclerosis using quantitative MRI morphometry and magnetic resonance spectroscopy. Brain 1996;119:715–22.

11. Pelletier D, Nelson SJ, Grenier D, et al. 3-D echo planar (1) HMRS imaging in MS: metabolite comparison from supratentorial vs. central brain. Magn Reson Imaging 2002;20:599–606.

12. Gonen O, Catalaa I, Babb JS, et al. Total brain N-acetylaspartate: a new measure of disease load in MS. Neurology 2000;54:15–9.

13. Caramanos Z, Narayanan S, Arnold DL. 1H-MRS quantification of tNA and tCr in patients with multiple sclerosis: a meta-analytic review. Brain 2005; 128:2483–506.

14. Arnold DL, Matthews PM, Francis G, et al. Proton magnetic resonance spectroscopy of human brain in vivo in the evaluation of multiple sclerosis: assessment of the load of disease. Magn Reson Med 1990;14:154–9.

15. Wolinsky JS, Narayana PA, Fenstermacher MJ. Proton magnetic resonance spectroscopy in multiple sclerosis. Neurology 1990;40:1764–9.

16. Arnold DL, De Stefano N, Narayanan S, et al. Proton MR spectroscopy in multiple sclerosis. Neuroimaging Clin N Am 2000;10:789–98.

17. Sajja BR, Wolinsky JS, Narayana PA. Proton magnetic resonance spectroscopy in multiple sclerosis. Neuroimaging Clin N Am 2009;19:45–58.

18. Davie CA, Hawkins CP, Barker GJ, et al. Serial proton magnetic resonance spectroscopy in acute multiple sclerosis lesions. Brain 1994;117:49–58.

19. De Stefano N, Matthews PM, Arnold DL. Reversible decreases in N-acetylaspartate after acute brain injury. Magn Reson Med 1995;34:721–7.

20. Urenjak J, Williams SR, Gadian DG, et al. Proton nuclear magnetic resonance spectroscopy unambiguously identifies different neural cell types. J Neurosci 1993;13:981–9.

21. Srinivasan R, Sailasuta N, Hurd R, et al. Evidence of elevated glutamate in multiple sclerosis using magnetic resonance spectroscopy at 3 T. Brain 2005;128:1016–25.

22. De Stefano N, Matthews PM, Antel JP, et al. Chemical pathology of acute demyelinating lesions and its correlation with disability. Ann Neurol 1995;38: 901–9.

23. Zaaraoui W, Rico A, Audoin B, et al. Unfolding the long-term pathophysiological processes following an acute inflammatory demyelinating lesion of multiple sclerosis. Magn Reson Imaging 2010;28: 477–86.

24. Narayana PA, Doyle TJ, Lai D, et al. Serial proton magnetic resonance spectroscopic imaging, contrast-enhanced magnetic resonance imaging, and quantitative lesion volumetry in multiple sclerosis. Ann Neurol 1998;43:56–71.

25. Tartaglia MC, Narayanan S, De Stefano N, et al. Choline is increased in pre-lesional normal appearing white matter in multiple sclerosis. J Neurol 2002;249:1382–90.

26. Silver NC, Lai M, Symms MR, et al. Serial magnetization transfer imaging to characterize the early evolution of new MS lesions. Neurology 1998;51: 758–64.

27. Filippi M, Rocca MA, Martino G, et al. Magnetization transfer changes in the normal appearing white matter precede the appearance of enhancing lesions in patients with multiple sclerosis. Ann Neurol 1998;43:809–14.

28. Rocca MA, Cercignani M, Iannucci G, et al. Weekly diffusion-weighted imaging of normal-appearing white matter in MS. Neurology 2000;55:882–4.

29. Werring DJ, Brassat D, Droogan AG, et al. The pathogenesis of lesions and normal-appearing white matter changes in multiple sclerosis: a serial diffusion MRI study. Brain 2000;123:1667–76.

30. Wuerfel J, Bellmann-Strobl J, Brunecker P, et al. Changes in cerebral perfusion precede plaque formation in multiple sclerosis: a longitudinal perfusion MRI study. Brain 2004;127:111–9.

31. Brex PA, Parker GJ, Leary SM, et al. Lesion heterogeneity in multiple sclerosis: a study of the relations between appearances on T1 weighted images, T1 relaxation times, and metabolite concentrations. J Neurol Neurosurg Psychiatry 2000; 68:627–32.

32. Hattingen E, Magerkurth J, Pilatus U, et al. Combined (1) H and (31) P spectroscopy provides new insights into the pathobiochemistry of brain damage in multiple sclerosis. NMR Biomed 2011; 24:536–46.

33. Piani D, Frei K, Do KD, et al. Murine brain macrophages induced NMDA receptor mediated neurotoxicity in vitro by secreting glutamate. Neurosci Lett 1991;133:159–62.

34. Mader I, Seeger U, Weissert R, et al. Proton MR spectroscopy with metabolite-nulling reveals elevated macromolecules in acute multiple sclerosis. Brain 2001;124:953–61.

35. Arnold DL, Matthews PM, Francis G, et al. Proton magnetic resonance spectroscopic imaging for metabolic characterization of demyelinating plaques. Ann Neurol 1992;31:235–41.

36. Mader I, Roser W, Kappos L, et al. Serial proton MR spectroscopy of contrast-enhancing multiple sclerosis plaques: absolute metabolic values over 2 years during a clinical pharmacological study. AJNR Am J Neuroradiol 2000;21:1220–7.

37. Rovira A, Pericot I, Alonso J, et al. Serial diffusion-weighted MR imaging and proton MR. AJNR Am J Neuroradiol 2002;23:989–94.

38. Narayanan S, Fu L, Pioro E, et al. Imaging of axonal damage in multiple sclerosis: spatial distribution of magnetic resonance imaging lesions. Ann Neurol 1997;41:385–91.

39. Fu L, Matthews PM, De Stefano N, et al. Imaging axonal damage of normal-appearing white matter in multiple sclerosis. Brain 1998;121:103–13.

40. Sarchielli P, Presciutti O, Pelliccioli GP, et al. Absolute quantification of brain metabolites by proton magnetic resonance spectroscopy in normal-appearing white matter of multiple sclerosis patients. Brain 1999;122:513–21.

41. Bjartmar C, Kinkel RP, Kidd G, et al. Axonal loss in normal-appearing white matter in a patient with acute MS. Neurology 2001;57:1248–52.

42. Tiberio M, Chard DT, Altmann DR, et al. Metabolite changes in early relapsing-remitting multiple sclerosis. A two year follow-up study. J Neurol 2006; 253:224–30.

43. Inglese M, Li BS, Rusinek H, et al. Diffusely elevated cerebral choline and creatine in relapsing-remitting multiple sclerosis. Magn Reson Med 2003;50:190–5.

44. He J, Inglese M, Li BS, et al. Relapsing-remitting multiple sclerosis: metabolic abnormality in nonenhancing lesions and normal-appearing white matter at MR imaging: initial experience. Radiology 2005;234:211–7.

45. Suhy J, Rooney WD, Goodkin DE, et al. 1H MRSI comparison of white matter and lesions in primary progressive and relapsing-remitting MS. Mult Scler 2000;6:148–55.

46. Narayana PA, Wolinsky JS, Rao SB, et al. Multicentre proton magnetic resonance spectroscopy imaging of primary progressive multiple sclerosis. Mult Scler 2004;10:S73–8.

47. Tourbah A, Stievenart JL, Abanou A, et al. Normal-appearing white matter in optic neuritis and multiple sclerosis: a comparative proton spectroscopy study. Neuroradiology 1999;41:738–43.

48. Fernando KT, McLean MA, Chard DT, et al. Elevated white matter myo-inositol in clinically isolated syndromes suggestive of multiple sclerosis. Brain 2004;127:1361–9.

49. Wattjes MP, Harzheim M, Lutterbey GG, et al. Axonal damage but no increased glial cell activity in the normal-appearing white matter of patients with clinically isolated syndromes suggestive of multiple sclerosis using high-field magnetic resonance spectroscopy. AJNR Am J Neuroradiol 2007;28:1517–22.

50. Gustafsson MC, Dahlqvist O, Jaworski J, et al. Low choline concentrations in normal-appearing white matter of patients with multiple sclerosis and normal MR imaging brain scans. AJNR Am J Neuroradiol 2007;28:1306–12.

51. Kapeller P, McLean MA, Griffin CM, et al. Preliminary evidence for neuronal damage in cortical grey matter and normal appearing white matter in short duration relapsing-remitting multiple sclerosis: a quantitative MR spectroscopic imaging study. J Neurol 2001;248:131–8.

52. Chard DT, Griffin CM, McLean MA, et al. Brain metabolite changes in cortical grey and normal-appearing white matter in clinically early relapsing-remitting multiple sclerosis. Brain 2002;125:2342–52.

53. Sarchielli P, Presciutti O, Tarducci R, et al. Localized (1)H magnetic resonance spectroscopy in mainly cortical gray matter of patients with multiple sclerosis. J Neurol 2002;249:902–10.

54. Wylezinska M, Cifelli A, Jezzard P, et al. Thalamic neurodegeneration in relapsing-remitting multiple sclerosis. Neurology 2003;60:1949–54.

55. Adalsteinsson E, Langer-Gould A, Homer RJ, et al. Gray matter N-acetyl aspartate deficits in secondary progressive but not relapsing-remitting multiple sclerosis. AJNR Am J Neuroradiol 2003;24:1941–5.

56. Inglese M, Liu S, Babb JS, et al. Three-dimensional proton spectroscopy of deep gray matter nuclei in relapsing-remitting MS. Neurology 2004;63:170–2.

57. Sastre-Garriga J, Ingle GT, Chard DT, et al. Metabolite changes in normal-appearing gray and white matter are linked with disability in early primary progressive multiple sclerosis. Arch Neurol 2005; 62:569–73.

58. Geurts JJ, Reuling IE, Vrenken H, et al. MR spectroscopic evidence for thalamic and hippocampal, but not cortical, damage in multiple sclerosis. Magn Reson Med 2006;55:478–83.

59. Sijens PE, Mostert JP, Oudkerk M, et al. 1H MR spectroscopy of the brain in multiple sclerosis subtypes with analysis of the metabolite concentrations in gray and white matter: initial findings. Eur Radiol 2006;16:489–95.

60. Van Au Duong M, Audoin B, Le Fur Y, et al. Relationships between gray matter metabolic abnormalities and white matter inflammation in patients at the very early stage of MS: a MRSI study. J Neurol 2007;254:914–23.

61. Caramanos Z, DiMaio S, Narayanan S, et al. (1) H-MRSI evidence for cortical gray matter pathology that is independent of cerebral white matter lesion load in patients with secondary progressive multiple sclerosis. J Neurol Sci 2009;282: 72–9.

62. Aboul-Enein F, Krssák M, Höftberger R, et al. Reduced NAA-levels in the NAWM of patients with MS is a feature of progression. A study with quantitative magnetic resonance spectroscopy at 3 tesla. PLoS One 2010;5:e11625.

63. Sharma R, Narayana PA, Wolinsky JS. Grey matter abnormalities in multiple sclerosis: proton magnetic resonance spectroscopic imaging. Mult Scler 2001;7:221–6.

64. Oguz KK, Kurne A, Aksu AO, et al. Assessment of citrullinated myelin by 1H-MR spectroscopy in early-onset multiple sclerosis. AJNR Am J Neuroradiol 2009;30:716–21.

65. Srinivasan R, Ratiney H, Hammond-Rosenbluth KE, et al. MR spectroscopic imaging of glutathione in the white and gray matter at 7 T with an application to multiple sclerosis. Magn Reson Imaging 2010; 28:163–70.

66. Choi I, Lee S, Denney DR, et al. Lower levels of glutathione in the brains of secondary progressive multiple sclerosis patients measured by 1H magnetic resonance chemical shift imaging at 3 T. Mult Scler 2011;17:289–96.

67. Mastrostefano R, Occhipinti E, Bigotti G, et al. Multiple sclerosis plaque simulating cerebral tumor: case report and review of the literature. Neurosurgery 1987;21:244–6.

68. Hunter SB, Ballinger WE Jr, Rubin JJ. Multiple sclerosis mimicking primary brain tumor. Arch Pathol Lab Med 1987;111:464–8.

69. Giang DW, Poduri KR, Eskin TA, et al. Multiple sclerosis masquerading as a mass lesion. Neuroradiology 1992;34:150–4.

70. Kurihara N, Takahashi S, Furuta A, et al. MR imaging of multiple sclerosis simulating brain tumor. Clin Imaging 1996;20:171–7.

71. Silva HC, Callegaro D, Marchiori PE, et al. Magnetic resonance imaging in five patients with a tumefactive demyelinating lesion in the central nervous system. Arq Neuropsiquiatr 1999;57: 921–6.

72. Zagzag D, Miller DC, Kleinman GM, et al. Demyelinating disease versus tumor in surgical neuropathology. Clues to a correct pathological diagnosis. Am J Surg Pathol 1993;17:537–45.

73. Given CA, Stevens BS, Lee C. The MRI appearance of tumefactive demyelinating lesions. AJR Am J Roentgenol 2004;182:195–9.

74. Ernst T, Chang L, Walot I, et al. Physiologic MRI of a tumefactive multiple sclerosis lesion. Neurology 1998;51:1486–8.

75. Law M, Meltzer DE, Cha S. Spectroscopic magnetic resonance imaging of a tumefactive demyelinating lesion. Neuroradiology 2002;44:986–9.

76. Saindane AM, Cha S, Law M, et al. Proton MR spectroscopy of tumefactive demyelinating lesions. AJNR Am J Neuroradiol 2002;23:1378–86.

77. Pandya HG, Wilkinson ID, Agarwal SK, et al. The nonspecific nature of proton spectroscopy in brain masses in children: a series of demyelinating lesions. Neuroradiology 2005;47:955–9.

78. Blasel S, Pfeilschifter W, Jansen V, et al. Metabolism and regional cerebral blood volume in autoimmune inflammatory demyelinating lesions mimicking malignant gliomas. J Neurol 2011;258: 113–22.

79. Tan HM, Chan LL, Chuah KL, et al. Monophasic, solitary tumefactive demyelinating lesion: neuroimaging features and neuropathological diagnosis. Br J Radiol 2004;77:153–6.

80. Cianfoni A, Niku S, Imbesi SG. Metabolite findings in tumefactive demyelinating lesions utilizing short echo time proton magnetic resonance spectroscopy. AJNR Am J Neuroradiol 2007;28:272–7.

81. Malhotra HS, Jain KK, Agarwal A, et al. Characterization of tumefactive demyelinating lesions using MR imaging and in-vivo proton MR spectroscopy. Mult Scler 2009;15:193–203.

82. Saini J, Chatterjee S, Thomas B, et al. Conventional and advanced magnetic resonance imaging in tumefactive demyelination. Acta Radiol 2011;52: 1159–68.

83. De Stefano N, Caramanos Z, Preul MC, et al. In vivo differentiation of astrocytic brain tumors and isolated demyelinating lesions of the type seen in multiple sclerosis using 1H magnetic resonance spectroscopic imaging. Ann Neurol 1998;44:273–8.

84. Hourani R, Brant LJ, Rizk T, et al. Can proton MR spectroscopic and perfusion imaging differentiate between neoplastic and nonneoplastic brain lesions in adults? AJNR Am J Neuroradiol 2008;29: 366–72.

85. Majós C, Aguilera C, Alonso J, et al. Proton MR spectroscopy improves discrimination between tumor and pseudotumoral lesion in solid brain masses. AJNR Am J Neuroradiol 2009;30:544–51.

86. Cucurella MG, Rovira A, Grivé E, et al. Serial proton spectroscopy, magnetization transfer ratio and T 2 relaxation in pseudotumoral demyelinating lesions. NMR Biomed 2002;15:284–92.

87. Henning A, Schär M, Kollias SS, et al. Quantitative magnetic resonance spectroscopy in the entire human cervical spinal cord and beyond at 3T. Magn Reson Med 2008;59:1250–8.

88. Marliani AF, Clementi V, Albini Riccioli L, et al. Quantitative cervical spinal cord 3T proton MR spectroscopy in multiple sclerosis. AJNR Am J Neuroradiol 2010;31:180–4.

89. Ciccarelli O, Wheeler-Kingshott CA, McLean MA, et al. Spinal cord spectroscopy and diffusion-based tractography to assess acute disability in multiple sclerosis. Brain 2007;130:2220–31.

90. Kendi AT, Tan FU, Kendi M, et al. MR spectroscopy of cervical spinal cord in patients with multiple sclerosis. Neuroradiology 2004;46:764–9.

91. Blamire AM, Cader S, Lee M, et al. Axonal damage in the spinal cord of multiple sclerosis patients detected by magnetic resonance spectroscopy. Magn Reson Med 2007;58:880–5.

92. Fu L, Wolfson C, Worsley KJ, et al. Statistics for investigation of multimodal MR imaging data and an application to multiple sclerosis patients. NMR Biomed 1996;9:339–46.

93. De Stefano N, Matthews PM, Narayanan S, et al. Axonal dysfunction and disability in a relapse of multiple sclerosis: longitudinal study of a patient. Neurology 1997;49:1138–41.

94. Davie CA, Barker GJ, Thompson AJ, et al. 1H magnetic resonance spectroscopy of chronic cerebral white matter lesions and normal appearing white matter in multiple sclerosis. J Neurol Neurosurg Psychiatry 1997;63:736–42.

95. Casanova B, Martínez-Bisbal MC, Valero C, et al. Evidence of Wallerian degeneration in normal appearing white matter in the early stages of relapsing-remitting multiple sclerosis: a HMRS study. J Neurol 2003;250:22–8.

96. De Stefano N, Narayanan S, Francis GS, et al. Evidence of axonal damage in the early stages of multiple sclerosis and its relevance to disability. Arch Neurol 2001;58:65–70.

97. De Stefano N, Matthews PM, Fu L, et al. Axonal damage correlates with disability in patients with relapsing-remitting multiple sclerosis. Results of a longitudinal magnetic resonance spectroscopy study. Brain 1998;121:1469–77.

98. Kapeller P, Brex PA, Chard D, et al. Quantitative 1H MRS imaging 14 years after presenting with a clinically isolated syndrome suggestive of multiple sclerosis. Mult Scler 2002;8:207–10.

99. Vrenken H, Barkhof F, Uitdehaag BM, et al. MR spectroscopic evidence for glial increase but not for neuro-axonal damage in MS normal-appearing white matter. Magn Reson Med 2005;53:256–66.

100. Kirov II, Patil V, Babb JS, et al. MR spectroscopy indicates diffuse multiple sclerosis activity during remission. J Neurol Neurosurg Psychiatry 2009;80:1330–6.

101. Zeller D, Kampe K, Biller A, et al. Rapid-onset central motor plasticity in multiple sclerosis. Neurology 2010;74:728–35.

102. Gonen O, Moriarty DM, Li BS, et al. Relapsing-remitting multiple sclerosis and whole-brain N-acetylaspartate measurement: evidence for different clinical cohorts initial observations. Radiology 2002;225:261–8.

103. Rigotti DJ, Gonen O, Grossman RI, et al. Global N-acetylaspartate declines even in benign multiple sclerosis. AJNR Am J Neuroradiol 2011;32:204–9.

104. Téllez N, Alonso J, Río J, et al. The basal ganglia: a substrate for fatigue in multiple sclerosis. Neuroradiology 2008;50:17–23.

105. Gadea M, Martínez-Bisbal MC, Marti-Bonmatí L, et al. Spectroscopic axonal damage of the right locus coeruleus relates to selective attention impairment in early stage relapsing-remitting multiple sclerosis. Brain 2004;127:89–98.

106. Pfueller CF, Brandt AU, Schubert F, et al. Metabolic changes in the visual cortex are linked to retinal nerve fiber layer thinning in multiple sclerosis. PLoS One 2011;6:e18019.

107. Parry A, Corkill R, Blamire AM, et al. Beta-interferon treatment does not always slow the progression of axonal injury in multiple sclerosis. J Neurol 2003;250:171–8.

108. Narayanan S, De Stefano N, Francis GS, et al. Axonal metabolic recovery in multiple sclerosis patients treated with interferon beta-1b. J Neurol 2001;248:979–86.

109. Sarchielli P, Presciutti O, Tarducci R, et al. 1H-MRS in patients with multiple sclerosis undergoing treatment with interferon beta-1a: results of a preliminary study. J Neurol Neurosurg Psychiatry 1998; 64:204–12.

110. Schubert F, Seifert F, Elster C, et al. Serial 1H-MRS in relapsing-remitting multiple sclerosis: effects of interferon-beta therapy on absolute metabolite concentrations. MAGMA 2002;14:213–22.

111. Khan O, Shen Y, Bao F, et al. Long-term study of brain 1H-MRS study in multiple sclerosis: effect of glatiramer acetate therapy on axonal metabolic function and feasibility of long-Term H-MRS monitoring in multiple sclerosis. J Neuroimaging 2008; 18:314–9.

112. Wolinsky JS, Narayana PA, O'Connor P, et al. Glatiramer acetate in primary progressive multiple sclerosis: results of a multinational, multicenter, double-blind, placebo-controlled trial. Ann Neurol 2007;61:14–24.

113. Sajja BR, Narayana PA, Wolinsky JS, et al. Longitudinal magnetic resonance spectroscopic imaging of primary progressive multiple sclerosis patients treated with glatiramer acetate: multicenter study. Mult Scler 2008;14:73–80.

114. De Stefano N, Filippi M, Miller D, et al. Guidelines for using proton MR spectroscopy in multicenter clinical MS studies. Neurology 2007;69:1942–52.

115. Menge T, Hemmer B, Nessler S, et al. Acute disseminated encephalomyelitis: an update. Arch Neurol 2005;62:1673–80.

116. Tenembaum S, Chitnis T, Ness J, et al. Acute disseminated encephalomyelitis. Neurology 2007; 68:S23–36.

117. Bizzi A, Uluğ AM, Crawford TO, et al. Quantitative proton MR spectroscopic imaging in acute disseminated encephalomyelitis. AJNR Am J Neuroradiol 2001;22:1125–30.

118. Gabis LV, Panasci DJ, Andriola MR, et al. Acute disseminated encephalomyelitis: an MRI/MRS longitudinal study. Pediatr Neurol 2004;30:324–9.

119. Küker W, Ruff J, Gaertner S, et al. Modern MRI tools for the characterization of acute demyelinating lesions: value of chemical shift and diffusion-weighted imaging. Neuroradiology 2004; 46:421–6.

120. Mader I, Wolff M, Nägele T, et al. MRI and proton MR spectroscopy in acute disseminated encephalomyelitis. Childs Nerv Syst 2005;21:566–72.

121. Ben Sira L, Miller E, Artzi M, et al. 1H-MRS for the diagnosis of acute disseminated encephalomyelitis: insight into the acute-disease stage. Pediatr Radiol 2010;40:106–13.

122. Harada M, Hisaoka S, Mori K, et al. Differences in water diffusion and lactate production in two different types of postinfectious encephalopathy. J Magn Reson Imaging 2000;11:559–63.

123. Balasubramanya KS, Kovoor JM, Jayakumar PN, et al. Diffusion-weighted imaging and proton MR spectroscopy in the characterization of acute disseminated encephalomyelitis. Neuroradiology 2007;49:177–83.

124. Pittock SJ, Weinshenker BG, Lucchinetti CF, et al. Neuromyelitis optica brain lesions localized at sites of high aquaporine 4 expression. Arch Neurol 2006;63:964–8.

125. Matsushita T, Isobe N, Matsuoka T, et al. Extensive vasogenic edema of anti-aquaporin-4 antibody-related brain lesions. Mult Scler 2009;15:1113–7.

126. Bichuetti DB, Rivero RL, de Oliveira EM, et al. White matter spectroscopy in neuromyelitis optica: a case control study. J Neurol 2008;255:1895–9.

127. Aboul-Enein F, Krssák M, Höftberger R, et al. Diffuse white matter damage is absent in neuromyelitis optica. AJNR Am J Neuroradiol 2010;31: 76–9.

128. de Seze J, Blanc F, Kremer S, et al. Magnetic resonance spectroscopy evaluation in patients with neuromyelitis optica. J Neurol Neurosurg Psychiatry 2010;81:409–11.

MR Spectroscopy in Brain Infections

Rakesh K. Gupta, MD*, Kamlesh J. Jobanputra, MD,
Abhishek Yadav, PhD

KEYWORDS

• Brain • MR spectroscopy • Infections • MR imaging • Neuro-infections

KEY POINTS

- Magnetic resonance spectroscopy forms a part of diagnostic sequences used for imaging brain infections. A quality spectrum can usually be obtained with point resolved spectroscopy using an echo time of 135 ms, which is usually sufficient for diagnostic purposes.
- The metabolites important in central nervous system infections are amino acids (valine, leucine, and isoleucine, 0.9 ppm), alanine (1.48 ppm), acetate (1.92 ppm), succinate (2.4 ppm), glycine (3.56 ppm), and trehalose (3.6-3.8 ppm).
- The presence of amino acids at 0.9 ppm usually differentiates abscesses from tumors. The ratio of acetete/succinate differentiates parasitic from pyogenic infections. Trehalose, if seen, is specific for fungal infections.
- Magnetic resonance spectroscopy is diagnostic in pyogenic abscesses and parasitic cysts. It may be helpful as a support to imaging in diagnosis and prognosis in other infections.

INTRODUCTION

Magnetic resonance spectroscopy (MRS) provides information about the metabolite profile of the tissue under investigation and has long been under the domain of biochemists and researchers. The technique has evolved into a clinical tool and with its use it is possible to obtain information on a routine clinical scanner in a reasonably short time. This development has resulted in its routine use in clinical practice. After the initial euphoria of MRS entering into the domain of clinical radiology and purported by few enthusiasts to be able to diagnose everything to the cynical observations of many radiologists that it "does not help at all when it is required and provides quality data when not required," it has come a long way. Although it has established itself as a strong adjunct, most of the diagnostic difficulties arise not because of the inherent limitations of the technique but because of the suboptimal acquisition, limited knowledge, and inadequate interpretation of the acquired data.

In this discourse, when sufficient although confusing data about role of spectroscopy in clinical imaging have accumulated, every attempt has been made to analyze and classify the role of MRS in central nervous system (CNS) infections.

BASIC REQUIREMENTS FOR ACQUISITION AND INTERPRETATION OF MRS DATA

Although the technical details have been described in the first and second articles in this issue, it should be re-emphasized that MRS is a part of the diagnostic MR imaging workup of the brain infection and is not a stand-alone investigation. The decision of performing MRS in a case of known or suspected infection depends on the results of the conventional MR imaging.

MR Section, Department of Radiodiagnosis, Sanjay Gandhi Postgraduate Institute of Medical Sciences, Raebareli Road, Lucknow, Uttar Pradesh 226014, India
* Corresponding author.
E-mail addresses: rgupta@sgpgi.ac.in; rakeshree1@gmail.com

Neuroimag Clin N Am 23 (2013) 475–498
http://dx.doi.org/10.1016/j.nic.2013.03.004
1052-5149/13/$ – see front matter © 2013 Elsevier Inc. All rights reserved.

As these patients are usually sick and cannot stand for long periods of time to image, single-voxel methods like Point RESolved Spectroscopy (PRESS) at intermediate echo time (TE) with a volume of 1 to 2 mL from the region of interest usually provides diagnostic quality data in a very short time. Besides the usual brain metabolites observed on MRS, metabolites of interest in CNS infections are summarized in **Table 1**.

Specific metabolites should be searched for from a good quality spectrum to make a clinical conclusion for the diagnosis of brain infections. Poor quality data should be disregarded and no attempt should be made to interpret it. The voxel should be placed within the center of the lesion to ensure uncontaminated spectrum that may confound the interpretation.

MRS IN BACTERIAL INFECTIONS
Pyogenic Abscess

Brain abscesses are characteristically defined as a focal suppurative process within the brain parenchyma. The abscesses result from cerebritis (1–9 days) to well-developed abscess (days 14 onwards).[1] The causative organisms are quite variable and may consist of aerobes, anaerobes, facultative anaerobes, and a mixture of facultative anaerobes and true anaerobes. Pus culture is usually considered the reference standard for identification of its causative agents.

The fully developed mature abscess with central liquefactive necrosis appears as hypointense on T-weighted and hyperintense on T2-weighted images. The abscess rim appears isointense or slightly hyperintense on T1-weighted and hypointense on T2-weighted images and shows rim enhancement on postcontrast T1-weighted images.[2] It is not always possible to differentiate pyogenic abscesses from other cystic intracranial mass lesions solely from conventional MR imaging features.[3,4]

In vivo MRS may help in suggesting the definitive diagnosis of pyogenic abscess among the various lesions with comparable imaging features.[5] The spectral pattern permits the differentiation of pyogenic abscess from tumors by demonstrating the presence of amino acid peak (0.9 ppm) consisting of cytosolic amino acids, namely, valine, leucine, and isoleucine, in the former.[3] The amino acids persist in varied concentrations even when the patient is on medical therapy and/or when pus is sterile on culture. The presence of cytosolic amino acids on MRS has been explained by the fact that pyogenic abscesses contain large amounts of neutrophils and proteins. The cytolysis of neutrophils results in the release of proteolytic enzymes that hydrolyze proteins into amino acids and thus contribute to MR spectrum.[6] Treatment-naive abscesses present a variety of spectral patterns depending on the type of causative bacteria responsible for the pathologic abnormality.[7] The abscess with true aerobes (*Nocardia asteroides* and *Pseudomonas aeruginosa*) shows peaks of cytosolic amino acids, lactate, alanine, and glycine (3.56 ppm), along with mobile lipid peaks at various chemical shifts (0.9, 1.3 ppm) (**Fig. 1**). The in vivo spectrum of abscess containing only anaerobic bacteria (*Bacteroides fragilis* group and *Peptostreptococcus sp*) is comparatively metabolically richer. In addition to the above-mentioned metabolites, the spectrum shows acetate (1.92 ppm) with or without succinate (2.4 ppm) (**Fig. 2**). When both peaks are present, acetate seems to be present in a higher concentration than succinate. The spectrum taken from the abscess containing facultative anaerobes (such as *Staphylococcus aureus*, *Escherichia coli*, *Streptococcus mirabilis*, *Klebsiella pneumoniae*, *Enterococcus fecalis*, *Streptococcus intermedius*) may show metabolite patterns similar

Table 1
Showing the summary of metabolites to be looked for in case of CNS infections

Metabolites	Resonance Peaks at (ppm)	Features
Amino acids (valine leucine and isoleucine)	0.9	Phase reversal at intermediate TE, seen in abscesses not in tumors
Lipid/lactate (Lip/lac)	0.9 to 1.4, 1.33	Lactate doublet shows phase reversal at intermediate TE, seen in anaerobic metabolism, abscesses as well as tumors.
Alanine	1.46	Phase reversal at intermediate TE.
Acetate	1.92	A/S ratio to differentiate parasitic from pyogenic abscess
Succinate	2.4	A/S: >1 in pyogenic and <1 in parasitic
Glycine	3.56	Seen in pyogenic abscesses
Trehalose	3.6 to 3.8	Disaccharide specific for fungal infections

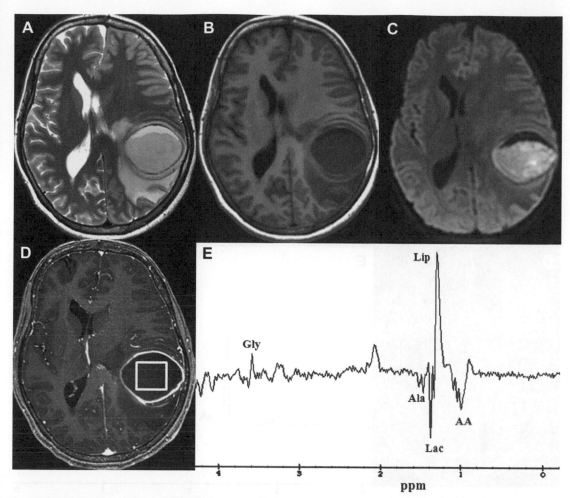

Fig. 1. Nocardia brain abscess in the left parieto-occipital region of a 26-year-old woman. Axial T2-weighted image (*A*) shows hyperintense lesion with peripheral hypointense rim and surrounding perifocal edema. Corresponding T1-weighted image (*B*) shows central hypointensity with isointense rim and hypointense edema. On DWI (*C*), the lesion shows central restricted diffusion consistent with an abscess cavity. Postcontrast T1-weighted image shows ring enhancement (*D*). In vivo ^{1}H MRS by using spin echo (SE) sequence (TR/TE/NEX 3000 ms/144 ms/128) from the center of the lesion shows peaks of AAs, 0.9 ppm; Ala, 1.46 ppm; Gly, 3.56 ppm; Lip/lac, 1.3 ppm; with contamination from the edematous brain parenchyma (*E*). Pus culture showed *Nocardia asteroides*.

to those of aerobic as well as anaerobic abscess. Facultative anaerobes when mixed with aerobes in abscess give a spectral pattern typical of aerobic bacteria growth. However, these bacteria in combination with anaerobes give the metabolite pattern of anaerobic abscess. The metabolism of facultative anaerobes is by definition flexible (ie, these are not restricted to their mode of metabolism). In the presence of oxygen, they follow the aerobic pathways for energy similar to aerobic bacteria; however, in oxygen-deficient conditions, they pursue anaerobic pathways.

In aerobic metabolism, the 2 molecules of pyruvate formed during glycolysis enter the tricarboxylic acid cycle and ultimately form carbon dioxide, water, and stored energy in the form of

adenosine triphosphate. Although succinate is an intermediate of the tricarboxylic acid cycle, its steady-state concentration is negligible and it is not seen in aerobic abscess. In contrast, in anaerobic abscess, the pyruvate undergoes anaerobic fermentation and is carboxylated to oxaloacetate and eventually transforms to malate. The malate is metabolized in mitochondria to form acetate and succinate.[3]

MRS helps to distinguish infective from noninfective lesions and may give information on the type of infective agent, which may guide the clinician to initiate appropriate antibiotic therapy, while the pus culture results are awaited.

A combination of in vivo MRS and diffusion-weighted imaging (DWI)/diffusion tensor imaging

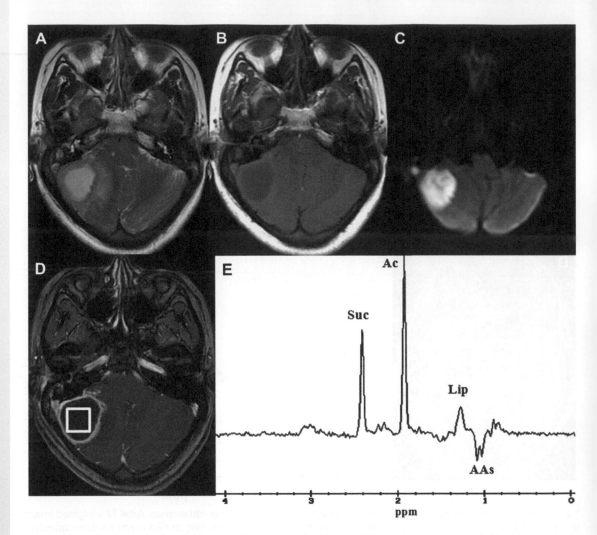

Fig. 2. Pyogenic abscess in the right cerebellar region of a 26-year-old woman. Axial T2-weighted image shows a well-defined hyperintense lesion with a hypointense wall and perifocal edema (*A*). The lesion appears hypointense on the axial T1-weighted image with isointense wall (*B*). On DWI (*C*), the lesion shows restricted diffusion with low ADC value on ADC map (not shown). Postcontrast T1-weighted image shows ring enhancement (*D*). In vivo ¹H MRS using SE sequence (TR/TE/NEX 3000 ms/144 ms/128) from the center of the lesion shows resonances of AAs, 0.9 ppm; Lip, 1.3 ppm; Ac, 1.9 ppm; and Suc, 2.4 ppm (*E*). Culture from pus grew *B fragilis*.

(DTI) has been used in the differential diagnosis of abscess from other intracranial cystic mass lesions.[8–11] It has been reported that demonstration of restricted diffusion on DWI with reduced apparent diffusion coefficient (ADC) is highly suggestive of brain abscesses; however, in the absence of restriction, in vivo MRS may help to distinguish brain abscess from other nonabscess lesions.[8] The viable inflammatory cells and bacteria have been thought to be responsible for restricted diffusion in brain abscess.[12] It may not always be possible to demonstrate amino acids, a hallmark of brain abscess, in all the cases. Typically staphylococcus abscess may not form amino acids

(Fig. 3), and in those cases, combining DWI and DTI may help in its definitive diagnosis.

Pyogenic Meningitis

Pyogenic meningitis has been defined as an inflammatory response to bacterial infection of the pia-arachnoid matter and the cerebrospinal fluid (CSF) of the subarachnoid space. The diagnosis of meningitis is usually made by CSF analysis using cytology, biochemistry, and culture.

MR is generally superior to computed tomography (CT) in demonstrating the distension of the subarachnoid space, which is reported to be an

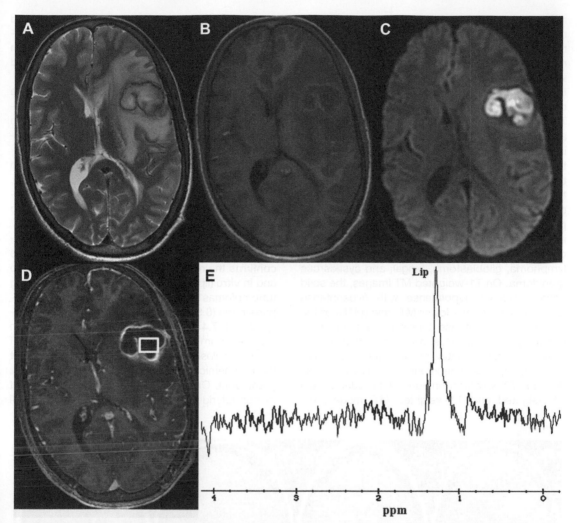

Fig. 3. Pyogenic abscess in the left fronto-parietal region of a 29-year-old man. Axial T2-weighted image shows a well-defined hyperintense lesion with a hypointense wall and perifocal edema (*A*). The lesion appears hypointense on the T1-weighted image with isointense wall (*B*). On DWI, lesion shows restriction in diffusion (*C*). Post-contrast T1-weighted image shows ring enhancement (*D*). In vivo ¹H MR spectroscopy using SE sequence (TR/TE/NEX 3000 ms/144 ms/128) from the center of the lesion shows only lipid (Lip) at 1.3 ppm (*E*). Culture from pus grew *S aureus*.

early finding in severe meningitis.[13] MRS has not yet been shown to be of much diagnostic value in patients with meningitis. In vivo proton MRS (¹H-MRS) in meningitis has reported normal levels of brain *N*-acetyl aspartate (NAA), creatine (Cr), choline (Cho), and inositol with mild elevation of Lactate (Lac).[14] Ex vivo MRS of CSF performed in proven cases of pyogenic meningitis has reported the peaks of cytosolic amino acids (0.9 ppm), Lac (1.33 ppm), alanine (1.47 ppm), acetate (1.92 ppm), and acetoacetate (2.24 ppm) along with reduced levels of glucose.[2] Anaerobic bacterial metabolism is likely to explain increased glucose consumption and consequently lactic acidosis in the CSF.

MRS IN TUBERCULAR INFECTIONS

Tuberculosis (TB) of the CNS is always secondary to TB elsewhere in the body and is caused by *Mycobacterium tuberculosis*.[15] The incidence of CNS TB has increased following the emergence of acquired immunodeficiency syndrome (AIDS).[16] TB causes a granulomatous inflammatory reaction, which may involve the meninges, causing TB meningitis, and/or brain parenchyma, causing tuberculoma or tuberculous abscess.

Tuberculoma

Tuberculoma is a space-occupying mass of granulomatous tissue.[15] The definitive diagnosis is necessary, as most tuberculomas respond to medical management. On MR imaging, tuberculoma's appearance varies depending on its stage of maturation (ie, whether noncaseating, caseating with solid or liquid center).[17] The noncaseating tuberculoma usually appears as hyperintense on T2-weighted and slightly hypointense on T1-weighted images. Metastases, lymphoma, and other infective granulomas also have similar imaging features.[18] On T1-weighted magnetization transfer (MT) imaging, the cellular component of the lesion appears brighter and is considered relatively specific for the disease (**Fig. 4**). The solid caseating tuberculoma appears isointense to hypointense on both T1-weighted and T2-weighted images. This T2 hypointense-appearing solid caseation often overlaps with imaging features of lymphoma, glioblastoma, fungal, and cysticercus granuloma. On T1-weighted MT images, the solid center appears hypointense with hyperintense rim. The significantly lower MT ratio (MTR) of the rim of T2 hypointense tuberculoma than cysticercus granuloma helps in its differentiation.[19,20] When the solid center of caseating lesion liquefies, it appears hyperintense with a hypointense rim on T2-weighted images with edema. On T1-weighted and T1-weighted MT images, the

peripheral hyperintense rim may be visualized beyond the T2 hypointensity and shows enhancement on postcontrast study. The lower MTR in different stages of tuberculoma is due to high lipid content present in the granuloma.

In vivo MRS may help in the differentiation of the tuberculoma with solid caseation from other nontuberculous lesions. In vivo, ex vivo, and in vitro MRS have been performed to fingerprint the metabolites of M $tuberculosis$ in tuberculomas.[21] In vivo MRS with stimulated echo acquisition mode sequence shows only lipid peaks at 0.9, 1.3, 2.0, 2.8, and 3.7 ppm, corresponding to terminal methyl group $[-(CH_3)]$, methylene group $-(CH_2)_n$, of CH_2CH fatty acyl chain, "CH-CH$_2$CH" of fatty acyl chain, and phosphoserine, respectively. Ex vivo MRS of the excised tuberculomas confirms the resonances seen in vivo. On ex vivo and in vitro (lipid extract) spectroscopy, caseating tuberculomas show peaks attributed to cyclopropane rings (0.5 and 0.1 ppm) and phenolic glycolipids (7.1–7.4 ppm). These peaks have also been reported from the lipid extracts of pure strain of M $tuberculosis$. Phenolic glycolipids represent the biochemical fingerprint of M $tuberculosis$ in a granuloma. One of the characteristic features of mycobacterium is the presence of a lipid-rich cell

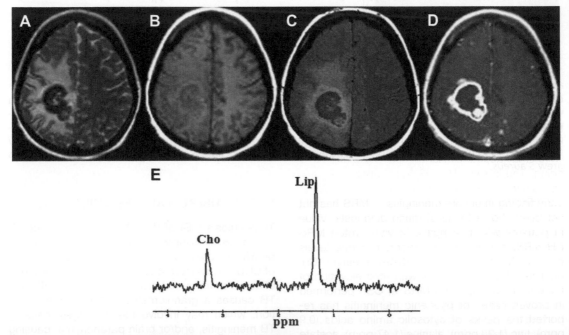

Fig. 4. Brain tuberculoma in the right parasagittal region of a 25-year-old man. Axial T2-weighted image shows predominantly hypointense lesion with surrounding edema (*A*). It appears isointense to hypointense on T1-weighted image (*B*). On magnetization transfer T1-weighted image it appears hypointense with peripherally hyperintense rim (*C*) that shows rim enhancement on postcontrast magnetization transfer of T1-weighted image (*D*). In vivo ^{1}H MRS using SE sequence (TR/TE/NEX 3000 ms/144 ms/128) from the center of the lesion shows resonances of Lip, 1.3 ppm, and Cho, 3.2 ppm (*E*). Histology confirmed it as tuberculous granuloma.

wall that contributes to the lipid peaks in tuberculomas. On perchloric acid extract of tuberculoma as well as cultured *M tuberculosis*, serine could also be demonstrated.

Although in vivo spectroscopy is known to show only lipid in T2 hypointense tuberculoma, the lesion with variegated appearance shows Cho at 3.22 ppm along with lipid (see **Fig. 4**). As these lesions show a large amount of cellularity and minimal solid caseation, the cellular regions appear brighter on T1-weighted MT imaging and show Cho peak on spectroscopy along with lipid. Predominance of cellularity in such variegated tuberculoma is responsible for prominent Cho peak and may cause difficulty in its differentiation from neoplastic lesions.[22]

Tuberculous Abscess

Tuberculous brain abscesses are the result of infection of *M tuberculosis*; tuberculous brain abscesses are relatively rare and form about 4% to 7% of the total CNS TB in developing countries. These abscesses on MR imaging generally appear as nonspecific large, solitary, and frequently multiloculated ring-enhancing lesions with surrounding edema and mass effect.[23] The rim of tuberculous abscesses shows significantly lower MTR values (19.89 ± 1.55) than that of pyogenic abscesses (24.81 ± 0.03) as the latter remain rich in protein content as compared with the former, which is loaded with high-lipid containing *M tuberculosis* bacilli.[24] Restriction on DWI with low ADC values has also been observed in tubercular abscesses and is considered to be the result of the presence of intact inflammatory cells in the pus.[12,25–27]

In vivo MRS has also been used for the differentiation of tuberculous abscesses from other lesions, such as pyogenic and fungal abscesses, which may appear similar on conventional MR imaging. The in vivo ^{1}H MRS from tuberculous abscess shows only Lac and lipid peaks (at 0.9 and 1.3 ppm), without any evidence of cytosolic amino acids (**Fig. 5**). MTR and amino acid peaks may help to discriminate pyogenic from tuberculous abscess.[24,25]

Tubercular Meningitis

Tuberculous meningitis is the most frequent manifestation of TB in the CNS. The incidence of tuberculous meningitis in a given community is proportional to the prevalence of tuberculous infection in general.[15] Diagnosis depends on CSF cytology and biochemistry depends on the detection of acid-fast bacilli in smear. However, because of the relatively low sensitivity of laboratory tests,

noninvasive imaging plays an important role in its diagnosis.

The imaging features in tuberculous meningitis largely depend on the stage at which MR imaging is performed. MR imaging in tuberculous meningitis may be normal in the early stages of disease, especially on noncontrast studies. MT is superior to conventional spin echo sequences for imaging the abnormal meninges, which are seen as hyperintense on precontrast T1-weighted MT images and enhance further on postcontrast T1-weighted MT images.[20] The visibility of the inflamed meninges on precontrast T1-weighted MT images with low MTR is very specific of tuberculous meningitis and differentiates it from other nontuberculous chronic meningitis.[19,20,28] Ex vivo spectroscopy of CSF has been attempted in this context.[29] High-resolution ex vivo MRS of CSF showed the Lac, acetate, and sugars along with the peaks from cyclopropyl rings (−0.5 to +0.5 ppm) and phenolic glycolipids (7.1 and 7.4 ppm); these have not been observed with pyogenic meningitis.

MRS IN FUNGAL INFECTIONS

Fungal infections of CNS are relatively rare in immunocompetent individuals, where they tend to be caused by pathogenic species such as *Cryptococcus*. Immunocompromised patients, however, are susceptible to invasive infection with a wider range of opportunist fungal pathogens, such as *Aspergillus* and *Candida*.[30]

Fungal Abscess

Both *Aspergillus* and *Candida* species can produce cerebral abscesses. The *Aspergillus* infection has been observed in immunocompromised patients. Two general patterns of infection are seen: (1) direct extension from the paranasal sinuses, eye, or middle ear leading to abscess in frontal or temporal lobe and (2) hematogenous spread with formation of multiple small abscesses at the junction of gray and white matter (WM).[31] The CSF findings are usually nonspecific. The presence of red blood cells in the CSF of a patient with brain abscess is suggestive of possible intracranial aspergillosis.[32]

On conventional MR imaging, the fungal abscess resembles pyogenic abscesses. The abscess core appears hyperintense with hypointense rim on T2-weighted images and hypointense core with isointense to minimally hyperintense rim on T1-weighted images. Postcontrast study shows rim enhancement.[33] It has been shown that the pyogenic abscesses have smooth and lobulated walls, whereas the tubercular abscesses have

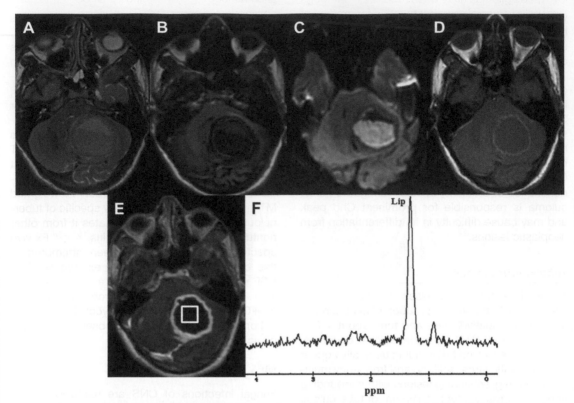

Fig. 5. Tubercular abscess in the left cerebellar hemisphere of a 45-year-old man. Axial T2-weighted image shows well-defined, round, heterogeneously hyperintense lesion with peripheral hypointense rim (A). On the T1-weighted image (B), the lesion is heterogeneously hypointense centrally with a peripheral isointense rim. DWI shows restriction in the dependent part of the cavity with low ADC (not shown), suggesting cellular debris (C). Magnetization transfer T1-weighted image shows T2 hypointense rim that appears hyperintense (D). Postcontrast T1-weighted image shows thick nodular rim enhancement (E). ^{1}H MRS from the center of the lesion shows predominant peak of lipid (Lip) at 1.3 ppm (F). Histology from the wall consistent with tubercular abscess. Pus culture was positive for M tuberculosis. (Reprinted from Gupta RK, Kumar S. Central nervous system tuberculosis. Neuroimage Clin N Am 2011;21:795–814; with permission.)

smooth, lobulated, or crenated walls with no intra-cavitary projections.[25] The fungal abscesses show intracavitary projections directed centrally from the wall without any contrast enhancement in these projections. These projections have not been shown in nonfungal abscesses and seem to be a characteristic feature of a fungal cause on conventional MR imaging. The wall and projections of the fungal abscesses show restricted diffusion on DWI with low ADC values; however, the cavity of the abscess may show high ADC values (Fig. 6).

The limited published data on in vivo ^{1}H MRS in fungal abscesses[25] showed cytosolic amino acids (valine, leucine, and isoleucine) and lactate along with multiple peaks between 3.6 and 4.0 ppm. These peaks have been assigned to trehalose sugar present in the fungal wall, confirmed with ex vivo high-resolution spectroscopy of aspirated material. Such sugar peaks have also been reported in cryptococcomas.[34,35] The presence of characteristic

sugar peaks from the fungal wall on in vivo spectrum may help in diagnosis in such cases.

Mucormycosis or phycomycosis is a fatal fungal infection of immunocompromised patients caused by the Mucor species. Predisposing factors include diabetes mellitus with ketoacidosis, naso-orbital necrotizing infection, and meningoencephalitis.[31] MR imaging shows parenchymal abnormalities in the basal ganglia, thalamus, and midbrain. The lesions appear hypointense on T1-weighted, T2-weighted, and fluid-attenuated inversion recovery (FLAIR) images with surrounding edema and enhance on postcontrast studies. In vivo MRS in mucormycosis showed lactate, alanine, acetate, succinate, and lipid peaks along with the peaks of NAA, Cr, and Cho.[36] An unassigned peak at 3.8 ppm was also present; ex vivo high-resolution studies may allow this to be characterized and provide a biochemical fingerprint for mucormycosis.

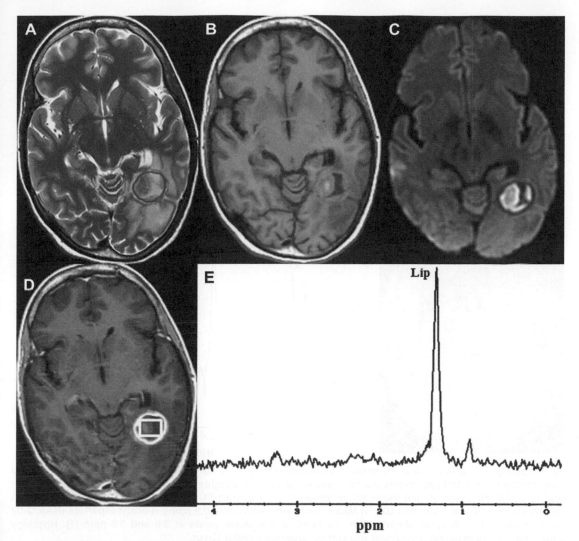

Fig. 6. Fungal abscess in left posterior temporal region of a 34-year-old woman. The lesion appears as a well-defined hyperintense mass with hypointense irregular wall and intracavitary projections on axial T2-weighted image with perilesional edema (*A*). Axial T1-weighted image shows hypointense core with isointense to hyperintense intracavitary projections (*B*). DWI shows restricted diffusion with hyperintense projections with hypointense cavity (*C*). It shows rim enhancement on postcontrast axial T1-weighted image (*D*). In vivo ¹H MRS shows lipid (Lip, 1.3 ppm) peak (*E*). Pus culture grew *Histoplasma capsulatum*.

Fungal Granuloma

Fungal granulomas are the space-occupying lesions caused by *Aspergillus* and *Cryptococcus* species and have been referred to as *Aspergillus granuloma* and *cryptoccoma*, respectively.

Aspergillus granuloma

On T2-weighted MR imaging, the *A granuloma* gives a heterogenous pattern of intensity (ie, hyperintense lesions mixed with hypointense foci). On T1-weighted images, the lesion is hypointense. On spectroscopy there is high Cho, low Cr, Lac, and low NAA (**Fig. 7**). Because the spectrum is completely nonspecific for the aspergillus granuloma, it does not help in its differentiation from other neoplastic and nonneoplastic mass lesions.[33]

Cryptococcosis

Cryptococcosis is the most common cause of CNS fungal infections in humans and is the most commonly identified fungal infection in the CNS in AIDS patients. It is a ubiquitous monomorphic fungus that primarily exists as encapsulated yeast and reproduces by budding.[33] A polysaccharide capsule surrounds the fungus. The cryptococcal

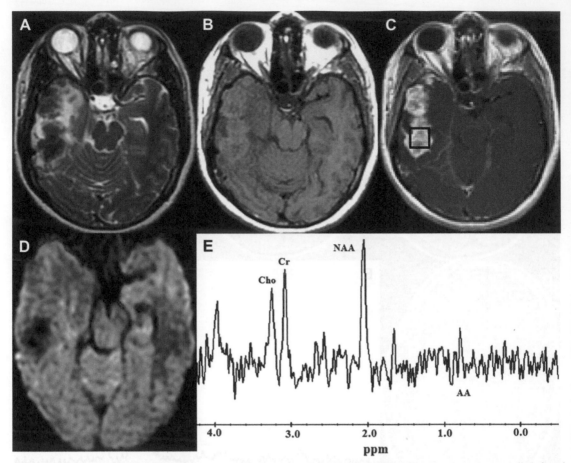

Fig. 7. Aspergillous granuloma in left temporal region of a 46-year-old man. The lesion appears as a well-defined hyperintense mass with hyperintense perifocal edema on axial T2-weighted image (*A*). It appears iso-intense on axial T1-weighted image (*B*) and shows enhancement on postcontrast T1-weighted image (*C*). DWI image does not show any diffusion restriction (*D*). ^{1}H MRS shows amino acids (AA, 0.9 ppm), N-acetyl aspartate (NAA, 2.02 ppm), creatine (Cr, 3.0 ppm), choline (Cho, 3.2 ppm), and multiple peaks at 3.6 and 3.8 ppm (*E*). Histology confirmed it as aspergillous granuloma and culture grew *Aspergillus flavus*.

infection results from inhalation or ingestion of fungus with the respiratory tract being the primary site of infection. It penetrates the meningeal vessel wall and colonizes the perivascular spaces, sheaths of fungi leading to pseudocyst formation, typically found in basal ganglia and subcortical areas. The proteolytic enzymes produced by the fungus may destroy the pial lining of the Virchow-Robin (VR) spaces so that cryptococci penetrate the parenchyma, causing meningoencephalitis. Another location is the choroid plexuses where Cryptococcus may cause the formation of voluminous masses.[37,38] Imaging findings on both CT and MR imaging are nonspecific in the case of cryptococcal meningitis. MR imaging may be negative or uncommonly show contrast enhancement. Several MR appearances have been described in CNS cryptococcosis in AIDS patients: dilated VR spaces,

cryptococcoma, and military enhancing nodules in parenchyma or leptomeningeal cisternal spaces and a mixed pattern. The dilated VR spaces filled with mucoid material, inflammatory cells, and organisms manifest on MR imaging as punctuate hyperintense round-oval lesions on T2-weighted images and hypointense on T1-weighted images and show no evidence of contrast enhancement or associated mass effect or perilesional edema. The cryptococcomas have variable appearances depending on the relative constituents of the lesions. The gelatinous pseudocysts or the nonreactive form of meningoencephaitis represent sequelae of cryptococcus colonization along the VR spaces or in the large perivascular spaces of the choroid plexus. They are usually hyperintense on T2-weighted and hypointense on T1-weighted images and may show contrast enhancement on postcontrast study. The lesions that are hyperintense on T2-weighted images and enhance after contrast administration characterize the granulomatous type of meningoencephalitis. These granulomas are preferentially located in the ependyma of choroid plexus and may cause localized ventricular dilatation.[39]

There are isolated reports of ^{1}H MRS in cases of intracerebral cryptococcal abscess and cryptococcomas. In vivo ^{1}H MRS shows variable Lac along with a decrease in NAA, Cho, and Cr.[40] Ex vivo ^{1}H MR spectroscopy has shown the presence of lipid/Lac and trehalose sugars in the regions of 3.42, 3.62, 3.83, and 5.17 ppm, which represent the polysaccharide capsule of cryptococcal yeast.[34]

Phaeohyphomycosis

Primary cerebral phaeohyphomycosis is a serious infection with poor prognosis. The infection may mimic a high-grade glial tumor on imaging. Biopsy and culture resolve the 2 entities. NAA/Cho ratio of approximately one on MRS may raise suspicion of an underlying pathologic abnormality other than glioma. Increased awareness of cerebral phaeohyphomycosis and careful analysis of MRS should encourage early biopsy and aggressive treatment to improve the outcome.[41]

MRS IN PARASITIC INFECTIONS
Neurocysticercosis

Neurocysticercosis, caused by the metacestodes of the tapeworm *Taenia solium*, is common in developing countries, and its frequency is also increasing in developed countries.[42] The natural history of neurocysticercosis and its clinical course are poorly understood. Clinical diagnosis of neurocysticercosis is most frequently based on enzyme-linked immunosorbent assay (ELISA) and enzyme-linked immunoelectrotransfer blot.[43]

Cysticercus cysts may remain viable for many years. Locations of cysts vary; they may be intracranial (parenchymal, ventricular, subarachnoid [cisternal]) or spinal. During the course of development, cysticercus cysts in the brain go through a cystic or vesicular stage, the viable stage; colloidal or granular stage, and the chronic calcified stage. MR imaging appearances vary with the different stages of degeneration of the cysts.[44] Cysts in the viable vesicular stage appear hyperintense on T2-weighted and hypointense on T1-weighted images, while the scolex is seen as an eccentrically placed nodule, hypointense on T2-weighted without perifocal edema and contrast enhancement. The colloidal stage cysts appear as hyperintense with isointense to hypointense rim on T2-weighted images, and with perifocal edema.

Often this stage undergoes rim enhancement on postcontrast study. On T1-weighted images, the cyst appears as a hypointense center with isointense periphery. In the nodular granular stage, the imaging feature simulates tuberculoma, small abscesses, and metastatic tumors and it appears isointense to the normal parenchyma on T1-weighted images and isointense to hypointense with or without surrounding edema on T2-weighted images. The lesion in the nodular calcified stage appears isointense to hypointense on T1-weighted images and hypointense on T2-weighted images. The calcification on imaging can be studied best by the use of gradient echo sequence with corrected phase imaging.[45] On phase-corrected gradient echo, the calcification appears bright.

In vivo and ex vivo MRS has been performed in a few studies of neurocysticercosis.[6,46] In vivo spectroscopy in neurocysticercosis shows peaks of cytosolic amino acids (valine, leucine, and isoleucine), Lac, alanine, succinate, NAA, Cr, and Cho (**Figs. 8** and **9**). The peaks of NAA, Cr, and Cho are assumed to be due to contamination from normal brain parenchyma within the voxel. Lac, alanine, succinate, and Cho peaks on ex vivo MRS of fluid aspirated from cerebral cysticercus cysts have been demonstrated.[47]

Ex vivo MRS of aspirated fluid also detected Cr in addition to the other metabolites. The presence of Cr in cysticercus cysts from humans and pigs helps in differentiating this from intracranial hydatid cysts.[48] It was observed that the fluid of degenerating cysticercus cysts (whether from humans or animals) is devoid of Cr, whereas the fluid from viable vesicular cysts contains Cr along with the other metabolites because of the presence of muscle fibers in the bladder wall and scolex of cysticercus cyst. In vivo spectroscopy may be of value in the large cysticercus cyst without visible scolex, where there is a large range of differential diagnosis including brain abscess and cystic metastases. In vivo MRS shows peaks of acetate, succinate, and Lac, and the presence of Cr depending on whether the lesion is in the vesicular or colloid stage.[47]

Echinococcosis (Hydatid Disease)

Echinococcosis, caused by metacestodes of the genus *Echinococcus*, is a zoonosis of worldwide distribution. The 2 common species *E granulosus* and *E multilocularis* cause cystic and alveolar echinococcosis, respectively. The endemic regions for cystic echinococcosis are the Middle East, India, South America, and Australia. The alveolar echinococcosis, although relatively rare, poses serious

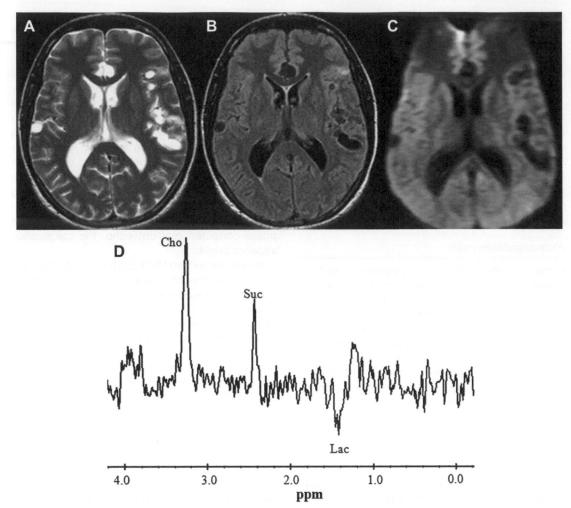

Fig. 8. Patient with multiple subarachnoid neurocysticercosis. On axial T2-weighted (*A*) and FLAIR (*B*) images, cystic lesions are seen in the left frontal and bilateral parietal lobes with hyperintensity to hypointensity. On DWI (*C*), the lesions show no restricted diffusion. ¹H MR spectrum shows peaks of choline (Cho) at 3.2 ppm, succinate (Suc) at 2.4 ppm, and lactate (Lac) at 1.3 ppm (*D*).

problems in colder areas, namely, Alaska, Central Europe, Turkey, Russia, and China. In the following section, only the cystic echinococcosis caused by *E granulosus* is discussed.

In *E granulosus*, the definitive hosts (with adult worms) are dogs, cats, and other canine species, whereas the intermediate hosts (with lesions due to larvae) are humans, sheep, camels, and other domestic animals. The cysts can be localized in any organ of the body; the commonest site is the liver. Intracranial involvement is seen in only about 2% of all the hydatid cases reported even in endemic areas.[49] Almost all the symptoms of the hydatid disease are due to the pressure effect on surrounding structures, resulting from distension, obstruction, erosion, or infection. The primary hydatid cysts, formed by the direct implantation of

larvae into neural parenchyma, are usually fertile and contain brood capsules and scolices, whereas secondary cysts, resulting from spontaneous or surgical rupture of primary cysts, are sterile and lack brood capsules.[50]

On MR imaging, it appears as a well-defined cystic mass, hypointense on T1-weighted, hyperintense on T2-weighted images with or without edema and may show rim enhancement on post-contrast studies. Where there is edema and enhancement, the hydatid cyst may resemble a pyogenic abscess.[51]

In vivo MRS from intracranial hydatid cysts shows Lac, alanine, acetate, succinate, and glycine peaks (**Fig. 10**).[6,52] Ex vivo high-resolution MRS of the aspirated fluid from the cyst confirms the in vivo assignments.

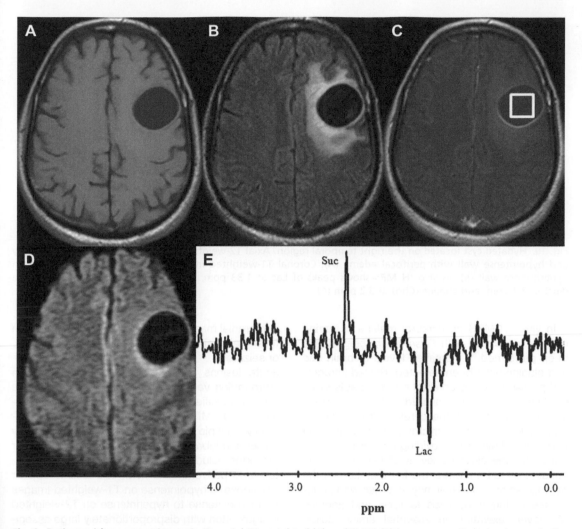

Fig. 9. Patient with neurocysticercosis. On axial T1-weighted (*A*) and FLAIR (*B*) images, a cystic lesion is seen in the left frontal lobe with thin ringlike peripheral enhancement on postcontrast T1-weighted image (*C*). On DWI (*D*), the lesion shows no restricted diffusion. ^{1}H MR spectrum obtained at TR/TE of 2000/270 shows succinate (Suc) peak assigned at 2.4 ppm, lactate (Lac) at 1.3 ppm (*E*).

On in vivo MRS, brain abscesses have prominent cytosolic amino acid peaks, and the acetate (A) to succinate (S) ratio is always more than one (A/S >1) if succinate is present. In contrast, in hydatid cysts cytosolic amino acids generally present at lower concentrations (barely detectable in vivo) and the A/S ratio is always less than one (A/S <1).[22] The same findings can be extended to other parasitic infections as well.

Furthermore, knowledge of whether a cyst is fertile is also valuable for planning surgery as the accidental rupture of fertile cysts during surgery results in disease recurrence. High-resolution MRS facilitates the differentiation of fertile and sterile hydatid cysts.[53,54] Two additional metabolites, malate (4.3 ppm) and fumarate (6.52 ppm), in the microscopically proven fertile hydatid cysts

of humans and sheep have been identified; these metabolites are not found in sterile cysts.[48] In the future, technological developments may allow these additional metabolites to be detected within vivo MRS and be of value in management.

Malaria

Cerebral malaria is a life-threatening complication in 2% of cases of *Plasmodium falciparum* infection.[55] Diffuse involvement of the brain in cerebral malaria patients leads to nonspecific neurologic presentations. The prognosis of human cerebral malaria is based on the continual lactic acidosis of brain and CSF; however, lumbar puncture may be hazardous because of cerebral swelling.

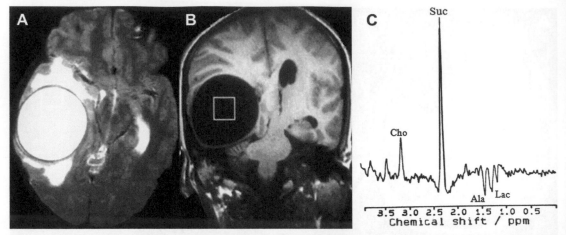

Fig. 10. Hydated cyst located on the right temporal region. Axial T2-weighted image shows hyperintense cavity and hypointense wall with perifocal edema (A). Coronal T1-weighted image shows hypointense cavity with hyperintense wall (B). In vivo ^{1}H MRS shows peaks of Lac at 1.33 ppm; alanine (ala) at 1.48 ppm, succinate (Suc) at 2.4 ppm, and choline (Cho) at 3.2 ppm (C).

In vitro ^{1}H MRS on cerebral malaria in murine models inoculated with *Plasmodium berghei* has been performed.[56] Increased levels of brain Lac and alanine have been detected. Raised intracranial pressure due to cerebral edema predisposes the tissue to ischemia, and adherence of parasitized erythrocytes to the cerebral microvascular endothelium leading to microvascular obstruction and regional hypoxia, providing a plausible explanation for the elevated levels of Lac. Alanine is considered to be a better marker than Lac for the hypoxia as the Lac level may also rise with an increase in tumor necrosis factor-α and anemia. Moreover, elevation in essential amino acids, such as valine, leucine, and isoleucine, has also been observed in experimental cerebral malaria. The concentration of usual brain metabolites NAA and Cho decreases significantly in the murine brain with cerebral malaria. The significant linear correlation between the time elapsed after infection and small progressive decrease in cell density/cell viability markers glycerophosphocholine and NAA has been reported. The metabolite information from in vivo spectroscopy is nonspecific for diagnostic purposes; however, it is possible that metabolites may provide noninvasive prognostic markers in known disease in the future.

Toxoplasmosis

Acquired cerebral toxoplasmosis is a parenchymal infection caused by *Toxoplasma gondii*, which occurs in the HIV population[57–62] and in other immunocompromised hosts.[63] In addition to being the most common opportunistic CNS infection in patients with AIDS, it is the most common cause of

intracranial mass lesions. It typically presents with fever, headache, confusion, focal neurologic signs, or seizures.[57,58] On noncontrast CT, acute or subacute lesions typically appear hypodense with surrounding vasogenic edema.[57] Chronic lesions appear calcified on CT, especially after treatment.[61] On MR imaging, lesions are most commonly multiple and affect the deep central gray nuclei and lobar gray-white junction.[48,54–59] Other locations include the posterior fossa, cerebral cortex, and periventricular WM. The lesions appear isointense to hypointense on T1-weighted images and hypointense to hyperintense on T2-weighted images often with disproportionately large associated edema. Rarely, nonedematous lesions without mass effect may be seen, especially in non-AIDS cases.[59] On T2-weighted imaging, the masses may be difficult to distinguish from the surrounding edema or a central isointense or hypointense core may be noted on T2-weighted images, giving a "target" appearance. The lesions characteristically enhance on postcontrast study.[62] Avid enhancement is the rule and ringlike or nodular enhancement patterns are most commonly noted, whereas smaller lesions may show a homogeneous pattern. However, fulminant involvement may occur despite a paucity of enhancement.[63] MR imaging plays a central role in monitoring the response to antibiotic therapy.[57–59,62] Toxoplasmosis is generally associated with an increase in Cho and decreases in NAA along with the presence of Lac/lipid peaks (Fig. 11). Toxoplasma lesions are difficult to differentiate from primary CNS lymphoma, commonly encountered in AIDS patients; however, no single method including MRS is known to resolve the diagnostic dilemma.

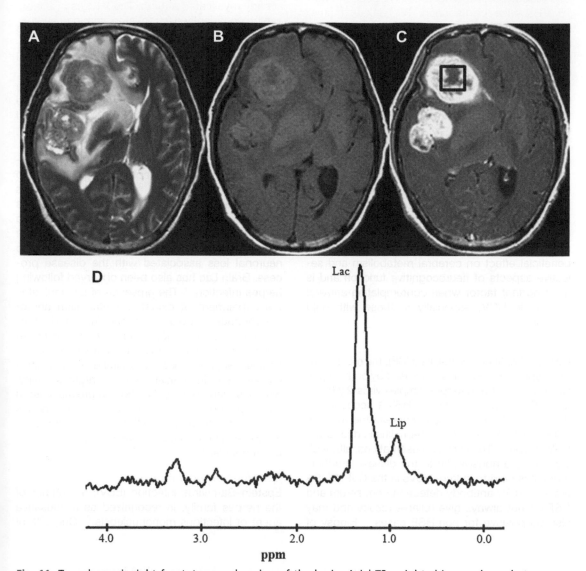

Fig. 11. Toxoplasmosis right frontotemporal region of the brain. Axial T2-weighted image shows heterogeneously hypointense lesion with surrounding edema (*A*). On T1-weighted image the lesion shows isointense to hyperintense signal intensity (*B*). Postcontrast T1-weighted image shows thick irregular ring-enhancing lesions (*C*). In vivo ^{1}H MRS at TR/TE of 2000/270 shows peaks of Lac/Lip at 1.33 ppm (*D*). Histology confirmed it as toxoplasmosis.

MRS IN VIRAL INFECTIONS, PARA-INFECTIOUS SYNDROMES

Viral infections may present as primary encephalitis because of direct viral attack on neural tissue, and para-infectious or postinfectious encephalitis because of systemic viral infection.[64] Viruses cause meningitis, encephalitis, meningoencephalitis, meningoencephalomyelitis, and myelitis.

Viral Infections

Hepatitis C virus
In recent years, many extrahepatic manifestations associated with chronic hepatitis C virus (HCV)

infection have been described in the absence of significant chronic liver disease, such as neuropsychologic symptoms and cryoglobulinemia.[65–67] The neuropsychologic findings most commonly observed include reduction in processing speed and working memory ability.[68,69] The other reported manifestations include HCV-induced vasculitis with involvement of CNS and peripheral nervous system,[70] including global encephalopathy, ischemic or hemorrhagic stroke,[71,72] and mononeuropathy multiplex.[70,73] Stroke may also occur because of HCV-related anticardiolipin antibody syndromes.[74] Neurologic complications of HCV infection other than hepatic encephalopathy are generally attributed to para-infectious phenomena. Another HCV-associated para-infectious phenomenon described is acute disseminated encephalomyelitis (ADEM). At least one case of HCV-RNA detection in vivo in human brain has been reported in the literature and there is a possibility that HCV is able to induce encephalitis caused by neurotrophism.

In vivo MRS shows an increase of Cho/Cr and myo-inositol/Cr ratios (**Fig. 12**). The levels of neurometabolite in the brain are significantly correlated with the extent of fatigue as measured by the fatigue impact scale score. The MRS findings suggest glial activation in response to the virus infection accompanied with neuroprotective mechanisms in HCV infection. Treatment has a beneficial effect on cerebral metabolism and selective aspects of neurocognitive function and is an important factor when contemplating antiviral therapy in HCV, especially in those with mild disease.

Herpes simplex encephalitis

Herpes simplex encephalitis (HSE), the most common type of encephalitis, is caused by both herpes simplex virus-1 and herpes simplex virus-2 (HSV-1 and HSV-2) types. However, HSV-1 accounts for 95% of all the HSE cases, whereas the majority (80%–90%) of neonatal encephalitis is due to the HSV-2 type.[75] The clinical presentations, although variable, are nonspecific to the disease. Furthermore, it is hard to culture HSVs in the CSF. ELISA tests used for antibody detection from serum and CSF do not always give reliable results and may also be positive for non-HSE cases.[76] Biopsy of

the brain tissue for herpes virus is 96% sensitive and 99% specific.[77] Herpes infection characteristically involves the medial temporal and frontal lobes.

MR imaging is the modality of choice for the diagnosis of HSE and is characterized as the high signal intensity in the temporal and frontal lobes on conventional T2-weighted images[78]; hemorrhagic changes may also be apparent. DWI is found to be superior to conventional imaging in patients with encephalitis with respect to delineation of the lesion.[79] There are few studies in the literature of MRS in HSE patients. Decreases in NAA peak resulting in reduction of NAA/Cr ratio have been reported (**Fig. 13**).[80,81] The depletion of NAA content in the brain has been ascribed to neuronal loss associated with the disease process. Brain Lac has also been observed following herpes infection.[78] The presence of Lac indicates the impairment of oxidative metabolism and/or macrophage activity. A longitudinal study performed in a case of HSE revealed that imaging returns to normal more rapidly than metabolites. The findings suggest that the imaging abnormalities caused by interstitial edema regress early, whereas neuronal dysfunction improves over a longer period.[82] The spectroscopic abnormalities are nonspecific and add little to the MR imaging; its role as a prognostic marker in the proven cases is not yet clear.

Epstein–Barr virus infection

Epstein–Barr virus infection (EBV), a member of the herpes family, is recognized as a causative agent of infectious mononucleosis.[75] Only 5% of

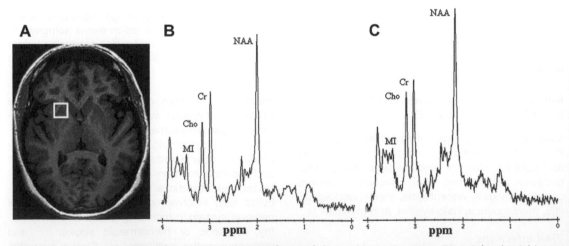

Fig. 12. A 28-year-old man with asymptomatic HCV detected during blood donation. T1-weighted axial image shows voxel location from which MRS data were obtained (*A*). In vivo ¹H MRS from the right basal ganglia with spin echo (SE) TE 35 ms shows increase in myo-inositol (mI, 3.56 ppm) (*B*) compared with age-matched control (*C*). Cho, choline; Cr, creatine; NAA, *N*-acetyl aspartate.

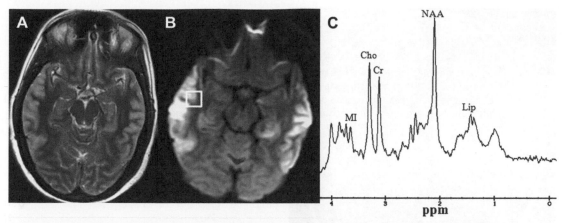

Fig. 13. Herpes simplex encephalitis. A 35-year-old woman presented with fever, loss of consciousness, and seizures for last 3 days. T2-weighted axial image shows hyperintensity involving both temporal lobes (*A*), more clearly visible on DWI (*B*). Note the asymmetrical involvement of medial temporal lobes. ^{1}H MRS (*C*) from the voxel in the right temporal lobe shows N-acetyl aspartate (NAA, 2.02 ppm), creatine (Cr, 3.0 ppm), myo-inositol (mI, 3.56 ppm) and increased choline (Cho 3.2 ppm) and free lipids (Lip).

the patients with infectious mononucleosis show CNS complications.[83] Laboratory investigation of CSF in patients with CNS complications usually shows increased lymphocytes and protein. The definite diagnosis is usually based on a four-fold rise in EBV-specific immunoglobulin M antibodies against viral capsid antigen in serum and positive polymerase chain reaction for EBV DNA in CSF.[84]

MR imaging shows symmetric low-intensity and high-intensity lesions of both basal ganglia (predominantly in the putamen) on T1-weighted and T2-weighted images, respectively, with no enhancement on postintravenous study.[78] Nonspecific clinical presentation and the variable occurrence of the lesions in different brain locations make the imaging diagnosis of EBV encephalitis difficult.[85] A recent study has reported reduced ADC in the splenium of the corpus callosum and parietal-occipital cortical areas of those normalized on 3 week follow-up.[86]

MRS findings from basal ganglia in patients with EBV have shown reduced NAA/Cr ratio with concomitant elevation in levels of excitatory amino acids, macromolecules, and myo-inositol.[85] Such nonspecific spectroscopic findings have also been observed in other viral encephalitis.

Subacute sclerosing panencephalitis

Subacute sclerosing panencephalitis (SSPE) is a slowly progressive, fatal, inflammatory disease of the CNS resultant from infection of the measles virus of the genus *Morbillivirus*, a subgroup of paramyxoviruses.[87] SSPE is one of the various manifestations produced by the measles viruses because of direct attack of the virus in the setup

of an altered immune status. Of the total patients having SSPE, 65% to 70% of the patients had a history of previous measles infection.

The diagnosis for SSPE is generally made by high antibody titer against measles virus along with mildly raised protein concentration and markedly high levels of gamma-globulin in CSF and blood. CT and MR imaging findings in SSPE are usually nonspecific. The lesions on conventional MR imaging appear hyperintense on T2-weighted images and hypointense on T1-weighted images.[78] The lesions are usually located in the posterior parietal, temporal, and occipital regions, corona radiata, and subcortical and deep WM. MR imaging sometimes remains inconclusive and shows a normal imaging pattern even when the disease is at an advanced stage on clinical examination. Elevated mean diffusivity and low fractional anisotropy values have been reported even in normal conventional MR imaging in patients with SSPE using diffusion and DTI.[88]

Spectroscopy data obtained from imaging abnormal-appearing and normal-appearing brain regions have shown markedly decreased to normal NAA, with slight increases in myo-inositol, Cho, and Lac, and normal Cr.[89] Depletion of NAA suggests neuronal dysfunction in SSPE. The increased Cho is probably caused by inflammation, and increased myo-inositol probably represents active gliosis (**Fig. 14**). Although the spectroscopic findings are nonspecific, it gives additional information regarding the extent of the disease in regions that appear normal on standard imaging sequences. Reductions in NAA and increase in myo-inositol are known to correlate with clinical severity.[90] ^{1}H MRS may be a useful

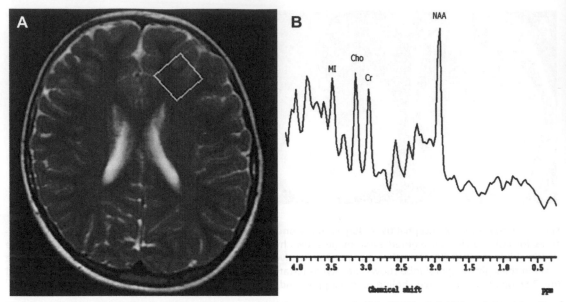

Fig. 14. A 6-year-old girl with stage II subacute sclerosing panencephalitis (SSPE). Axial T2-weighted localizer image (2875/120) shows a 2 × 2 × 2-cm voxel placed in the left FSWM (A). ¹H MR spectrum (single voxel, PRESS; 2000/31/256) shows a normal NAA/Cr ratio and increased Cho/Cr and MI/Cr ratios (B). (*From* Alkan A, Sarac K, Kutlu R, et al. Early- and late-state subacute sclerosing panencephalitis: chemical shift imaging and single-voxel MR spectroscopy. AJNR Am J Neuroradiol 2003;24:501–6; with permission. Copyright © 2003, American Society of Radiology.)

measure of disease severity and progression in SSPE.

Human immunodeficiency virus encephalopathy

Direct effects of human immunodeficiency virus (HIV) infection of the brain are referred to as HIV encephalopathy. Such HIV-related brain disease is thought to occur in 2 stages. The first stage occurs subclinically at the time of initial HIV infection,[91] characterized by small (<1 cm) multifocal WM lesions. These multifocal WM lesions are localized areas of hyperintensity on T2-weighted images throughout the cerebral WM, seen in one-third of seropositive asymptomatic patients, which remain unchanged over time and are thought to represent gliosis caused by primary HIV infection.[92] The next stage of HIV infection in the brain is characterized by progressive subacute encephalitis and brain atrophy, also known as the AIDS dementia complex. Both MR imaging and CT can effectively screen for cerebral atrophy, present in virtually all patients with clinically significant HIV encephalopathy.[93–95] Central atrophy (ventricular enlargement) predominates over cortical atrophy (sulcal prominence).[96] Neuroimaging pathologic correlation has shown that the lesions are isointense to mildly hypointense on T1-weighted images, and markedly hyperintense on T2-weighted images. The lack of significant hypointensity on T1-weighted images

is helpful in differentiating HIV encephalopathy from progressive multifocal leukoencephalopathy. Lesions typically begin in the periventricular WM and centrum semiovale with sparing of the subcortical U-fibers. The lesions are most commonly symmetric, "fluffy," or "cotton-like" and are poorly circumscribed, typically becoming confluent and diffuse. Mass effect or enhancement is typically absent. MRS may show a decreased NAA/Cr ratio in the frontal gray matter of patients with early-stage symptomatic HIV encephalopathy.[97] WM lesions of HIV encephalopathy are characterized by increased myo-inositol, increased Cho (**Fig. 15**), and decreased NAA.[98] These neurochemical changes offer the ability to monitor noninvasively therapeutic effects of antiviral therapy.[98,99]

The NAA/Cr ratio is significantly lower in progressive multifocal leukoencephalopathy and lymphoma than in HIV encephalopathy and toxoplasmosis. All patients show a significant increase in the Cho/Cr ratio regardless of lesion subtype. The presence of a lipid peak is more common in lymphomas (71%) than in other HIV subgroups. A Lac peak is common in progressive multifocal leukoencephalopathy, but uncommon in other HIV subgroups. Thus, MRS of the WM shows a high sensitivity in detecting brain involvement in HIV-related diseases including HIV encephalopathy. The pattern may have partial specificity for lesion subtype, especially in the presence of

Seronegative Control (46-year-old male)   HIV+ Normal Cognition (49-year-old male)   HAND (48-year-old male)

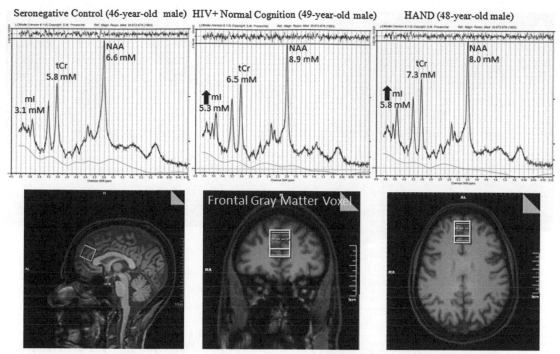

Fig. 15. ¹H MR spectrum obtained from a 3 T MR scanner (TR/TE = 3000/30 ms). In the medial frontal gray matter (anterior cingulate) region, both HIV subjects with normal cognition or with HIV-associated neurologic disorder (HAND) show elevated (*arrow*) myo-inositol (mI) compared with the seronegative control subject. (*Courtesy of* Dr Linda Chang, MD, Professor, Department of Medicine, John A. Burns School of Medicine, University of Hawaii, Honolulu, Hawaii.)

marked decreased NAA or increased Lac or lipid peaks. MRS is more sensitive than conventional MR imaging in detecting HIV-related brain injury in asymptomatic individuals.

Para-infectious Encephalopathy

The 2 main forms of para-infectious encephalopathies are ADEM and acute necrotizing encephalopathy (ANE).[100]

The most common virus associated with ADEM is measles, followed by rubella, chicken pox, EBV infection, and mumps. The changes of ADEM remain localized mainly in the WM and the inflammation of myelin and associated demyelination are the major findings of the disease.

MR imaging of ADEM patients demonstrates disseminated T2-weighted hyperintensity in the deep and subcortical WM of the cerebral hemispheres as well as in the cerebellar WM, midbrain, and brainstem.[78,100,101] The postcontrast study shows variable enhancement of the lesions.

On MR imaging, ANE lesions are characterized by hyperintensity in the bilateral thalamic regions on conventional T2-weighted images and DWI. The calculated ADC value from ADEM is higher than ANE. It has been observed that ADEM patients recover faster on steroids with the ADC

values falling rapidly to the normal values as compared with ANE patients.

There is a single study in which MRS was performed in patients with ADEM and ANE.[100] Lac is present in both cases; however, ADEM shows (**Fig. 16**) higher Lac levels than ANE. Similarly, more marked reduction in NAA/Cr has been observed in ADEM as compared with ANE. MRS findings in ADEM and ANE are nonspecific and are not useful for its diagnosis. MRS may however be useful for monitoring treatment response in ADEM and ANE patients.

Restricted diffusion has been reported in the acute stage of ADEM in contrast to the subacute stage of the disease.[102] Reduced NAA ratio with an increase in the Cho/Cr ratio has been observed in the subacute stage, whereas there is not much of a change in metabolites in the acute stage.[102] The identification of the restricted diffusion along with unchanged metabolite ratios in the earlier stage may help in staging the disease. DWI and in vivo MRS findings in infants with ANE show that marked decrease in ADC is associated with severe brain damage and poor clinical outcome.[103] DWI and in vivo MRS may provide useful information not only for diagnosis but also for severity assessment and clinical outcome of ANE.

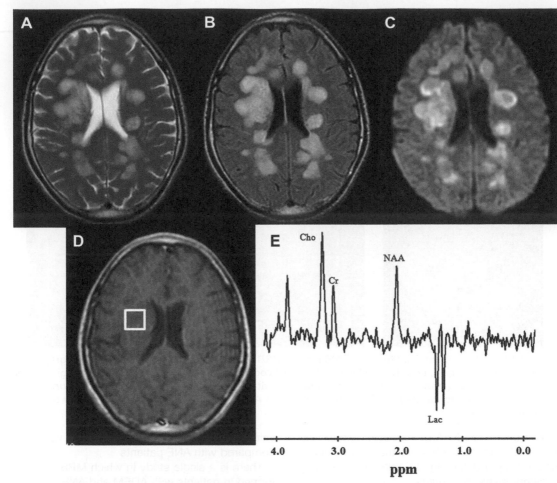

Fig. 16. Acute demyelinating encephalomyelitis in a 8-year-old boy. Axial T2-weighted (*A*) and T2-FLAIR image (*B*) show multiple confluent hyperintensities in bilateral periventricular and subcortical white matter. DWI shows diffusion restriction with high signal intensity on DWI (*C*). Postcontrast T1-weighted image shows no enhancement of these lesions (*D*). In vivo ^{1}H MR spectrum obtained shows reduction in the NAA (2.02 ppm), increases in choline (Cho), with lactate (Lac) at 1.33 ppm and creatine (Cr) at 3.0 ppm (*E*).

SUMMARY

MR spectroscopy, when combined with routine diagnostic imaging, may provide specific information especially in brain abscess and parasitic infection, which may help in its definitive diagnosis. However it may have a supportive role in the diagnosis and management of other CNS infections. These considerations may be useful in guiding the clinical radiologists in imaging the patients with known or suspected CNS infections.

REFERENCES

1. Britt RH, Enzmann DR, Yeager AS. Neuro-pathological and computerized tomographic findings in experimental brain abscess. J Neurosurg 1981; 55:590–603.

2. Venkatesh SK, Gupta RK. Pyogenic infections. In: Gupta RK, Lufkin RB, editors. MR imaging and spectroscopy of central nervous system infection. New York: Kluwer Academic/Plenum Publishers; 2001. p. 57–93.

3. Kim SH, Chang KH, Song IC, et al. Brain abscess and brain tumor: discrimination with in vivo H-1 MR spectroscopy. Radiology 1997;204:239–45.

4. Sudhakar KV, Agarwal S, Rashid MR, et al. MRI demonstration of haemorrhage in the wall of a brain abscess: possible implications for diagnosis and management. Neuroradiology 2001; 43:218–22.

5. Shukla-Dave A, Gupta RK, Roy R, et al. Prospective evaluation of in vivo proton MR spectroscopy in differentiation of similar appearing intracranial cystic lesions. Magn Reson Imaging 2001;19: 103–10.

6. Gupta RK, Chang KH. Parasitic infections. In: Gupta RK, Lufkin RB, editors. MR imaging and spectroscopy of central nervous system infection. New York: Kluwer Academic/Plenum Publishers; 2001. p. 205–39.

7. Garg M, Gupta RK, Husain M, et al. Etiological categorization of brain abscesses with in vivo proton MR spectroscopy. Radiology 2004;230:893–9.

8. Mishra AM, Gupta RK, Jaggi RS, et al. Role of diffusion-weighted imaging and in vivo proton magnetic resonance spectroscopy in the differential diagnosis of ring-enhancing intracranial cystic mass lesions. J Comput Assist Tomogr 2004;28:540–7.

9. Lai PH, Ho JT, Chen WL, et al. Brain abscess and necrotic brain tumor: discrimination with proton MR spectroscopy and diffusion-weighted imaging. AJNR Am J Neuroradiol 2002;23:1369–77.

10. Lai PH, Hsu SS, Ding SW, et al. Proton magnetic resonance spectroscopy and diffusion-weighted imaging in intracranial cystic mass lesions. Surg Neurol 2007;68(Suppl 1):S25–36.

11. Nath K, Agarwal M, Ramolla M, et al. Role of diffusion tensor imaging (DTI) and in vivo proton MR spectroscopy (PMRS) in the differential diagnosis of cystic intracranial mass lesions. Magn Reson Imaging 2009;27(2):198–206.

12. Mishra AM, Gupta RK, Saksena S, et al. Biological correlates of diffusivity in brain abscess. Magn Reson Med 2005;54:878–85.

13. Zimmerman RA, Bilaniuk LT, Sze G. Intracranial infection. In: Brant-Zawadzki M, Norman D, editors. Magnetic resonance imaging of the central nervous system. New York: Raven Press; 1987. p. 235–57.

14. Shawl S. Neurologic evaluation of patient with acute bacterial meningitis. Neurol Clin 1995;13:549–77.

15. Tandon PN, Pathak SN. Tuberculosis of the central nervous system. In: Spillane JD, editor. Tropical neurology. New York: Oxford University Press; 1973. p. 37–62.

16. Hopewell PC. Overview of clinical tuberculosis. In: Bloom BR, editor. Tuberculosis: pathogenesis, protection, and control. Washington, DC: American Society of Microbiology; 1994. p. 25–46.

17. Gupta RK, Pandey R, Khan EM, et al. Intracranial tuberculomas: MRI signal intensity correlation with histopathology and localized proton spectroscopy. Magn Reson Imaging 1993;11:443–9.

18. Gupta RK, Husain N, Kathuria MK, et al. Magnetization transfer MR imaging correlation with histopathology in intracranial tuberculomas. Clin Radiol 2001;56:656–63.

19. Gupta R. Magnetization transfer MR imaging in central nervous system infections. Indian J Radiol Imaging 2002;12:51–8.

20. Gupta RK, Kathuria MK, Pradhan S. Magnetization transfer MR imaging in CNS tuberculosis. AJNR Am J Neuroradiol 1999;20:867–75.

21. Gupta RK, Roy R, Dev R, et al. Finger printing of Mycobacterium tuberculosis in patients with intracranial tuberculomas by using in vivo, ex vivo, and in vitro magnetic resonance spectroscopy. Magn Reson Med 1996;36:829–33.

22. Garg M, Gupta RK. MR spectroscopy in intracranial infection. In: Gillard J, Waldman A, Barker P, editors. Clinical MR neuroimaging diffusion, perfusion and spectroscopy. Cambridge, UK: Cambridge university press ; 2005. p. 380–406.

23. Farrar DJ, Flanigan TP, Gordon NM, et al. Tuberculous brain abscess in a patient with HIV infection: case report and review. Am J Med 1997;102:297–301.

24. Gupta RK, Vatsal DK, Husain N, et al. Differentiation of tuberculous from pyogenic brain abscesses with in vivo proton MR spectroscopy and magnetization transfer MR imaging. AJNR Am J Neuroradiol 2001;22:1503–9.

25. Luthra G, Parihar A, Nath K, et al. Comparative evaluation of fungal, tubercular, and pyogenic brain abscesses with conventional and diffusion mr imaging and proton MR Spectroscopy. AJNR Am J Neuroradiol 2007;28:1332–8.

26. Gupta RK, Prakash M, Mishra AM, et al. Role of diffusion weighted imaging in differentiation of intracranial tuberculoma and tuberculous abscess from cysticercus granulomas—a report of more than 100 lesions. Eur J Radiol 2005;55:384–92.

27. Reddy JS, Mishra AM, Behari S, et al. Role of diffusion-weighted imaging in the differential diagnosis of intracranial cystic mass lesions: a report of 147 lesions. Surg Neurol 2006;66:246–50.

28. Kamra P, Azad R, Prasad KN, et al. Infectious meningitis: prospective evaluation with magnetization transfer MRI. Br J Radiol 2004;77:387–94.

29. Gupta RK. Tuberculosis and other non-tuberculous bacterial graunulomatous infections. In: Gupta RK, Lufkin RB, editors. MR imaging and spectroscopy of central nervous system infection. New York: Kluwer Academic/Plenum Publishers; 2001. p. 95–145.

30. Satishchandra P, Sharma GR. Fungal infections of the nervous system. In: Garg RK, Kar AM, Agarwal A, et al, editors. Reviews in tropical neurology. Lucknow (India): Shivam Arts; 2002. p. 111–24.

31. Sepkowitz K, Armstrong D. Space-occupying fungal lesions. In: Scheld WM, Whitley RJ, Durack DT, editors. Infections of the central nervous system. Philadelphia: Lippincott-Raven Press; 1997. p. 741–62.

32. Meyer RD, Young LS, Armstrong D, et al. Aspergillosis complicating neoplastic disease. Am J Med 1973;54:6–15.

33. Kathuria MK, Gupta RK. Fungal infections. In: Gupta RK, Lufkin RB, editors. MR imaging and spectroscopy of central nervous system infection. New York: Kluwer Academic/Plenum Publishers; 2001. p. 177–203.

34. Dzendrowskyi T, Himmelreich U, Malik R, et al. Distinction between cerebral Cryptococcomas, Staphylococcus aureus infections and tumours in an animal model. Proc Int Soc Mag Res Med 2000;8:173.

35. Himmelreich U, Dzendrowoskyj TE, Allen C, et al. Cryptococcomas distinguished from gliomas with MR spectroscopy: an experimental rat and cell culture study. Radiology 2001;220:122–8.

36. Siegal JA, Cacayorin ED, Nassif AS, et al. Cerebral mucormycosis: proton MR spectroscopy and MR imaging. Magn Reson Imaging 2000;18:915–20.

37. Andreula CF, Burdi N, Carella A. CNS cryptococcosis in AIDS: spectrum of MR findings. J Comput Assist Tomogr 1993;13:1477–86.

38. Bowen BC, Post MJD. Intra cranial infections. In: Atlas SW, editor. Magnetic resonance imaging of the brain and spine. New York: Raven Press; 1991. p. 501–38.

39. Tien RD, Chu PK, Hesselink JR, et al. Intracranial cryptococcosis in immunocompromised patients: CT and MR findings in 29 cases. AJNR Am J Neuroradiol 1991;12(2):283–9.

40. Chang L, Miller BL, McBride D, et al. Brain lesions in patients with AIDS: H-1 MR spectroscopy. Radiology 1995;197(2):525–31.

41. Hauck EF, McGinnis M, Nauta HJ. Cerebral phaeohyphomycosis mimics high-grade astrocytoma. J Clin Neurosci 2008;15:1061–6.

42. Garg RK, Kar AM. Neurocysticercosis: diagnosis and treatment in special situations. In: Singh G, Prabhakar S, editors. Taenia solium cysticercosis from basic to clinical science. New York: CAB International; 2002. p. 281–7.

43. Garcia HH, Gilman RH, Catacora M, et al. Serologic evolution of neurocysticercosis patients after antiparasitic therapy. Cysticercosis working group in Peru. J Infect Dis 1997;175:486–9.

44. Sharda D, Chawla S, Gupta RK. Imaging and spectroscopy of neurocysticercosis. In: Singh G, Prabhakar S, editors. Taenia solium cysticercosis from basic to clinical science. New York: CAB International; 2002. p. 311–27.

45. Chawla S, Gupta RK, Kumar R, et al. Demonstration of scolex in calcified cysticercus lesion using gradient echo with or without corrected phase imaging and its clinical implications. Clin Radiol 2002;57:826–34.

46. Pandit S, Lin A, Gahbauer H, et al. MR spectroscopy in neurocysticercosis. J Comput Assist Tomogr 2001;25:950–2.

47. Chawla S, Gupta RK, Husain N, et al. Prediction of viability of neurocysticercosis with proton magnetic resonance spectroscopy and its correlation with histopathology. Life Sci 2004;74:1081–92.

48. Garg M, Chawla S, Prasad KN, et al. Differentiation of hydatid cyst from cysticercus cyst by proton MR spectroscopy. NMR Biomed 2002;15:320–6.

49. Rudman MA, Khaffai S. CT of cerebral hydatid disease. Neuroradiology 1988;30:496–9.

50. Önal Ç, Barlas O, Orakdögen M, et al. Three unusual cases of intracranial hydatid cyst in the pediatric age group. Pediatr Neurosurg 1997;26:208–13.

51. Nurchi G, Floris F, Montaldo C, et al. Multiple cerebral hydatid disease: case report with magnetic resonance imaging study. Neurosurgery 1992;30:436–8.

52. Kohli A, Gupta RK, Poptani H, et al. In vivo proton magnetic resonance spectroscopy in a case of intracranial hydatid cyst. Neurology 1995;45:562–4.

53. Garg M, Gupta RK, Prasad KN, et al. Fertility assessment of hydatid cyst by proton MR spectroscopy. J Surg Res 2002;106:196–201.

54. Kingsley PB, Shah TC, Woldenberg R. Identification of diffuse and focal brain lesions by clinical magnetic resonance spectroscopy. NMR Biomed 2006;19:435–62.

55. Marsden PD, Bruce-Chwatt IJ. Cerebral malaria. In: Hornabrook RW, editor. Tropics on tropical neurology. Philadelphia: Devis; 1975. p. 29–44.

56. Sanni LA, Rae C, Maitiland A, et al. Is ischemia involved in the pathogenesis of murine cerebral malaria? Am J Pathol 2001;159:1105–11.

57. Porter SB, Sande MA. Toxoplasmosis of the central nervous system in the acquired immunodeficiency syndrome. N Engl J Med 1992;327:1643–8.

58. Luft BJ, Hafner R, Korzun AH, et al. Toxoplasmic encephalitis in patients with the acquired immunodeficiency syndrome. N Engl J Med 1993;329:995–1000.

59. Laissy JP, Soyer P, Parlier C, et al. Persistent enhancement after treatment for cerebral toxoplasmosis in patients with AIDS: predictive value for subsequent recurrence. AJNR Am J Neuroradiol 1994;115:1773–8.

60. Issakhanian M, Chang L, Cornford M, et al. HIV-2 infection with cerebral toxoplasmosis and lymphomatoid granulomatosis. J Neuroimaging 2001;11:212–6.

61. Revel MP, Grey F, Brugieres P, et al. Hyperdense CT foci in treated AIDS toxoplasmosis encephalitis: MR and pathologic correlation. J Comput Assist Tomogr 1992;16:372–5.

62. Ramsey R, Gean AD. Neuroimaging of AIDS I. Central nervous system toxoplasmosis. Neuroimaging Clin N Am 1997;7:171–86.

63. Ionita C, Wasay M, Balos L, et al. MRI in toxoplasmosis encephalitis after bone marrow transplantation: paucity of enhancement despite

fulminant disease. AJNR Am J Neuroradiol 2004; 25:270–3.

64. Cassady KA, Whitley RJ. Pathogenesis and pathophysiology of viral infections of the central nervous system. In: Scheld WM, Whitley RJ, Durack DT, editors. Infections of the central nervous system. Philadelphia: Lippincott-Raven Press; 1997. p. 7–22.

65. Jamal MM, Soni A, Quinn PG, et al. Clinical features of hepatitis C-infected patients with persistently normal alanine transaminase levels in the Southwestern United States. Hepatology 1999;30: 1307–11.

66. Forton DM, Allsop JM, Main J, et al. Evidence for a cerebral effect of the hepatitis C virus. Lancet 2001;358:38–9.

67. Agnello V, De Rosa FG. Extrahepatic disease manifestations of HCV infection: some current issues. J Hepatol 2004;40:341–52.

68. Hilsabeck RC, Perry W, Hassanein TI. Neuropsychological impairment in patients with chronic hepatitis C. Hepatology 2002;35:440–6.

69. Weissenborn K, Krause J, Bokemeyer M, et al. Hepatitis C virus infection affects the brain- evidence from psychometric studies and magnetic resonance spectroscopy. J Hepatol 2004;41:845–51.

70. Dore GJ, Correll PK, Li Y, et al. Changes to AIDS dementia complex in the era of highly active antiretroviral therapy. AIDS 1999;13:1249–53.

71. Tozzi V, Balestra P, Bellagamba R, et al. Persistence of neuropsychologic deficits despite long-term highly active antiretroviral therapy in patients with HIV-related neurocognitive impairment: prevalence and risk factors. J Acquir Immune Defic Syndr 2007;45:174–82.

72. Larussa D, Lorenzini P, Cingolani A, et al. Highly active antiretroviral therapy reduces the age-associated risk of dementia in a cohort of older HIV-1-infected patients. AIDS Res Hum Retroviruses 2006;22:386–92.

73. Thein HH, Maruff P, Krahn MD, et al. Improved cognitive function as a consequence of hepatitis C virus treatment. HIV Med 2007;8:520–8.

74. Navia BA, Cho ES, Petito CK, et al. The AIDS dementia complex: II. Neuropathology. Ann Neurol 1986;19:525–35.

75. Tien RD, Felsberg GJ, Osumi AK. Herpesvirus infections of the CNS: MR findings. Am J Roentgenol 1993;161:167–76.

76. Lakeman FD, Whitley RJ. Diagnosis of herpes simplex encephalitis: application of polymerase chain reaction to cerebrospinal fluid from brain-biopsied patients and correlation with disease. J Infect Dis 1995;171:857–63.

77. Morawetz RB, Whitley RJ, Murphy DM. Experience with brain biopsy for suspected herpes encephalitis: review of forty consecutive cases. Neurosurgery 1983;12:654–7.

78. Gupta RK, Lufkin RB. Viral infections. In: Gupta RK, Lufkin RB, editors. MR Imaging and spectroscopy of central nervous system infection. New York: Kluwer Academic/Plenum Publishers; 2001. p. 147–75.

79. Tsuchiya K, Katase S, Yoshino A, et al. Diffusion-weighted MR imaging of encephalitis. Am J Roentgenol 1999;173:1097–9.

80. Demaerel P, Wilms G, Robberecht W, et al. MRI and herpes simplex encephalitis. Neuroradiology 1992;32:490–3.

81. Samann PG, Schiegel J, Muller G, et al. Serial proton MR spectroscopy and diffusion imaging findings in HIV-related herpes simplex encephalopathy. AJNR Am J Neuroradiol 2003;24:2015–9.

82. Takanashi J, Sugita K, Ishii M, et al. Longitudinal MR imaging and proton MR spectroscopy in herpes simplex encephalitis. J Neurol Sci 1997;149: 99–102.

83. Silverstein A, Steinberg G, Nathanson M. Nervous system involvement in infectious mononucleosis: the heralding and or major manifestation. Arch Neurol 1972;26:353–8.

84. Ross JP, Cohen JI. Epstein–Barr virus. In: Scheld WM, Whitley RJ, Durack DT, editors. Infections of the central nervous system. Philadelphia: Lippincott-Raven Press; 1997. p. 117–27.

85. Cecil KM, Jones BV, Williams S, et al. CT, MRI and MRS of Epstein–Barr virus infection: case report. Neuroradiology 2000;42:619–22.

86. Hagemann G, Mentzel HJ, Weisser H, et al. Multiple reversible MR signal changes caused by Epstein-Barr virus encephalitis. AJNR Am J Neuroradiol 2006;27:1447–9.

87. Parameshwaran K, Radhakrishnan K. Subacute sclerosing panencephalitis. In: Kar AM, Shukla R, Agarwal A, et al, editors. Reviews in tropical neurology. Lucknow (India): Shivam Arts; 2002. p. 30–40.

88. Trivedi R, Gupta RK, Agarawal A, et al. Assessment of white matter damage in subacute sclerosing panencephalitis using quantitative diffusion tensor MR imaging. AJNR Am J Neuroradiol 2006;27: 1712–6.

89. Salvan AM, Confort-Gouny S, Cozzone PJ, et al. In vivo cerebral proton MRS in a case of subacute sclerosing panencephalitis. J Neurol Neurosurg Psychiatry 1999;66:547–55.

90. Aydin K, Tatli B, Ozkan M, et al. Quantification of neurometabolites in subacute sclerosing panencephalitis by 1H-MRS. Neurology 2006;67:911–3.

91. Sidtis JJ, Price RW. Early HIV-1 infection and the AIDS dementia complex. Neurology 1990;40: 323–6.

92. Trotot PM, Gray F. Neuroimaging of AIDS I. Diagnostic imaging contribution in the early stages of HIV infection of the brain. Neuroimaging Clin N Am 1997;7:243–60.

93. Chrysikopoulos HS, Press GA, Grafe MR, et al. Encephalitis caused by human immunodeficiency virus: CT and MR imaging manifestations with clinical and pathologic correlation. Radiology 1990;175:185–91.

94. Post MJ, Tate LG, Quencer RM, et al. CT, MR, and pathology in HIV encephalitis and meningitis. AJR Am J Roentgenol 1988;151:373–80.

95. Heyes MP, Ellis RJ, Ryan L, et al, HNRC Group. HIV Neurobehavioral Research Center. Elevated cerebrospinal fluid quinolinic acid levels are associated with region-specific cerebral volume loss in HIV infection. Brain 2001;124: 1033–42.

96. Hawkins CP, McLaughlin JE, Kendall BE, et al. Pathological findings correlated with MRI in HIV infection. Neuroradiology 1993;35:264–8.

97. Navia BA, Gonzalez RG. Functional imaging of the AIDS dementia complex and the metabolic pathology of the HIV-1 infected brain. Neuroimaging Clin N Am 1997;7:431–45.

98. Chang L, Ernst T, Leonido-Yee M, et al. Highly active antiretroviral therapy reverses brain metabolite abnormalities in mild HIV dementia. Neurology 1999;53:782–9.

99. Simone IL, Federico F, Tortorella C, et al. Localised 1H-MR spectroscopy for metabolic characterisation of diffuse and focal brain lesions in patients infected with HIV. J Neurol Neurosurg Psychiatry 1998;64:516–23.

100. Harada M, Hisaoka S, Mori K, et al. Difference in water diffusion and lactate production in two different types of postinfectious encephalopathy. J Magn Reson Imaging 2000;11:559–63.

101. Caldemeyer KS, Smith RR, Harris TM, et al. MRI in acute disseminated encephalomyelitis. Neuroradiology 1994;36:216–20.

102. Balasubramanya KS, Kovoor JME, Jayakumar PN, et al. Diffusion-weighted imaging and proton MR spectroscopy in the characterization of acute disseminated encephalomyelitis. Neuroradiology 2007;49:177–83.

103. Goo HW, Choi CG, Yoon CH, et al. Acute necrotizing encephalopathy: diffusion MR imaging and localized proton MR spectroscopic findings in two infants. Korean J Radiol 2003;4:61–5.

Pediatric Brain Tumors

Lara A. Brandão, MD[a,b,*], Tina Young Poussaint, MD[c]

KEYWORDS

• MR • MR spectroscopy • Pediatric • Brain tumor

KEY POINTS

- Pediatric brain tumors are the most common solid tumor in children and the leading cause of death in this patient population.
- Magnetic resonance spectroscopy (MRS) enables the radiologist to identify tumor tissue, to grade tumors, to differentiate tumor types, to distinguish active tumor from radiation necrosis or scar tissue, to guide stereotactic biopsy sites, and to determine early response to treatment.
- MRS may provide prognostic information used to guide therapy early on in the patient's treatment, effectively improving outcomes and minimizing side effects.
- Taurine has been established as an important biomarker in distinguishing medulloblastomas (the most common posterior fossa neoplasm in children) from other common pediatric brain tumors, such as cerebellar astrocytomas.
- In spite of being grade I tumors, pilocytic astrocytomas typically show significantly elevated choline (Cho) peaks, Cho/NAA and Cho/creatine ratios, along with reduced NAA and creatine peaks and presence of lactate on MR spectroscopy.
- The presence of high myo-inositol (mI) levels strongly suggests a diagnosis of ependymoma.
- In the brainstem glioma, a citrate peak can be demonstrated at approximately 2.6 ppm and can be used to follow tumor progression.
- Studies have suggested that mI level could be used as a marker for tumor grading in astrocytoma, whereas higher levels could be found in low-grade (grade II) astrocytoma compared with higher-grade astrocytoma or glioblastoma.
- Choroid plexus papillomas (CPP) typically demonstrate significantly elevated myo-inositol peak, low creatine, and decreased choline when compared with choroid plexus carcinomas (CPC).
- MRS may provide additional information in cases in which the differential diagnosis by neuroimaging is difficult, such as tumor versus infection, tumor versus tumefactive demyelinating lesions, and tumor versus radiation necrosis.

INTRODUCTION

Second only to leukemia as the most prevalent malignancy of childhood, the brain tumor is the most common solid tumor among children, significantly surpassing other types of solid tumors (eg, sarcomas, carcinomas, and lymphoma) as the leading cause of death in the pediatric patient population.[1,2]

Proton nuclear magnetic resonance spectroscopy (1H-MRS), a noninvasive, in vivo technique that provides additional metabolic diagnostic indices beyond anatomic information, has been extensively used to evaluate brain tumors.

Funding Sources: None.
Conflict of Interest: None.
a Clínica Felippe Mattoso, Av. Das Américas 700, sala 320, Barra Da Tijuca, Rio De Janeiro CEP-22640-100, Brazil;
b Clínica IRM - Ressonância Magnética, Rua Capitão Salomão 44-Humaitá, Rio de Janeiro 22271040, Brazil;
c Division of Neuroradiology, Department of Radiology, Boston Children's Hospital, Harvard Medical School, 300 Longwood Avenue, Boston, MA 02115, USA
* Corresponding author.
E-mail address: larabrandao.rad@terra.com.br

Neuroimag Clin N Am 23 (2013) 499–525
http://dx.doi.org/10.1016/j.nic.2013.03.003
1052-5149/13/$ – see front matter © 2013 Elsevier Inc. All rights reserved.

Magnetic resonance spectroscopy (MRS) enables the radiologist to identify tumor tissue, to grade tumors, to differentiate tumor types, to distinguish active tumor from radiation necrosis or scar tissue, to guide stereotactic biopsy sites, and to determine early response to treatment.[3–16]

Several studies have demonstrated that most tumors have decreased N-acetyl-aspartate (NAA) (neuronal/oligodendrocytic marker), stable creatine (Cr), except in instances of energy failure (tumor necrosis), and increased choline (Cho) (increased membrane turnover, cellularity).[6,15,17]

Compared with long echo-time (TE) spectroscopy, short TE spectroscopy enables the detection of additional metabolites that are characterized by a shorter T2 relaxation time at an improved signal-to-noise ratio (SNR), including, among others, taurine (Tau), glutamine plus glutamate (Glx), myo-inositol plus glycine (mI + gly), and alanine (Ala).[18] These metabolites have demonstrated some utility in the diagnosis of specific tumor histology.[18,19]

In this article, we discuss posterior fossa tumors, supratentorial parenchymal and extraparenchymal tumors, and pineal region tumors. We also describe the differential diagnosis of focal brain lesions that may resemble brain tumors.

POSTERIOR FOSSA TUMORS
Medulloblastoma

Medulloblastoma (MB), a highly malignant neoplasm, is the most common posterior fossa neoplasm in children, representing 15% to 20% of all pediatric brain tumors and 30% to 40% of posterior fossa neoplasms.[6,20–24] The tumor usually arises at the midline within the vermis and exhibits growth into the fourth ventricle.[25–30]

On computed tomography (CT), the tumor is usually characterized as hyperdense, and on T2 images, as isointense to hypointense compared with gray matter (**Fig. 1A**).[27] These imaging findings are likely secondary to high cell density and high nuclear-to-cytoplasmic ratio.[20]

Apparent diffusion coefficient (ADC) values are significantly lower in MBs than in all other posterior fossa tumors (P<.001) related to high cell density (see **Fig. 1B**).[8,20,31,32]

Typical spectral findings

Cho On MRS, MBs usually demonstrate a significant elevation of the Cho peak related to the high cell density and elevated Cho/Cr and Cho/NAA ratios, reflecting its malignant nature (see **Fig. 1C**).[2,6,7,17] High Cho has been previously reported as a characteristic finding of primitive neuroectodermal tumors (PNETs).[25,33]

In a study by Carles Majós and colleagues,[33] significantly elevated levels in Cho peak were used to distinguish PNET from non-PNET tumors with a high degree of accuracy (94%). Elevation of the Cho peak is useful in distinguishing between MB and L'Hermitte-Duclos disease (LDD), as MBs occasionally present with a laminated appearance, and with no contrast enhancement, may mimic LDD. The Cho peak is typically elevated in patients with MB when compared with patients with LDD.[24]

Tau Spectra with a short TE show a significantly elevated Tau concentration at 3.3 ppm in patients with MB when compared with other tumors (see **Fig. 1C**).[3,7,18,19,34,35] Further, at a TE of 30 ms, the Tau peak projects above the

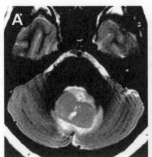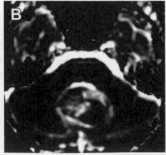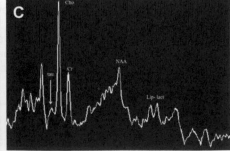

Fig. 1. Medulloblastoma: 27-year-old woman presenting with 2-month history of dizziness and nausea. There is a solid lesion in the posterior fossa, located in the midline and growing into the fourth ventricle. The lesion is T2 hypointense to normal cerebellar parenchyma (*A*) and has restricted diffusion on the apparent diffusion coefficient map (*B*). MRS (*C*) demonstrates significant elevation of the Cho peak, reduction of the NAA and Cr peaks, along with some Lips and lactate. Of note is the Tau peak (tau) at 3.3 ppm, next to the Cho peak. There is also some elevation of the Glx peak (*arrow*).

baseline; whereas, at a TE of 144 ms, the Tau peak occurs below the baseline.[3]

Tau has been established as an important biomarker in distinguishing MBs from other common pediatric brain tumors, such as cerebellar astrocytomas.[3,7,34,36,37] Although higher Tau levels are associated with increased cellular proliferation and tumoral aggressiveness,[3,7,18,32,38] decreased ADC combined with elevated levels of Cho and Tau, often suggest more significant malignancy in MBs.[18]

Glutamine and glutamate In a study of 60 children with untreated brain tumors, Panigrahy and colleagues[7] measured the highest glutamate (Glu) concentrations in pineal germinoma and in MB (see **Fig. 1**C). Specifically, the MB, pineal germinoma, and astrocytoma showed mean Glx concentrations *above the mean* in all tumors; whereas, Glx concentration was low in both the choroid plexus papilloma and carcinoma. The quantitation of these metabolites proved useful in separating either MB or astrocytoma from the choroid plexus papilloma.[7]

Ala Ala levels, when elevated, are readily detectable in specific diseases, including meningioma, glioblastoma, and MBs.[3,39] Consistent with this, Panigrahy and colleagues[7] report the highest mean Ala concentration among posterior fossa tumors in MBs.

Lipids Prominent lipid (Lip) resonances were observed in some, but not all, spectra of malignant MB (see **Fig. 1**C).[3,7] In an in vitro, high-resolution analysis of the lipid content in the tissue serum and cerebrospinal fluid (CSF) of patients with primary brain tumors, Srivastava and colleagues[40] demonstrated that proton MRS of the lipid extract of serum (blood specimen collected before the surgical procedure) and surgically discarded tissue had a *significantly* larger number of total cholesterol–containing and Cho-containing phospholipids in patients with MB and glioblastoma multiforme as compared with healthy subjects. This study supports the role of Lip estimation in CSF and tissue serum as a complementary diagnostic tool for evaluating pediatric brain tumors preoperatively.

Lactate High lactate (Lac) values are usually found in the spectra (see **Fig. 1**C).[2,6,7,17]

Final considerations

Prognosis Although significant differences exist between the metabolite profiles of metastatic and localized MB at presentation, localized tumors with metabolite profiles similar to those that have metastasized are at increased risk of relapse (**Table 1**).[41] Metastatic tumors, for example, are characterized by higher total Cho (tCho), which is consistent with increased cell turnover and tumor growth, a finding substantiated by a significant positive correlation between tCho and the Ki67 index.[41]

Tau is present in both metastatic and localized tumors, although higher levels are typically found in metastatic tumors, which is consistent with previous findings in neuroblastoma (ie, Tau is a reliable biomarker for more aggressive subtypes of neural tumors).[41–43] The fact that higher mobile Lip levels are observed in localized tumors may also reflect a higher proportion of nonviable tumor in these cases.

Therapeutic response MRS may be used to assess therapeutic response in patients with MB. If an elevation of the Cho peak is seen within the margins of the surgical bed, residual or recurrent tumor should be considered (**Fig. 2**). In cases in which the patient has received radiation therapy (RT), the extent of disease must be carefully interpreted. Specifically, a transient elevation of the Cho peak may be seen and a follow-up should be performed to distinguish RT effects from tumor recurrence.[2,17]

Late chemotherapy/radiotherapy effects In a study evaluating the neuro-metabolic alterations in pediatric survivors of posterior fossa tumors, Rueckriegel and colleagues[44] demonstrated that concentrations of NAA were significantly decreased in the respective white ($P<.0001$) and gray matters ($P<.0001$) of patients with MB compared with NAA levels in healthy controls. Further incremental decreases of metabolite concentrations in patients with MB compared with concentrations found in patients with pilocytic astrocytoma (PA) may point to additional harm caused by irradiation and chemotherapy.

Metastases Metastases from MB will present with the same spectral abnormalities as those described for the primary tumor. After chemotherapy,

Table 1
Metastatic versus localized medulloblastoma

Metastatic Medulloblastoma	Localized Medulloblastoma
Higher total choline	Higher mobile lipids
Higher taurine	Higher lactate
	Lower creatine

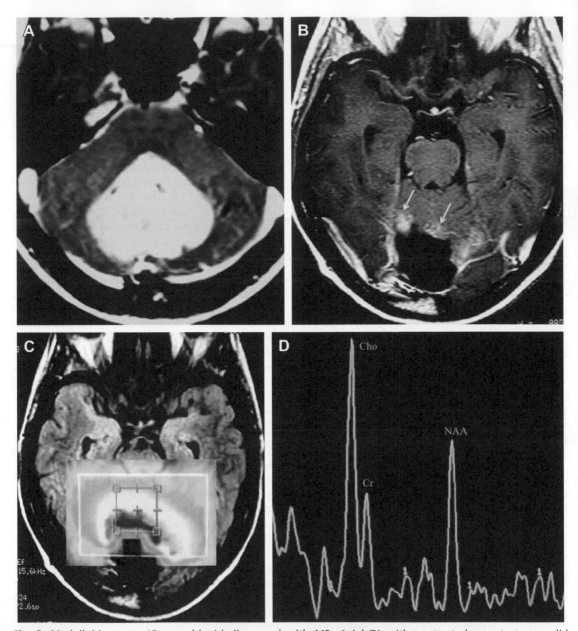

Fig. 2. Medulloblastoma: 15-year-old girl diagnosed with MB. Axial T1 with contrast demonstrates a solid enhancing lesion in the midline, growing into the fourth ventricle (*A*). The lesion was resected (*B*) but some enhancing nodules are demonstrated in the anterior margin of the surgical cavity that may represent radiation change or residual tumor (*arrows*). Multivoxel MRS (*C, D*) demonstrates a significant elevation of the Cho, Cho/Cr and Cho/NAA ratios in the area of enhancement, suggesting residual tumor.

MRS and diffusion may help assess therapeutic response.[2,45,46]

Atypical Teratoid/Rhabdoid Tumor

Children with atypical teratoid/rhabdoid tumors (ATRTs) of infancy and childhood present at a younger age than those with MB, with the median age at diagnosis 2 to 4 years.[6,47] (The median age for diagnosis of MB is about 6 years). Girls are more affected than boys, and most ATRTs (94%) are intra-axial, occurring in the infratentorial compartment in 47% of cases.[48]

Neuroimaging characteristics of ATRT (Fig. 3A–C) can be similar to those of MB in the posterior fossa; to germ-cell tumors; and to PNETs when

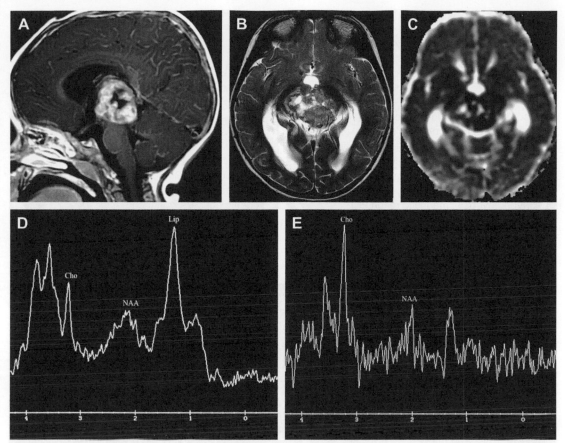

Fig. 3. ATRT: 14-month-old boy with vomiting. There is a heterogeneous enhancing pineal region mass (*A*). The solid portions of the lesion are T2 hypointense to normal parenchyma (*B*) and present with restricted diffusion on the ADC map (*C*). Spectra obtained with short (*D*) and long echo time (TE) (*E*) demonstrate a prominent Cho peak along with reduction of the NAA. Notice also a prominent Lip peak in the spectra obtained with short TE (*D*).

arising in the supratentorial compartment.[8,49,50] however, the prognosis is worse than that typically associated with MB.[49–53]

Typical spectral findings

MRS shows elevated Cho and reduced NAA as well as a prominent Lip peak (see **Fig.** 3D–E). However, there are no reports in the literature that quantify these changes or address the presence or size of Tau peaks.[6]

Final considerations

To differentiate these tumors from MBs, we should consider the following.

Location ATRTs tend to be more lateral in location and may compromise the cerebello pontine angle.

Heterogeneity ATRTs tend to be more heterogeneous in signal intensity when compared with MBs. Hemorrhage and blood products may be seen.

Cerebellar Astrocytoma

Cerebellar pilocytic astrocytoma (CPA), one of the most common posterior fossa tumors (second only to MB), is often diagnosed as a juvenile PA, with excellent survival after gross total surgical resection.[2,6,54–56] The differential diagnosis between CPA and MBs is crucial, however, because treatment and prognosis differ completely. The diagnosis is made by the following neuroimaging characteristics.

T2 characteristics

The enhancing solid component of CPA (**Figs.** 4B and 5B) is typically hyperintense on T2 images (see **Figs.** 4A and 5A) compared with the normal cerebellar parenchyma.[2,6] By contrast, the solid component of MBs is usually isointense or hypointense (see **Fig.** 1A) to normal cerebellar parenchyma on T2 images. However, higher-grade astrocytomas may manifest lower signal intensity on T2-weighted images, effectively mimicking MBs.[6]

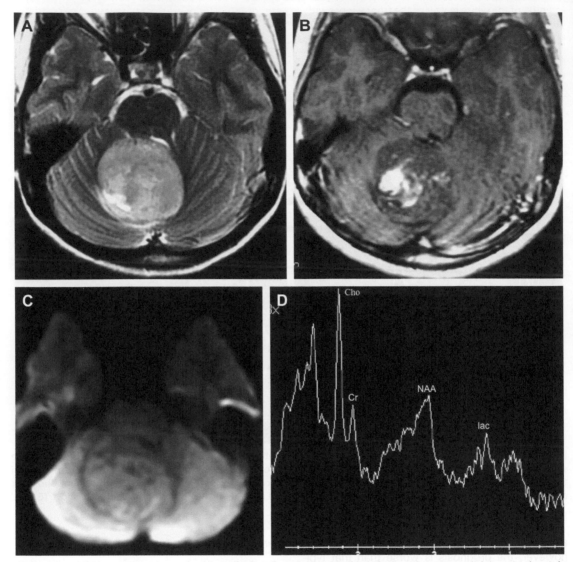

Fig. 4. Pilocytic astrocytoma: 11-year-old girl with 4-month history of headache. There is a solid mass in the right cerebellum with T2 hyperintense signal (*A*) and patchy enhancement on the T1 image with gadolinium (*B*). The lesion is isointense on the diffusion trace image (*C*). MRS (*D*) demonstrates reduction of NAA and Cr peaks, significant elevation of the Cho peak, and presence of lactate. There is no Tau peak.

Diffusion characteristics

The solid component of the CPA has greater ADC values (see **Figs. 4**C and **5**C) than do other cerebellar tumors, such as ependymoma, ATRT, and MB (see **Fig. 1**B).[2,32]

MRS

The Tau peak, considered very characteristic of MBs, is not typically demonstrated in PAs.[36]

Typical spectral findings

Cho Increases in tCho may be reliably correlated with the grade of a glioma; however, tCho is not an effective or accurate biomarker for grade I PAs that show a wide range of tCho values, including those demonstrating a marked increase. In fact, high Cho content and Cho/Cr and Cho/NAA ratios are consistently demonstrated in CPA despite the benign clinical course for tumors of this type (see **Figs. 4**D and **5**D, E).[2,4,6,17,57]

Lac Apart from tumor necrosis, there are several possible reasons for elevated Lac levels in this histologically benign tumor (see **Figs. 4**D and **5**D, E), including an abnormal number (or dysfunction

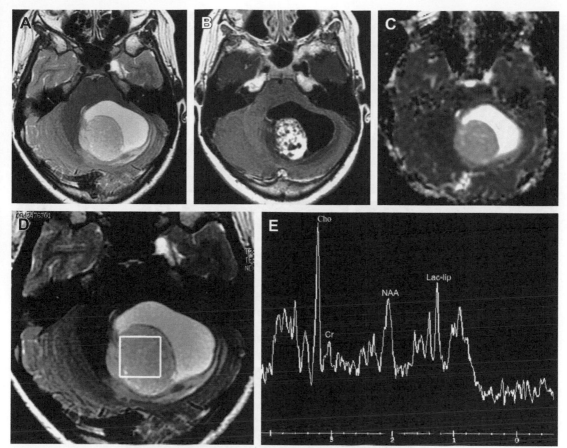

Fig. 5. Nine-year-old girl with 4-month history of headache, neck pain, vomiting, ataxia, nystagmus, and papilledema. There is a cystic-solid left cerebellar PA. The solid component of the lesion is T2 hyperintense (*A*) and there is heterogeneous enhancement (*B*). There is no restricted diffusion on the ADC map image (*C*). MRS (*D, E*) demonstrates significant elevation of the Cho peak, presence of Lips and Lac, and reduction of the NAA and Cr peaks.

of) mitochondria, which could interfere with oxidative phosphorylation and electron transport, alterations in proportional oxygen delivery, oxygen extraction or usage by the tumor, or anaerobic glycolysis by tumor cells.[57]

Cr In a study of untreated pediatric brain tumors, Panigrahy and colleagues[7] demonstrated that Cr was significantly reduced in PA (see **Figs. 4**D and **5**D, E), thereby distinguishing tumors of this type from all other posterior fossa tumors (*P*>.000001). Schneider and colleagues[58] also found that total creatine (tCr) was significantly reduced in circumscribed PA, clearly distinguishing them from other tumors.

Final consideration

Posterior fossa compared with suprasellar PAs Interestingly, some investigators have reported significant differences in the spectral composition between the cerebellar and suprasellar PAs, with significantly higher ml and glutamate/glutamine peaks in suprasellar tumors, and a trend toward lower Cr in cerebellar tumors.[6,59,60] However, Panigrahy and colleagues[7] have shown no differences between the spectroscopic patterns of supratentorial and infratentorial PA.

Further, there have been no significant differences identified in MRS profiles between pediatric and adult PAs.[58]

Ependymoma

Ependymomas are the fourth most common posterior fossa tumors in children following MB, cerebellar astrocytoma, and brainstem glioma.[2,20] The most important imaging finding in identifying an ependymoma is extension of the tumor through the fourth ventricular outflow foramina (**Fig. 6**A, B)[6]; however, this feature is not entirely pathognomonic, as some MBs may extend through the

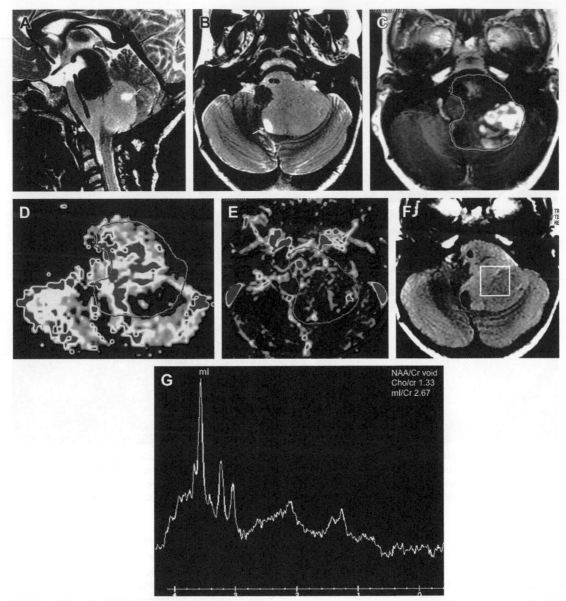

Fig. 6. Three-year-old boy diagnosed with ependymoma. Sagittal (*A*) and axial T2 (*B*) images demonstrate a solid mass extending from the fourth ventricle laterally to the foramina of Luschka on the left, engulfing the basilar and vertebral arteries. There is also inferior extension into the upper cervical canal through the foramina of Magendie. A cystic component is demonstrated in the posterior aspect of the tumor (*A, B, arrow*). There is heterogeneous enhancement (*C*), and elevation of the capillary density on the cerebral blood volume perfusion map (*D*). There is no increased permeability in the lesion (*E*). MRS (*F, G*) demonstrates a significant elevation of the ml peak. There is also some elevation of the Cho peak, along with reduction of the NAA peak.

fourth ventricular exit foramina. In addition, they usually show more bulbous extension and restricted diffusion rather than small amounts of tissue through the foramina that is characteristic of an ependymoma.[20,61]

Punctate calcification is demonstrated in 50% of ependymoma cases on CT.[6] These tumors are heterogeneous on magnetic resonance (MR) imaging (see **Fig. 6**), reflecting a combination of solid tumor, cyst, calcification, necrosis, edema, or hemorrhage.[62]

When performed, perfusion MR of ependymoma generally demonstrates markedly elevated cerebral blood volume (CBV) (see **Fig. 6**D) and, unlike many other glial neoplasms, poor return to baseline that may be attributable to fenestrated blood vessels and an incomplete blood brain barrier (BBB).[63–65] In the authors' experience, some ependymomas demonstrate significantly high permeability while no significant elevation of the permeability is demonstrated in other cases (see Fig. 6E).

Typical spectral findings

MRS shows considerable heterogeneity.[6]

mI Short echo spectra (TE = 30 ms) show low to very high mI (see Fig. 6F, G), although never as high as in choroid plexus papillomas (CPPs) (Fig. 7).[6,7,59]

In a study by Harris and colleagues,[59] the presence of high mI levels strongly suggests a diagnosis of ependymoma when short TE is used at 1.5 T. Ependymomas and infiltrative low-grade gliomas show higher levels of mI compared with MBs and PAs.[58]

Cr Harris and colleagues[59] suggest that ependymomas have higher Cr levels than do astrocytomas and MBs.

Glx Schneider and colleagues[18] also demonstrated that ependymomas are characterized by an elevation in mI and Glx.

Brainstem Glioma

Brainstem tumors represent 10% to 20% of all central nervous system (CNS) tumors in childhood.[2] Most brainstem gliomas are diffuse and involve the pons.[6] Diagnosis is based on the characteristic changes on MR imaging of diffuse T2 hyperintense expansion of the brainstem without biopsy (Fig. 8).[2]

Single voxel MRS (SV-MRS) is usually selected over chemical shift imaging (CSI) to evaluate brainstem gliomas. This ensures that the quality of individual tumor spectra is not adversely affected by unavoidable compromises accompanying CSI

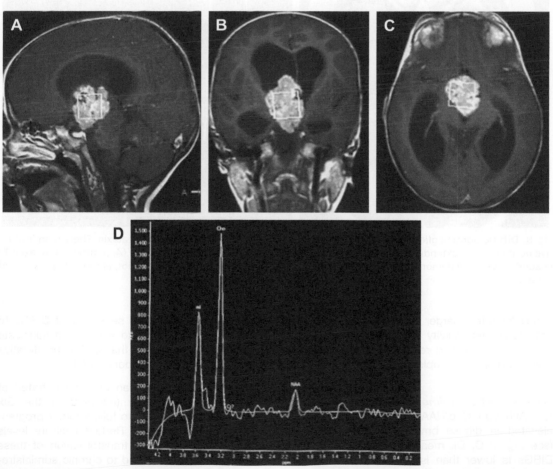

Fig. 7. CPP: 23-month-old girl presenting with signs of increased intracranial pressure. There is a solid enhancing mass located in the third ventricle (A–C). MRS (D) demonstrates elevation of the Cho and mI peaks.

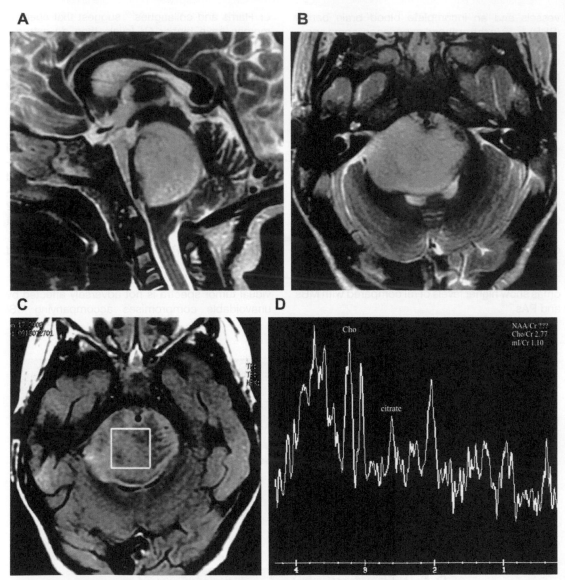

Fig. 8. Diffuse pontine glioma: 4-year-old girl with 3-month history of strabismus and ataxia. There is an infiltrative pontine lesion extending superiorly to the midbrain and inferiorly to the medulla (*A*, sagittal and *B*, axial T2 images). MRS (*C*, *D*) demonstrates elevation of the Cho peak, Cho/Cr and Cho/NAA ratios, along with presence of citrate.

acquisitions from larger volumes. In addition, the processing and quality control of CSI are more time consuming, and require the expertise of a skilled MR spectroscopist.[66]

Typical spectral findings

Cho Although Cho/NAA and Cho/Cr ratios are elevated in diffuse brainstem gliomas (DIBGs) (see **Fig. 8** C, D), mean tCho concentration in DIBGs is lower than is mean tCho in normal-appearing brainstems in controls. This may be an indicator of low membrane turnover and may

explain, in part, the low sensitivity of DIBGs to RT. Total Cho could also serve as a surrogate marker to identify tumors that are less proliferative but also less likely to respond to RT.[66]

Citrate A citrate peak can be demonstrated at approximately 2.6 ppm (adjacent to the Glx peak) and can be used to follow tumor progression (see **Fig.** 8D).[67–69] Reduced citrate levels may indicate malignant transformation of these tumors, or may be related to chronic administration of steroids, RT, and/or chemotherapy.[68] Although the citrate signal is most prominent and most often observed in DIBGs, it is also noted in other common pediatric brain tumors and in the developing brain of infants younger than 6 months.[69]

Final considerations
Low-grade versus high-grade pontine gliomas The spectral pattern in pontine gliomas is related to aggressiveness. Proton MRS and perfusion imaging may be useful in differentiating low-grade (usually focal) pontine tumors, which have lower Cho peaks and lower blood volumes, from high-grade tumors in which the Cho/Cr ratio is usually higher.

Malignant transformation Available literature suggests that at least a subset of diffuse pontine gliomas is histologically low grade (World Health Organization [WHO] grade II) at initial clinical presentation, but rapidly evolve into high-grade neoplasms, with most found to be glioblastoma multiforme at postmortem examination.[69–75] This finding is consistent with a very high rate of mortality: 90% of patients succumb within 2 years after initial diagnosis.[66,76–78]

Some studies suggest that MRS might be a useful early predictor of disease progression, preceding clinical and radiological deterioration.[66,76,77] Metabolic changes indicative of malignant transformation include increased levels of tCho, decreased metabolite ratios of NAA/tCho and Cr/tCho, and increased levels of Lips. In addition, a significant reduction in the "apparent" citrate levels may also be associated with malignant transformation.[69]

Therapeutic response MRS may be used in estimating therapeutic response or tumor progression.[76,77] Using multivoxel MRS (MV-MRS), Laprie and colleagues[76] followed 8 patients with diffuse pontine glioma in a series of studies from diagnosis to the time of response to RT and found that Cho:NAA values decreased, followed by an increase at the time of relapse.

In a study by Thakur and colleagues,[77] 2 pediatric patients with diffuse pontine tumors showed clinical improvements following RT; however, MRS showed an overall increase in Cho/Cr and Cho/NAA ratios, indicating tumor progression. Although these findings seem contradictory, the disease did, in fact, progress in both patients. There is now evidence from 3 independent studies that MRS identifies subjects with progressing disease and impending relapse several months before clinical manifestations of the illness.[76–78] This finding could be important for assessing the efficacy of novel treatment strategies in individual patients early on in the plan of care.

SUPRATENTORIAL TUMORS
Astrocytoma

Pilocytic astrocytomas (PAs) are the most common glial tumors in children. They are typically well demarcated with T2 signal abnormality roughly equivalent to the amount of gadolinium enhancement. Occasionally, these tumors present with an associated cyst. Supratentorial astrocytomas are most commonly located in the optic/hypothalamic region (Fig. 9), but can also be found in the brain parenchyma (Fig. 10).

Typical spectral findings
In spite of being grade I tumors, these lesions typically show significantly elevated Cho peaks, Cho/NAA and Cho/Cr ratios, along with reduced NAA and Cr peaks and presence of Lac on MRS (see Figs. 9D, E and 10).

Final considerations
Diffuse WHO grade II astrocytoma versus WHO grade I PA Using normalized concentrations of tCho and tCr, Schneider and colleagues[58] recently investigated whether in vivo proton MRS could differentiate between WHO grade I PA and diffuse, fibrillary WHO grade II astrocytoma (DA) in children. This study found that tCr showed a trend toward lower values in PA compared with DA and that increased tCr concentrations are typical for DA but not for PA. Thus, tCr seems to be a more important indicator than tCho in distinguishing PA from DA. Normalized concentrations of tCho are not, therefore, a reliable tool for reaching a differential diagnosis between PA and DA.

Another characteristic of diffuse infiltrative low-grade astrocytomas (grade II) is elevated mI peak at 1.5 T with TE of 35 ms (Fig. 11), which may also help to differentiate them from PAs (see Figs. 9 and 10) and MBs.[7,8,18,58]

Other studies have suggested that mI level could be used as a marker for tumor grading in astrocytoma, whereas higher levels could be found in low-grade (grade II) astrocytoma compared with higher-grade astrocytoma or glioblastoma.[18,79,80] The fact that the concentration of pooled mI is lowest in the more aggressive tumors is not surprising, however. The higher membrane turnover in malignant tumors results in a higher conversion of the MRS-visible portion of mI into phosphatidylinositol, which is a membrane-bound phospholipid and therefore no longer visible on MR spectra.[45,81]

Outcome An outcome-based comparison of grade II astrocytomas established that lesions with aggressive behavior within 2 years after diagnosis had significantly higher levels of citrate than did stable tumors.[82] Moreover, this study

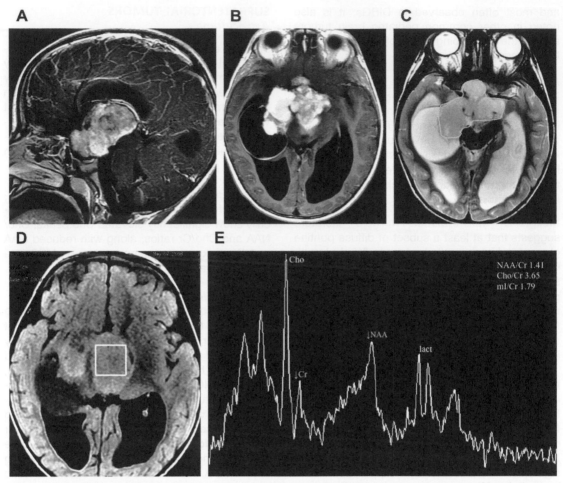

Fig. 9. Chiasmatic-hypothalamic astrocytoma: 3-year-old girl presenting with 6-month history of headaches and 3-month history of strabismus. There is a solid-cystic mass in the hypothalamic-chiasmatic region, presenting with significant enhancement (*A*, sagittal and *B*, axial T1 with contrast). The solid portion of the tumor is hyperintense on T2 and FLAIR images (*C, D*). The spectra (*E*), demonstrates a significant elevation of the Cho peak, Cho/NAA and Cho/Cr ratios, along with reduction of the NAA and Cr peaks. There is also elevation of lactate.

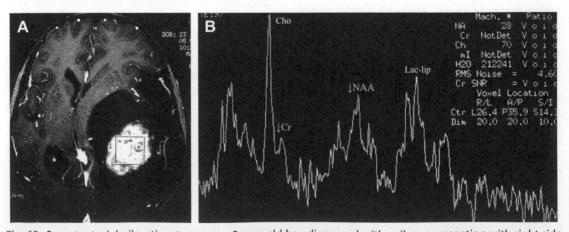

Fig. 10. Supratentorial pilocytic astrocytoma: 9-year-old boy diagnosed with epilepsy, presenting with right-side hemiparesis. There is a large mass in the left cerebral hemisphere, presenting with a solid enhancing component and peripherally located cysts (*A*). Spectroscopy (*B*) demonstrates significant elevation of the Cho peak along with reduction of the NAA and Cr peaks. There is also elevation of Lac and Lips.

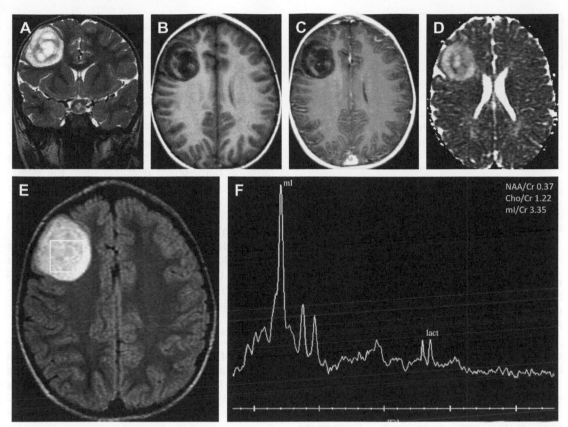

NAA/Cr 0.37
Cho/Cr 1.22
mI/Cr 3.35

Fig. 11. Grade II frontal astrocytoma: 5-year-old boy with vomiting. There is a solid mass in the right frontal lobe, hyperintense on T2 and FLAIR images (*A, E*), and predominantly hypointense on T1 (*B*), with no enhancement (*C*). There is no restricted diffusion on the ADC map (*D*). The striking elevation of mI peak in the spectra (*F*) is very suggestive of a grade II astrocytoma. Diagnosis was confirmed after surgical resection.

identified prominent citrate as a metabolic feature that distinguishes aggressive pediatric astrocytomas from stable astrocytomas. It appears prominent citrate may be an early, sensitive indicator for pediatric grade II astrocytomas destined for aggressive behavior, and, as such, may prove useful for noninvasive patient stratification. However, citrate was not specific for poor outcome, as it was not detectable in a significant percentage of the high-grade astrocytomas. A significant disparity in NAA levels was also noted between aggressive low-grade astrocytomas and indolent low-grade astrocytomas, although to a much lesser degree than was seen in citrate levels.

Stratification of astrocytomas outside the pons remains a significant challenge in pediatric neuro-oncology; thus, early identification of astrocytomas destined for malignant progression is critical to achieving optimal patient management.

Pilomyxoid astrocytomas versus PAs Pilomyxoid astrocytomas (PMAs) appear as low-grade tumors sharing imaging features similar to those of PAs. However, PMAs demonstrate a more variable clinical course and tend to behave more aggressively than PAs, with a decreased duration of disease-free survival and higher mortality rates.[83–85]

MRS patterns of PMA differ substantially from those of PA. For example, Cirak and colleagues[86] found a similar elevation in Cho/Cr ratios between PMA and PA, but reported an increase in Cho concentration in the intratumoral region of PA compared with Cho levels in the intratumoral region of PMA. The investigators attributed this elevation to the more cellular components in PA compared with the myxoid background of PMA. In another study, Morales and colleagues[83] found similar Cho/Cr ratios in the intratumoral regions of both PMA and PA, with a slightly elevated ratio in PMA. Using a long TE, these investigators also identified an elevation in Cho/Cr ratios in the peritumoral regions of PMA compared with PA, reflecting the more aggressive and infiltrative behavior of the former tumor. In addition, Morales and colleagues[83] also noted

Table 2
PMA versus PA

PMA	PA
Higher Cho/Cr in the tumor	Lower Cho/Cr in the tumor
Higher peritumoral Cho/Cr	No peritumoral elevation of the Cho/Cr
Lower ml/Cr in the tumor	Higher ml/Cr in the tumor

Abbreviations: Cho, choline; Cr, creatine; ml, myo-inositol; PA, pilocytic astrocytoma; PMA, pilomyxoid astrocytoma.
Data from Komotar RJ, Burger PC, Carson BS, et al. Pilocytic and pilomyxoid hypothalamic/chiasmatic astrocytomas. Neurosurgery 2004;54:72–9.

a decrease in the ml/Cr ratios of PMAs compared with PAs, which is likely the result of the more aggressive and invasive behavior of PMAs (**Table 2**).

Supratentorial ependymomas represent 40% of all ependymomas.[2] MR imaging shows large, heterogeneous tumors in a peritrigonal location; however, the tumors may be intraventricular or subcortical. The heterogeneity results from the combination of solid tumor, intratumoral calcification, cysts, and, occasionally, hemorrhage (**Fig. 12**).[2,6,20]

The spectra of anaplastic supratentorial ependymomas will demonstrate significant reduction of NAA, Cr, and ml peaks, along with elevation of the Cho peak, Cho/Cr, and Cho/NAA ratios (see **Fig. 12**B, C). Elevation of the ml peak may be demonstrated in grade II ependymomas and is considered characteristic.[59]

Supratentorial PNETs

PNETs are found in younger children with a mean age of 5 years.[4] PNETs are highly cellular tumors composed of 90% to 95% of undifferentiated cells.[6] The molecular characteristics of supratentorial PNETs differ significantly from those of MBs.[87]

The most typical MR appearance of a PNET is that of a large, apparently sharply marginated mass that can be located either in the cerebral hemisphere (**Fig. 13**) or in the lateral ventricle. Solid portions of the tumor show reduced diffusion on diffusion weighted imaging (DWI) and increased blood volume on perfusion studies.[2]

MRS demonstrates significant elevation of the Cho peak along with reduced NAA and elevated Lips and Lac (see **Fig. 13**C). The differential diagnosis should include high-grade glioma, ependymomas, and ATRT.

Supratentorial ATRTs

Supratentorial ATRTs are included in the group of embryonal tumors of the CNS together with MBs and PNETs.[6,88] In the presence of an aggressive intracranial tumor, a diagnosis of ATRT must always be considered in children younger than 2 years, even if the location is unusual. The main differential diagnosis remains PNET and ependymoma, and the definitive diagnosis can be established only on biopsy.[89]

ATRT and PNET can have the same CT and MR imaging findings.[53] Further complicating diagnosis, ATRT cannot be differentiated from PNET with DWI, perfusion MR imaging, or spectroscopy.[90,91] Supratentorial ATRT will present with

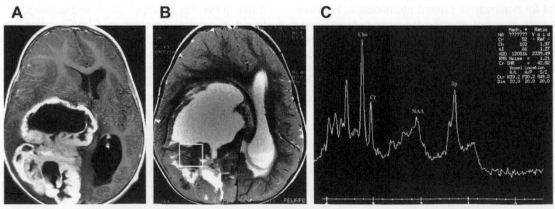

Fig. 12. Supratentorial anaplastic ependymoma: 1-year-old girl with fever, irritability, and hemiparesis on the left. There is a large lesion in the right frontal and parietal lobes with heterogeneous enhancement (*A*). Spectra (*B, C*) demonstrates elevation of the Cho peak, presence of Lips, along with reduction of the NAA and Cr peaks.

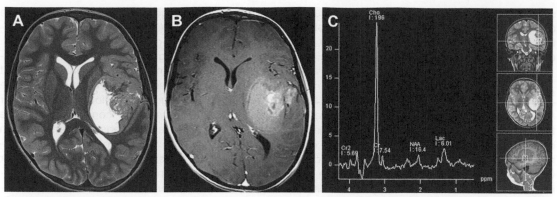

Fig. 13. Supratentorial PNET. Axial T2 image (*A*) demonstrates a large heterogeneous mass in the left frontal and temporal lobes. The solid portion is T2 hypointense secondary to high cell density. There is heterogeneous enhancement (*B*). Spectra (*C*) obtained with TE of 144 ms demonstrates a prominent Cho peak, along with reduction of all other metabolites.

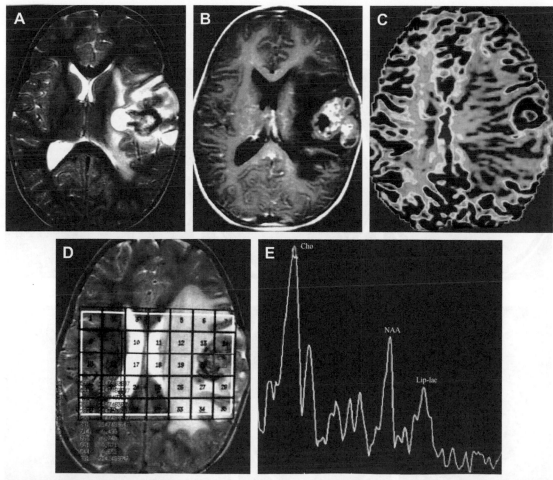

Fig. 14. Anaplastic oligodendroglioma: 4-year-old boy who presented with 4 episodes of seizure 1 year earlier. New seizure in the past month. There is a heterogeneous mass in the left frontal lobe presenting with cysts and calcification (*A*-axial T2) and heterogeneous enhancement (*B*). There is also a high vascular density (*C*, CBV map), which can be seen in low-grade and high-grade oligodendrogliomas. MRS (*D*, *E*) demonstrates reduction of the NAA peak, a significant elevation of the Cho peak, and presence of Lips and Lac, compatible with the malignant behavior of anaplastic oligodendrogliomas.

similar imaging features and a spectral pattern closely resembling that found in the posterior fossa (ie, with elevated levels of Cho and decreased levels of NAA).[89]

Oligodendroglial Tumor

Although oligodendroglial tumors constitute 5% to 7% of brain tumors in the general population, oligodendrogliomas are rare in children. A diagnosis of oligodendroglioma may be considered when a tumor develops in the frontal lobe, and is associated with calcification, cysts, and limited or absent contrast-enhancement. These features separate oligodendroglial tumors from most astrocytomas.[6]

Spectral pattern is directly related to tumor grade, with higher Cho and higher Cho/Cr and

Cho/NAA ratios generally noted in the more anaplastic regions (**Fig. 14**) as compared with ratios found in lower-grade tumors (**Fig. 15**).

When evaluating oligodendrogliomas for recurrence, it is important to remember that both high-grade (see **Fig. 14C**) and low-grade (see **Fig. 15D**) oligodendrogliomas have similar blood volumes, which is consistent with the increased microvessel density seen in both high-grade and low-grade oligodendroglial tumors.[92–94] However, Cho is significantly higher in high-grade than in low-grade oligodendrogliomas; the presence of Lac or Lip also correlates with high tumor grade (see **Fig. 14E**).[94] Proton MRS is thus viewed as superior to dynamic susceptibility-weighted perfusion imaging in evaluating oligodendroglial tumor recurrence.[6]

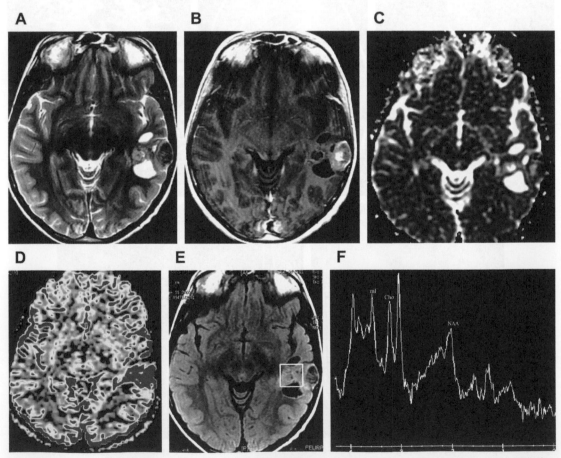

Fig. 15. Low-grade oligodendroglioma: 10-year-old boy with seizures since the age of 5, amnesia, and headaches. At that time he was diagnosed with a glial tumor. Recently the seizures were getting worse. A new MR image demonstrates a solid mass in the left temporal lobe presenting with cystic components (*A*) and enhancement (*B*). There is no restricted diffusion (*C*, ADC-map). There is elevation of the capillary density (*D*, CBV map). MRS (*E, F*) demonstrates that the mI peak is higher than the Cho peak, suggesting a low-grade lesion.

Neuronal and Mixed Neuronal-glial Tumors

Neuronal and mixed neuronal-glial tumors are characterized by neuronal and glial differentiation. Tumors in this category include gangliocytoma, ganglioglioma, dysembrioplastic neuroepithelial tumor (DNET), central neurocytoma, paraganglioma, and cerebellar liponeurocytoma.[62]

DNET

DNET is a benign tumor associated with intractable seizures occurring in children and young adults. These tumors are located cortically and usually associated with cortical dysplasia. Tumor calcification may be present in about one-third of the affected patients.[6]

Proton MRS of DNETs shows no significant difference of metabolite ratios from normal cortex other than the mI/Cr ratio, which may be elevated.[95]

Desmoplastic neuroepithelial tumors (desmoplastic infantile ganglioglioma/desmoplastic astrocytomas of infancy)

The desmoplastic infantile ganglioglioma (DIG) and desmoplastic astrocytomas of infancy (DACI) are very similar tumors seen primarily in infants and young children.[6] Patients with DIGs and DACIs (most often grouped together as desmoplastic neuroepithelial tumors) typically present in infancy with macrocephaly or partial complex seizures, with the median reported age of presentation at about 5 months. Large cysts and a solid cortical component are typical (Fig. 16). T2 isointensity of the solid component (see Fig. 16B) is useful in differentiating these tumors from PAs.

The MRS findings are mainly characterized by elevation of the mI peak, consistent with the benign clinical course of these lesions (see Fig. 16D).

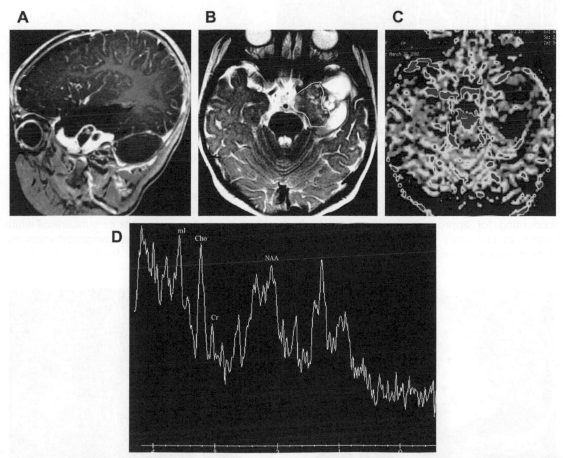

Fig. 16. Desmoplastic astrocytoma: 7-month-old girl with seizures. There is a superficially located mass in the left temporal lobe, with large cysts and peripheral "plaquelike" enhancement (A). The solid portion of the lesion is isointense on T2 (B). There is no elevation of the CBV (C), compatible with the benign clinical course of these tumors. MRS (D) demonstrates reduction of the NAA and Cr peaks, discrete elevation of the Cho peak, and a significant elevation of the mI peak.

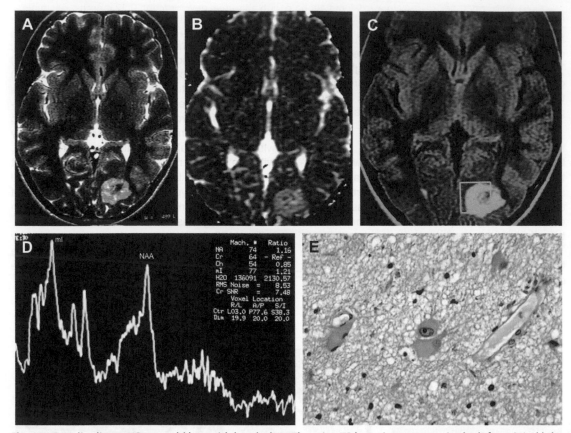

Fig. 17. Ganglioglioma: 13-year-old boy with headaches. There is a T2 hyperintense mass in the left occipital lobe, presenting with small foci of calcification with low signal intensity within it (A). There is no restricted diffusion (B, ADC map). MRS (C, D) demonstrates reduction of the NAA peak and significant elevation of the mI peak. Pathology (E) confirmed the diagnosis of ganglioglioma (hematoxilin-eosin). (*Courtesy of* Sergio Romano, MD.)

Gangliogliomas and gangliocytomas

Gangliogliomas and gangliocytomas are rare, accounting for approximately 3% of all brain tumors in children[6]; half of affected patients present with seizures. The tumor may be solid (Fig. 17), cystic with a mural nodule, or have the appearance of many small cysts. When located in the cortex or subcortical white matter, gangliogliomas and gangliocytomas are difficult to differentiate from astrocytomas,

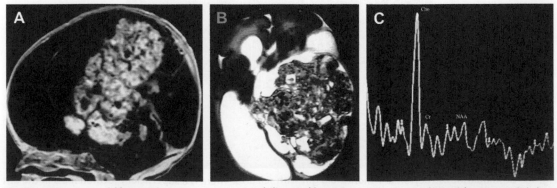

Fig. 18. CPC: 1-year-old boy with macrocephaly, irritability, and loss of appetite. Sagittal T1 with contrast (A) demonstrates a large enhancing mass compromising the left ventricle at the level of the atria. The mass is very heterogeneous on T2 (B). MRS (C) demonstrates significant reduction of the NAA, Cr, and mI peaks along with a prominent elevation of the Cho peak.

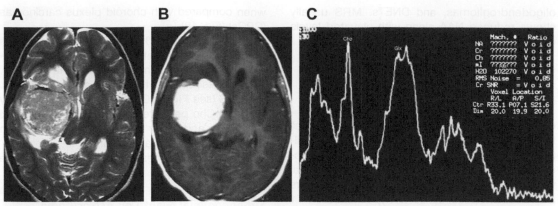

Fig. 19. Meningioma: 4-year-old girl with headaches, vomiting, and strabismus. There is a right sphenoid wing meningioma predominantly isointense on T2 (*A*), presenting with striking enhancement (*B*). MRS (*C*) demonstrates elevation of the Cho peak, Glx, and presence of Ala at 1.4 ppm.

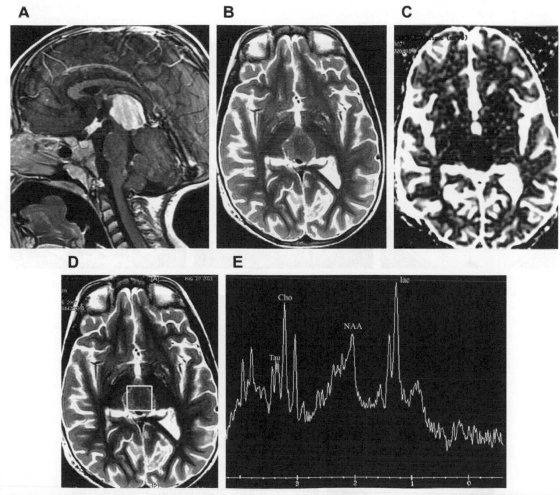

Fig. 20. Germinoma: 3-year-old boy with headaches, vomiting, drowsiness, and irritability. There is an enhancing mass in the pineal gland and suprasellar region (*A*), mildly T2 hypointense (*B*), with restricted diffusion (*C*, ADC map), compatible with high cellular density. The spectra (*D, E*) demonstrates reduction of the NAA peak, a Lac doublet at 1.3 ppm, and elevation of the Cho peak consistent with a high cellular tumor. Notice also a Tau peak next to the Cho peak.

oligodendrogliomas, and DNETs. MRS usually shows reduced NAA along with elevated levels of mI peak (see **Fig. 17C, D**).

SUPRATENTORIAL EXTRAPARENCHYMAL TUMORS
Choroid Plexus Tumors

Choroid plexus tumors represent 2% to 4% of all brain tumors in children.[2] Choroid plexus papillomas (CPPs) are well-circumscribed intraventricular masses that usually arise in the lateral ventricle, commonly in the trigone. These tumors are most often isointense to hypointense on T1 and hyperintense on T2; and they generally present with significant enhancement on MR imaging. MRS typically demonstrates significantly elevated mI peak, low Cr, and decreased Cho (see **Fig. 7**)

when compared with choroid plexus carcinomas (CPCs) (**Fig. 18**).[7,96]

CPCs represent 20% to 40% of choroid plexus tumors.[2] They are heterogeneous on MR imaging, extend beyond the margins of the ventricle, and are associated with edema and mass effect. On MRS (see **Fig. 18C**), they have a significantly elevated Cho peak, reduced mI peak compared with CPP, and lower Cr and Cr/tCr ratios than do other pediatric brain tumors.[96]

Prominent Lip resonances may also be observed in CPC.

Subependymal Giant Cell Astrocytoma

Subependymal giant cell astrocytoma (SEGA) is associated with tuberous sclerosis and may cause obstruction when located at the foramen of Monro.

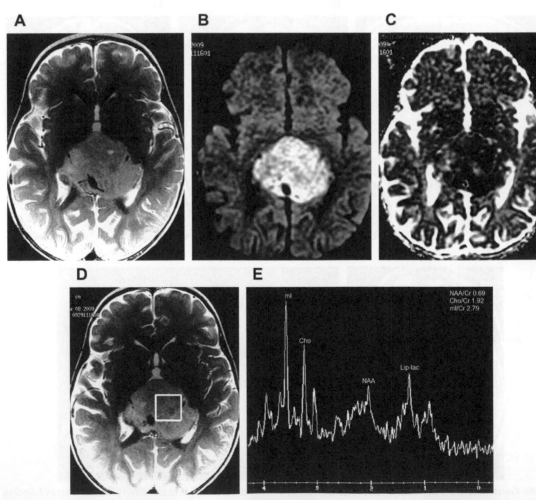

Fig. 21. Pineoblastoma: 20-month-old girl with difficulty walking and loss of motor skills. There is a solid pineal mass, T2 hypointense (*A*) presenting with restricted diffusion (*B, C*), indicating high cell density. Spectroscopy (*D, E*) demonstrates reduction of the NAA and Cr peaks, a significant elevation of the Cho peak, along with presence of Lips and lactate. Of note is elevation of the mI peak.

The MRS of SEGA is usually noisy, with high mI + gly at short TE being the most prominent finding.[97]

Meningioma

Meningiomas have a low incidence rate in children; and depending on the series, constitute approximately 1.0% to 7.7% of all CNS tumors.[98–101] Further; there is an increased association of meningiomas with NF-2 as well as in children who have had previous cranial irradiation.

Although meningiomas are readily diagnosed based on MR imaging features, the diagnosis may be confirmed by presence of Ala, which has been reported in many meningiomas.[102,103] Common spectral findings include significant elevation of Cho, modest elevation of the Glx peak, evidence of free Lips, and the presence of Ala (Fig. 19). The Cho peak is usually very high and should not suggest malignancy. Shah and colleagues[97] report that in cases of ventricular meningioma, high Glx may be seen.

PINEAL REGION TUMORS
Germ Cell Tumors

The CT appearance of germinoma is that of an isodense to hyperdense well-marginated mass.

On MRI, these tumors are usually isointense compared with cortical gray matter on T1 and T2 (Fig. 20).[6] They typically, although not always, demonstrate reduced diffusivity (see Fig. 20C).[104] MRS usually demonstrates evidence of a high cell density lesion characterized by elevated Cho peak (see Fig. 20D, E).

Tau is observed consistently in pineal germinoma, but at a lower concentration than in MBs. Glutamate may also be elevated.[7] Several studies suggest that increased Tau is associated with an increased cellular proliferation and tumoral aggressiveness.[3,7,18,38]

Pineal Parenchymal Tumors

Pineocytomas and pineoblastomas are tumors that arise from pineal parenchymal cells. Both

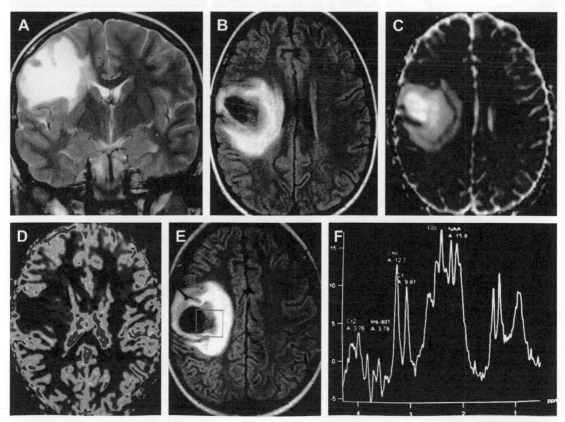

Fig. 22. Focal demyelination: 8-year-old boy with seizures in the left limb. There is a large right frontal mass presenting with high signal intensity on T2 (A). On FLAIR (B) small vessels can be seen within the lesion, suggesting perivenular demyelination. There is restricted diffusion in the periphery of the lesion (C, ADC-map) and no elevation of the CBV (D). The spectra (E, F) demonstrates a prominent Glx peak, more consistent with demyelination than tumor.

tumor types are considerably less common in children than pineal germ cell tumors.[6] Pineoblastomas are primitive, small round cell tumors that are highly cellular and are best classified as PNETs, grade IV embryonal tumors.

Harris and colleagues[105] recently reported that the MRS features of pineoblastoma include high Lips, reduced NAA, and elevated Cho peaks (**Fig. 21**). In addition, elevation of the ml peak may be seen occasionally.

DIFFERENTIAL DIAGNOSIS FOR FOCAL BRAIN TUMORS

MRS may provide additional information in cases in which the differential diagnosis by neuroimaging is difficult.

Tumor Versus Infection

In the case of a rim-enhancing lesion, to differentiate between a necrotic tumor and an abscess,

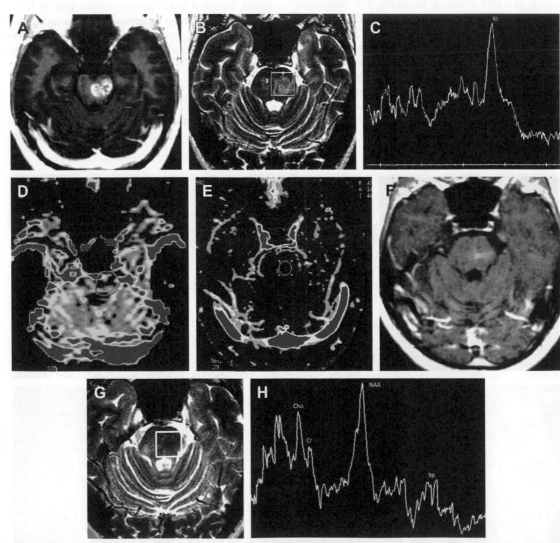

Fig. 23. Radiation Necrosis: 27-year-old man status post craniopharyrngioma resection at the age of 11 years and RT, now presenting with paresthesias in the inferior limbs and right arm as well as vertigo and dizziness. An outside MR was suggestive of pontine glioma. There is a left pontine lesion with irregular enhancement (A). MRS (B, C) demonstrates a prominent Lip peak and no elevation of the Cho, suggesting radiation necrosis. The CBV (D) is reduced and there is no increased permeability within the lesion (E), further suggesting radiation necrosis. Ten months after steroid therapy, the lesion had almost disappeared (F, axial with contrast, and G, axial T2), confirming the diagnosis of posttreatment changes. MRS (H) shows the Lip peak has reduced dramatically and normal metabolites can now be demonstrated.

the voxel should be placed within the cystic-necrotic area.[106] Presence of acetate, succinate, and amino acids, such as valine, alanine, and leucine, in the core of the lesion has high sensitivity for pyogenic abscess.[106,107]

Tumor Versus Pseudotumoral Demyelinating Plaque

A large masslike isolated inflammatory lesion may be seen in acute episodes of demyelination. During the acute phase of demyelination, Cho levels are usually elevated, and increased Lac and Lips are often seen in the setting of inflammatory infiltrates (**Fig. 22**).[9,108] Thus, increased Cho signal is believed to result from increased levels of myelin breakdown products, and short echo spectroscopy may likewise show increased glutamate and glutamine in demyelinating plaques, helping to distinguish inflammatory lesions from brain tumors.[109]

Tumor Versus Radiation Necrosis

MRS of radiation necrosis has shown the presence of a high Lip-dominant peak, low NAA peak, and a lower Cho peak compared with metastasis or glioblastoma (**Fig. 23**). The Lip-dominant peak may reflect the presence of the necrotic part of radiation necrosis. Fulham and colleagues[110–112] reported that a high lactate-dominant peak was observed in subacute radiation necrosis.

SUMMARY

Pediatric brain tumors are the most common solid tumor in children and the leading cause of death in this patient population. Yet, in spite of a high rate of incidence and mortality, our ability to reach rapid and definitive diagnoses has been historically impeded by (1) an inadequate grasp of the vast range of differential diagnoses that are possible in the setting of a suspected pediatric brain tumor, and (2) inadequate mastery of the precise imaging features of these numerous intracranial tumors and tumorlike conditions.

The primary objective of this article was to, first, briefly describe the most common brain tumors affecting children and adolescents, and, second, to offer a detailed overview of their respective imaging features on 1H-MRS, a noninvasive, in vivo imaging technique that provides additional metabolic diagnostic indices *beyond* anatomic information that is typically generated with conventional MR imaging. Indeed, with the introduction of advanced MRS, the neuroradiologist now has the tools needed to exploit a body of imaging information, including the precise histology and metabolic

profile of each lesion: information that is essential to understanding suggestive tumor characteristics and to developing appropriate differential diagnoses. For example, the metabolic information obtained from MRS can be used to complement standard MR imaging as an additional predictor of tumor aggressiveness. MRS also has the ability to differentiate tumors by identifying the various characteristics reflected in several metabolites, such as NAA; stable Cr, Cho; Tau; Glx; mI + gly; and Ala. MRS may also may provide prognostic information used to guide therapy early on in the patient's treatment, effectively improving outcomes and minimizing side effects, both in the short and long term.

Pediatric brain tumor type, then, forms the organizational basis of this article, from which various imaging features on MRS are defined, lesions are differentiated from one another, and differential diagnoses are developed. Once equipped with this critical information, clinicians will be enabled to make firm diagnoses, leading, in turn, to improved disease management, better patient outcomes, and enhanced quality of life in the setting of brain tumors of childhood.

REFERENCES

1. Gurney J, Smith M, Bunin G. CNS and miscellaneous intracranial and intraspinal neoplasms. In: Cancer Incidence and Survival among Children and Adolescents: United States SEER Program 1975-1995. NIH Publication No. 99-4649. In: Ries L, smith M, Gurney J, editors. National Cancer Institute SEER Program. Bethesda (MD): NIH Publication; 1999. p. 51–63.

2. Poussaint TY. Pediatric brain tumors. In: Newton HB, Jolesz FA, editors. Handbook of neuro-oncology neuroimaging. New York: Elsevier; 2008. p. 469–84.

3. Tong Z, Yamaki T, Harada K, et al. In vivo quantification of the metabolites in normal brain and brain tumors by proton MR spectroscopy using water as an internal standard. Magn Reson Imaging 2004; 22:1017–24.

4. Hwang JH, Egnaczyk GF, Ballard E, et al. Proton MR spectroscopic characteristics of pediatric pilocytic astrocytomas. AJNR Am J Neuroradiol 1998; 19:535–40.

5. Poussaint TY, Rodriguez D. Advanced neuroimaging of pediatric brain tumors: MR diffusion, MR perfusion, and MR spectroscopy. Neuroimaging Clin N Am 2006;16:169–92.

6. Barkovich AJ, Raybaud C. Intracranial, orbital and neck masses of childhood. In: Pediatric Neuroimaging. 5th edition. Philadelphia: Lippincott Williams & Wilkins and Wolters Kluwer; 2012. p. 637–711.

7. Panigrahy A, Krieger I, Gonzalez G, et al. Quantitative short echo time 1H-MR spectroscopy of untreated pediatric brain tumors: preoperative diagnosis and characterization. AJNR Am J Neuroradiol 2006;27:560–72.

8. Wang Z, Sutton LN, Cnaan A, et al. Proton MR spectroscopy of pediatric cerebellar tumors. AJNR Am J Neuroradiol 1995;16:1821–33.

9. Sutton LN, Wang Z, Gusnard D, et al. Proton magnetic resonance spectroscopy of pediatric brain tumors. Neurosurgery 1992;31:195–202.

10. Lazareff JA, Bockhorst KH, Curran J, et al. Pediatric low-grade gliomas: prognosis with proton magnetic resonance spectroscopic imaging. Neurosurgery 1998;43:809–17.

11. Lazareff JA, Olmstead C, Bockhorst KH, et al. Proton magnetic resonance spectroscopic imaging of pediatric low-grade astrocytomas. Childs Nerv Syst 1996;12:130–5.

12. Horska A, Ulug AM, Melhem ER, et al. Proton magnetic resonance spectroscopy of choroid plexus tumors in children. J Magn Reson Imaging 2001; 14:78–82.

13. Tzika AA, Vigneron DB, Dunn RS, et al. Intracranial tumors in children: small single-voxel proton MR spectroscopy using short and long-echo sequences. Neuroradiology 1996;38:254–6.

14. Girard N, Wang ZJ, Erbetta A, et al. Prognostic value of proton MR spectroscopy of cerebral hemisphere tumors in children. Neuroradiology 1998; 40:121–5.

15. Arle JE, Morriss C, Wang ZJ, et al. Prediction of posterior fossa tumor type in children by means of magnetic resonance image properties, spectroscopy, and neural networks. J Neurosurg 1997; 86:755–61.

16. Dezortova M, Hajek M, Cap F, et al. Comparison of MR spectroscopy and MR imaging with contrast agent in children with cerebral astrocytomas. Childs Nerv Syst 1999;15:408–12.

17. Brandão L, Domingues R. Intracranial neoplasms. In: McAllister L, Lazar T, Cook RE, editors. MR spectroscopy of the brain. Philadelphia: Lippincott Williams & Wilkins; 2003. p. 130–67.

18. Schneider JF, Gouny C, Viola A, et al. Multiparametric differentiation of posterior fossa tumors in children using diffusion-weighted imaging and short echo-time 1H-MR spectroscopy. J Magn Reson Imaging 2007;26:1390–8.

19. Panigrahy A, Nelson M, Blüml S. Magnetic resonance spectroscopy in pediatric neuroradiology: clinical and research applications. Pediatr Radiol 2010;40:3–30.

20. Barkovich A. Pediatric neuroimaging. 4th edition. Philadelphia: Lippincott Williams & Wilkins; 2005.

21. Nagel BJ, Palmer LS, Reddick WE, et al. Abnormal hippocampal development in children with medulloblastoma treated with risk-adapted irradiation. AJNR Am J Neuroradiol 2004;25: 1575–82.

22. Khong P, Kwong DL, Chan GC, et al. Diffusion-tensor imaging for the detection and quantification of treatment-induced white matter injury in children with medulloblastoma: a pilot study. AJNR Am J Neuroradiol 2003;24:734–40.

23. Kovantikaya A, Panigrahy A, Krieger MD, et al. Untreated pediatric primitive neuroectodermal tumor in vivo: quantification of taurine with MR spectroscopy. Radiology 2005;236:1020–5.

24. Annette C, Akinwandea D, Paynerb TD, et al. Medulloblastoma mimicking Lhermitte-Duclos disease on MRI and CT. Clin Neurol Neurosurg 2009;111: 536–53.

25. Bourgouin PM, Tampieri D, Grahovac SZ, et al. CT and MR imaging findings in adults with cerebellar medulloblastoma: comparison with findings in children. AJR Am J Roentgenol 1992;159:609–12.

26. Koci TM, Chiang F, Mehringer CM, et al. Adult cerebellar medulloblastoma: imaging features with emphasis on MR findings. AJNR Am J Neuroradiol 1993;14:929–39.

27. Meyers SP, Kemp SS, Tarr RW. MR imaging features of medulloblastomas. AJR Am J Roentgenol 1992;158:859–65.

28. Rollins N, Mendelshon D, Mulne A, et al. Recurrent medulloblastoma: frequency of tumor enhancement on Gd-DTPA MR imaging. AJNR Am J Neuroradiol 1990;11:583–7.

29. Zerbini C, Gelber RD, Weinberg D, et al. Prognostic factors in medulloblastoma, including DNA ploidy. J Clin Oncol 1993;11:616–22.

30. Kuhl J. Modern treatment strategies in medulloblastoma. Childs Nerv Syst 1998;14:2–5.

31. Rumboldt Z, Camacho DL, Lake D, et al. Apparent diffusion coefficients for differentiation of cerebellar tumors in children. AJNR Am J Neuroradiol 2006; 27:1362–9.

32. Yamasaki F, Kurisu K, Satoh K, et al. Apparent diffusion coefficient of human brain tumors at MR imaging. Radiology 2005;235:985–91.

33. Majós C, Alonso J, Aguilera C, et al. Adult primitive neuroectodermal tumor: proton MR spectroscopic findings with possible application for differential diagnosis. Radiology 2002;225:556–66.

34. Majós C, Aguilera C, Cós M, et al. In vivo proton magnetic resonance spectroscopy of intraventricular tumors of the brain. Eur Radiol 2009;19: 2049–59.

35. Jouanneau E, Tovar RA, Desuzinges C. Very late frontal relapse of medulloblastoma mimicking a meningioma in an adult. Usefulness of 1H magnetic resonance spectroscopy and diffusion-perfusion magnetic resonance imaging for preoperative diagnosis: case report. Neurosurgery 2006;58:E789–90.

36. Moreno-Torres A, Martínez-Pérez I, Baquero M, et al. Taurine detection by proton magnetic resonance spectroscopy in medulloblastoma: contribution to noninvasive differential diagnosis with cerebellar astrocytoma. Neurosurgery 2004;55: 824–9.

37. Wilke M, Eidenschink A, Muller-Weihrich S, et al. MR diffusion imaging and 1H spectroscopy in a child with medulloblastoma: a case report. Acta Radiol 2001;42:39–42.

38. Peeling J, Sutherland G. High-resolution 1H NMR spectroscopy studies of extracts of human cerebral neoplasms. Magn Reson Med 1992;24:123–6.

39. Michaelis T, Merboldt KD, Bruhn H, et al. Absolute concentrations of metabolites in the adult human brain in vivo: quantification of localized proton MR spectra. Radiology 1993;187:219–27.

40. Srivastava NK, Pradhan S, Gowda N, et al. In vitro, high-resolution 1H and 31P NMR based analysis of the lipid components in the tissue, serum, and CSF of the patients with primary brain tumors: one possible diagnostic view. NMR Biomed 2010;23: 113–22.

41. Peet AC, Daviesa NP, Lee R, et al. Magnetic resonance spectroscopy suggests key differences in the metastatic behaviour of medulloblastoma. Eur J Cancer 2007;43:1037–44.

42. Lindskog M, Kogner P, Ponthan F, et al. Non invasive estimation of tumour viability in a xenograft model of human neuroblastoma with proton magnetic resonance spectroscopy (1H MRS). Br J Cancer 2003;88:478–85.

43. Peet AC, Wilson M, Levine B, et al. 1H NMR spectroscopy identifies differences in choline metabolism related to the MYCN oncogene in neuroblastoma. Proc Intl Soc Mag Reson Med 2005;13:2489.

44. Rueckriegel SM, Driever PH, Bruhn H. Supratentorial neurometabolic alterations in pediatric survivors of posterior fossa tumors. Int J Radiat Oncol Biol Phys 2012;82(3):1135–41.

45. Pope WB, Kim HJ, Huo J, et al. Recurrent glioblastoma multiforme: ADC histogram analysis predicts response to bevacizumab treatment. Radiology 2009;252:182–9.

46. Al Sayyari A, Buckley R, McHenery C, et al. Distinguishing recurrent primary brain tumor from radiation injury: a preliminary study using a susceptibility-weighted MR imaging–guided apparent diffusion coefficient analysis strategy. AJNR Am J Neuroradiol 2010;31:1049–54.

47. Ertan Y, Sezak M, Turhan T, et al. Atypical teratoid/rhabdoid tumor of the central nervous system: clinicopathologic and immunohistochemical features of four cases. Childs Nerv Syst 2009;25:707–11.

48. Meyers SP, Khademian ZP, Biegel JA, et al. Primary intracranial atypical teratoid/rhabdoid tumors of infancy and childhood: MRI features and patient outcomes. AJNR Am J Neuroradiol 2006;27: 962–71.

49. Oka H, Scheithauer BW. Clinicopathological characteristics of atypical teratoid/rhabdoid tumor. Neurol Med Chir 1999;39:510–8.

50. Rorke LB, Packer RJ, Biegel JA. Central nervous system atypical teratoid/rhabdoid tumors in infancy and childhood: definition of an entity. J Neurosurg 1996;85:56–65.

51. Arslanoglu A, Aygun N, Tekhtani D, et al. Imaging findings of CNS atypical teratoid/rhabdoide tumors. AJNR Am J Neuroradiol 2004;25:476–80.

52. Lee WK, Choi CG, Lee JH. Atypical teratoid/rhabdoid of the cerebellum: report of two infantile cases. AJNR Am J Neuroradiol 2004;25:481–3.

53. Moeller KK, Coventry S, Jernigan S, et al. Atypical teratoid/rhabdoid tumor of the spine. AJNR Am J Neuroradiol 2007;28:593–5.

54. Gjerris F, Klinken L. Long-term prognosis in children with benign cerebellar astrocytoma. J Neurosurg 1978;49:179–84.

55. Pencalet P, Maixner W, Sainte-Rose C, et al. Benign cerebellar astrocytomas in children. J Neurosurg 1999;90:265–73.

56. Campbell JW, Pollack IF. Cerebellar astrocytomas in children. J Neurooncol 1996;28:223–31.

57. Porto L, Kieslich M, Franz K, et al. Spectroscopy of untreated pilocytic astrocytomas: do children and adults share some metabolic features in addition to their morphologic similarities? Childs Nerv Syst 2010;26:801–6.

58. Schneider JF, Viola A, Confort-Gouny S, et al. Infratentorial pediatric brain tumors: the value of new imaging modalities. J Neuroradiol 2007;34:49–58.

59. Harris L, Davies N, MacPherson L, et al. The use of short-echo time 1H MRS for childhood with cerebellar tumors prior to histopathological diagnosis. Pediatr Radiol 2007;37:1101–9.

60. Harris L, Davies N, MacPherson L, et al. Magnetic resonance spectroscopy in the assessment of pilocytic astrocytomas. Eur J Cancer 2008;44: 2640–7.

61. Blaser SI, Harwood-Nash DC. Neuroradiology of pediatric posterior fossa medulloblastoma. J Neurooncol 1996;29:23–34.

62. Kleihues P, Cavenee WK. World Health Organization classification of tumors: pathology and genetics of tumors of the central nervous system. Lyon (France): IARC Press; 2000.

63. Yuh EL, Barkovich AJ, Gupta N. Imaging of ependymomas: MRI and CT. Childs Nerv Syst 2009; 25:1203–13.

64. Uematsu Y, Hirano A, Llena JF. Electron microscopic observations of blood vessels in ependymoma. No Shinkei Geka 1988;16:1235–42 [in Japanese].

65. Chen CJ, Tseng YC, Hsu HL, et al. Imaging predictors of intracranial ependymomas. J Comput Assist Tomogr 2004;28:407–13.

66. Panigrahy A, Nelson MD Jr, Finlay JL, et al. Metabolism of diffuse intrinsic brainstem gliomas in children. Neuro Oncol 2008;10:32–44.

67. Lobel U, Sedlacik J, Reddick WE, et al. Quantitative diffusion-weighted and dynamic susceptibility-weighted contrast-enhanced perfusion MR imaging analysis of T2 hypointense lesion components in pediatric diffuse intrinsic pontine glioma. AJNR Am J Neuroradiol 2011;32:315–22.

68. Chen HJ, Panigrahy A, Dhall G, et al. Apparent diffusion and fractional anisotropy of diffuse intrinsic brain stem gliomas. AJNR Am J Neuroradiol 2010;31:1879–85.

69. Seymour ZA, Panigrahy A, Finlay JL, et al. Citrate in pediatric CNS tumors? AJNR Am J Neuroradiol 2008;29:1006–11.

70. Pan E, Prados M, Gupta N, et al, editors. Pediatric CNS tumors, vol. 3. Berlin, Heidelberg: Springer-Verlag; 2004. p. 49–61.

71. Farmer JP, Montes JL, Freeman CR, et al. Brainstem gliomas. A 10-year institutional review. Pediatr Neurosurg 2001;34:206–14.

72. Freeman CR, Farmer JP. Pediatric brain stem gliomas: a review. Int J Radiat Oncol Biol Phys 1998;40:265–71.

73. Mandell LR, Kadota R, Freeman C, et al. There is no role for hyperfractionated radiotherapy in the management of children with newly diagnosed diffuse intrinsic brainstem tumors: results of a pediatric oncology group phase III trial comparing conventional vs. hyperfractionated radiotherapy. Int J Radiat Oncol Biol Phys 1999;43:959–64.

74. Nelson MD, Soni D, Baram TZ. Necrosis in pontine gliomas: radiation induced or natural history? Radiology 1994;191:279–82.

75. Yoshimura J, Onda K, Tanaka R, et al. Clinicopathological study of diffuse type brainstem gliomas: analysis of 40 autopsy cases. Neurol Med Chir (Tokyo) 2003;43:375–82.

76. Laprie A, Pirzkall A, Haas-Kogan DA, et al. Longitudinal multivoxel MR spectroscopy study of pediatric diffuse brainstem gliomas treated with radiotherapy. Int J Radiat Oncol Biol Phys 2005;62:20–31.

77. Thakur SB, Karimi S, Dunkel IJ, et al. Longitudinal MR spectroscopic imaging of pediatric diffuse pontine tumors to assess tumor aggression and progression. AJNR Am J Neuroradiol 2006;27:806–9.

78. Hargrave D, Bartels U, Bouffet E. Diffuse brainstem glioma in children: critical review of clinical trials. Lancet Oncol 2006;7:241–8.

79. Castillo M, Smith JK, Kwock L. Correlation of myoinositol levels and grading of cerebral astrocytomas. AJNR Am J Neuroradiol 2000;21:1645–9.

80. Howe FA, Barton SJ, Cudlip SA, et al. Metabolic profiles of human brain tumors using quantitative in vivo 1H magnetic resonance spectroscopy. Magn Reson Med 2003;49:223–32.

81. Cheng LL, Chang IW, Louis DN, et al. Correlation of high-resolution magic angle spinning proton magnetic resonance spectroscopy with histopathology of intact human brain tumor specimens. Cancer Res 1998;58:1825–32.

82. Bluml S, Panigrahy A, Laskov M, et al. Elevated citrate in pediatric astrocytomas with malignant progression. Neuro Oncol 2011;13:1107–17.

83. Morales H, Kwock L, Castillo M. Magnetic resonance imaging and spectroscopy of pilomyxoid astrocytomas: case reports and comparison with pilocytic astrocytomas. J Comput Assist Tomogr 2007;31:682–7.

84. Komotar RJ, Burger PC, Carson BS, et al. Pilocytic and pilomyxoid hypothalamic/chiasmatic astrocytomas. Neurosurgery 2004;54:72–9.

85. Fernandez C, Figarella-Branger D, Girard N, et al. Pilocytic astrocytomas in children: prognostic factors a retrospective study of 80 cases. Neurosurgery 2003;53(3):544–53.

86. Cirak B, Horska A, Barker PB, et al. Proton magnetic resonance spectroscopic imaging in pediatric pilomyxoid astrocytoma. Childs Nerv Syst 2005;21:404–9.

87. Ellison DW. Childhood medulloblastoma: novel approaches to the classification of a heterogeneous disease. Acta Neuropathol 2010;120(3):305–16.

88. Louis D, Ohgaki H, Wiestler O, et al. The 2007 WHO classification of tumors of the central nervous system. Acta Neuropathol 2007;114:97–109.

89. Bing F, Nugues F, Grand S, et al. Primary intracranial extra-axial and supratentorial atypical rhabdoid tumor. Pediatr Neurol 2009;41:453–6.

90. Gauvain KM, McKinstry RC, Mukherjee P, et al. Evaluating pediatric brain tumor cellularity with diffusion-tensor imaging. AJR Am J Roentgenol 2001;177:449–54.

91. Law M, Kazmi K, Wetzel S, et al. Dynamic susceptibility contrast- enhanced perfusion and conventional MR imaging findings for adult patients with cerebral primitive neuroectodermal tumors. AJNR Am J Neuroradiol 2004;25:997–1005.

92. Cha S, Tihan T, Crawford F, et al. Differentiation of low grade oligodendrogliomas from low grade astrocytomas by using quantitative blood volume measurements derived from dynamic susceptibility contrast-enhanced MR imaging. AJNR Am J Neuroradiol 2005;26:266–73.

93. Jenkinson MD, Smith TS, Joyce KA, et al. Cerebral blood volume, genotype and chemosensitivity in oligodendroglial tumors. Neuroradiology 2006;48:703–13.

94. Xu M, See SJ, Ng WH, et al. Comparison of magnetic resonance spectroscopy and perfusion-weighted imaging in presurgical grading of oligodendroglial tumors. Neurosurgery 2005;56:919–26.

95. Bulakbasi N, Kocaoglu M, Sanal TH, et al. Dysembrioplastic neuroepithelial tumors: proton MR spectroscopy, diffusion and perfusion characteristics. Neuroradiology 2007;49:805–12.

96. Krieger MD, Panigrahy A, McComb JG, et al. Differentiation of choroid plexus tumors by advanced magnetic resonance spectroscopy. Neurosurg 2005;18:E4.

97. Shah T, Jayasundar R, Singh VP, et al. In vivo MRS study of intraventricular tumors. J Magn Reson Imaging 2011;34(5):1053–9.

98. Drake JM, Hendrick EB, Becker LE, et al. Intracranial meningiomas in children. Pediatr Neurosci 1985;12:134–9.

99. Kolluri VR, Reddy DR, Reddy PK, et al. Meningiomas in childhood. Childs Nerv Syst 1987;3:271–3.

100. Longstreth WT, Dennis LK, McGuire VM, et al. Epidemiology of intracranial meningioma. Cancer 1993;72:639–48.

101. Erdinçler P, Lena G, Sarioglu AC, et al. Intracranial meningiomas in children: review of 29 cases. Surg Neurol 1998;49:136–41.

102. Demir MK, Iplikcioglu AC, Dincer A, et al. Single voxel proton MR spectroscopy findings of typical and atypical intracranial meningiomas. Eur J Radiol 2006;60:48–55.

103. Rutten I, Raket D, Francotte N, et al. Contribution of NMR spectroscopy to the differential diagnosis of a recurrent cranial mass 7 years after irradiation for a pediatric ependymoma. Childs Nerv Syst 2006;22:1475–8.

104. Akinwande AD, Ying J, Momin Z, et al. Diffusion weighted imaging characteristics of primary central nervous system germinoma with histopathologic correlation: a retrospective study. Acad Radiol 2009;16:1356–65.

105. Harris LM, Davies NP, Wilson S, et al. Short echo time single voxel 1H magnetic resonance spectroscopy in the diagnosis and characterization of pineal tumors in children. Pediatr Blood Cancer 2011;57:972–7.

106. Pal D, Bhattacharyya A, Husain M, et al. In vivo proton MR spectroscopy evaluation of pyogenic brain abscesses: a report of 194 cases. AJNR Am J Neuroradiol 2010;31:360–6.

107. Lai PH, Ho JT, Chen WL, et al. Brain abscess and necrotic brain tumor: discrimination with proton MR spectroscopy and diffusion-weighted imaging. AJNR Am J Neuroradiol 2002;23(8):1369–77.

108. Bizzi A, Ulug AM, Crawford TO, et al. Quantitative proton MR spectroscopic imaging in acute disseminated encephalomyelitis. AJNR Am J Neuroradiol 2001;22:1125–30.

109. Cianfoni A, Niku S, Imbesi SG, et al. Metabolite findings in tumefactive demyelinating lesions utilizing short echo time proton magnetic resonance spectroscopy. AJNR Am J Neuroradiol 2007;28:272–7.

110. Fulham MJ, Bizzi A, Dietz MJ, et al. Mapping the brain tumor metabolites with proton MR spectroscopic imaging: clinical relevance. Radiology 1992;185:675–86.

111. Tzika AA, Cheng LL, Goumnerova L, et al. Biochemical characterization of pediatric brain tumors by using in vivo and ex vivo magnetic resonance spectroscopy. J Neurosurg 2002;96:1023–31.

112. Warren KE, Frank JA, Black JL, et al. Proton magnetic resonance spectroscopic imaging in children with recurrent primary brain tumors. J Clin Oncol 2000;18:1020–6.

Adult Brain Tumors
Clinical Applications of Magnetic Resonance Spectroscopy

Lara A. Brandão, MD[a,b,]*, Mauricio Castillo, MD[c]

KEYWORDS

- Proton magnetic resonance spectroscopy (H-MRS) • Adult brain tumors • Tumor histology
- Tumor grade • Tumor extension • Tumor progression • Therapeutic response
- Differential diagnosis

KEY POINTS

- Proton magnetic resonance spectroscopy (H-MRS) may be helpful in suggesting tumor histology and tumor grade and may better define tumor extension and the ideal site for biopsy compared with conventional magnetic resonance imaging.
- Combining H-MRS with other advanced imaging techniques such as diffusion-weighted imaging, perfusion-weighted imaging, and permeability maps improves diagnostic accuracy for intraaxial brain tumors.
- Short echo time allows for recognition of more metabolites than long echo time, which is important for differential diagnosis of brain masses and grading tumors.
- Higher choline (Cho) levels and lower myoinositol (Myo)/creatine (Cr) ratio are seen in more malignant tumors compared with lower-grade tumors.
- Lactate is directly related to tumor grade in adult brain tumors. However, lactate is found in essentially all pediatric brain tumors regardless of histologic grade.
- Gliomas are often invasive and show increased Cho levels in surrounding tissues, which may be used to distinguish these lesions from metastases.
- When lipids and lactate are found in a solid lesion, lymphoma should be suggested.
- A prominent lipid peak is seen in lymphomatosis cerebri, whereas a significant increase in Myo is characteristic of gliomatosis cerebri.
- A significant increase in the Cho peak and the presence of lipids and lactate are commonly seen in pilocytic astrocytoma, a grade I tumor.
- Typically, higher levels of Cho occur in grade III gliomas; whereas, in glioblastoma multiforme, the Cho levels may be much lower as a result of necrosis.
- If the Cho/N-acetylaspartate ratio is increased outside the area of enhancement, tumor infiltration can be diagnosed.
- An increase in Cho-containing compounds after radiation therapy may be seen in radiation necrosis misclassified as tumors.
- H-MRS in specific cases improves the accuracy and level of confidence in differentiating neoplastic from nonneoplastic masses.

Funding Sources: None.
Conflict of Interest: L.A. Brandão: None. M. Castillo: Editor in Chief, *American Journal of Neuroradiology*.
[a] Clínica Felippe Mattoso, Av. Das Américas 700, sala 320, Barra da Tijuca, Rio de Janeiro 30112011, Brazil;
[b] Clínica IRM- Ressonância Magnética, Rua Capitão Salomão 44 Humaitá, Rio de Janeiro 22271040, Brazil;
[c] Division of Neuroradiology, Department of Radiology, University of North Carolina School of Medicine, Room 3326, Old Infirmary Building, Manning Drive, Chapel Hill, NC 27599-7510, USA
* Corresponding author. Clínica Felippe Mattoso, Av. Das Américas 700, sala 320, Barra da Tijuca, Rio de Janeiro, CEP 30112011, Brazil.
E-mail address: larabrandao.rad@terra.com.br

neuroimaging.theclinics.com

INTRODUCTION

Localized proton magnetic resonance spectroscopy (H-MRS) of the human brain, first reported more than 20 years ago,[1–3] is a mature methodology used clinically worldwide for evaluation of brain tumors.[4] H-MRS may help with differential diagnosis, histologic grading, degree of infiltration, tumor recurrence, and response to treatment mainly when radiation necrosis develops and is indistinguishable from tumor by conventional magnetic resonance (MR) imaging.[5] Combining H-MRS with other advanced imaging techniques such as diffusion-weighted (DW) imaging, perfusion-weighted (PW) imaging, and permeability maps improves diagnostic accuracy for intraaxial brain tumors.[6–8]

TECHNIQUE
Short Echo Time Versus Long Echo Time

Different H-MRS parameters may be optimized and 1 of the most relevant is echo time (TE).[9] Short TE allows for recognition of more metabolites than long TE, which is important for differential diagnosis of brain masses and grading tumors. For example, myoinositol (Myo), a marker for low-grade gliomas, is only seen on short TE acquisitions.[5]

Multivoxel MRS Versus Single-Voxel MRS

A key consideration for brain tumor evaluations is their metabolic inhomogeneity. Multivoxel (MV) techniques, also called chemical shift imaging (CSI),[10] simultaneously record spectra from multiple regions and therefore map the spatial distribution of metabolites.[11] MV H-MRS provides smaller volumes of interest compared with single-voxel (SV), avoiding sampling error. For these reasons, high-resolution MV MRS such as MRS imaging is often favored for evaluating brain tumors.[5,12] Nevertheless, SV H-MRS has some advantages compared with MV techniques.[13] SV H-MRS is quicker and easier to obtain in standard clinical settings, providing the opportunity to obtain more than 1 spectrum (ie, spectra at 2 different TEs) in a reasonable amount of time. Evaluating spectra at both short and long TE improves the level of accuracy in differentiating focal brain lesions.[13] SV H-MRS provides better quality spectra compared with MRS imaging. The authors recommend that both techniques be used in the evaluation of brain masses (Fig. 1).

SPECTRAL PATTERN OF TUMORS

The spectral pattern of intracranial tumors may vary according to histology and malignancy grade and is discussed here.[14–18]

Reduction in N-Acetylaspartate Levels and in N-Acetylaspartate/Creatine Ratio

Reduction in N-acetylaspartate (NAA) levels and NAA/creatine (Cr) ratio is observed in tumors, indicating decreased viability and number of neurons (see Fig. 1; Fig. 2). The reader should bear in mind that in low-grade gliomas, the spectral pattern might be similar to that of normal brain (Fig. 3).[19] Absence of NAA in an intraaxial tumor generally implies an origin outside the central nervous system (metastasis) (Fig. 4) or a highly malignant tumor that has destroyed all neurons in that location (Fig. 5).[5]

Decreased Cr Levels

Decrease in Cr may occur, representing energy failure in aggressive malignant neoplasms (see Figs. 1 and 2).

Increase in Choline Levels and in Choline/NAA and Choline/Cr Ratios

An increase in choline (Cho) levels is shown by an increase in the Cho/NAA or Cho/Cr ratio, rather than its absolute concentration. Increased Cho is associated with higher turnover in the cell membrane and higher cell density resulting from proliferation of tumor cells (see Figs. 1 and 2).[20,21] In tumors, Cho levels correlate with the degree of malignancy and are linearly correlated with cell density (the inverse of what is seen with the apparent diffusion coefficient [ADC]) instead of the proliferative index. Higher Cho levels are seen in more malignant tumors (see Figs. 1 and 2) and lower levels in lower-grade tumors (see Fig. 3). Cho is usually higher in the center of a solid mass and decreases peripherally. Cho is consistently low in necrotic areas (see Fig. 5).[5]

Myo

Myo is a glial marker because it is primarily synthesized in glial cells, almost only in astrocytes. The Myo/Cr ratio is usually higher in lower-grade (see Fig. 3) than in higher-grade tumors (see Fig. 2).[22]

Lactate Peak

Increased lactate levels are likely the result of anaerobic glycolysis, although they can also be due to insufficient blood flow leading to ischemia or necrosis.[23,24] Lactate is directly related to tumor grade in adult brain tumors, with higher peaks seen in higher-grade tumors (see Fig. 2). However, lactate is found in essentially all pediatric brain tumors regardless of histologic grade.

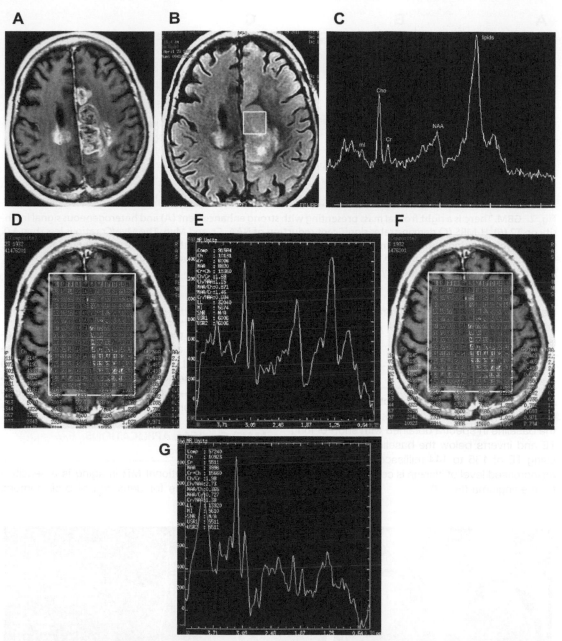

Fig. 1. MV MRS versus SV-MRS. A 79-year-old man presenting with right side hemiparesis of 1 month duration, seizures, and speech difficulties. There is a heterogeneously enhancing mass in the left frontal and parietal lobes, crossing the midline, surrounding the right lateral ventricle posteriorly (*A*) with extensive necrosis compatible with a GBM. SV-MRS (*B, C*) provides a good quality spectrum and demonstrates a significant increase of the lipid peak, increase of Cho and reduction of NAA, Cr, and Myo peaks. Spectra obtained from the left parietal region (*D, E*) demonstrate increased Cho and Cho/Cr and Cho/NAA ratios and a significant increase in the lipid peak compatible with extensive necrosis. MV MRS allows different areas to be evaluated at the same time. In the left frontal region (*F, G*), the main abnormality is an increase in the Cho peak. Cho, choline; Cho/Cr, choline/creatine; Cho/NAA, choline/N-acetyl-aspartate; Cr, creatine; MV MRS, multivoxel magnetic resonance spectroscopy; Myo, myo-inositol; NAA, N-acetyl-aspartate; SV MRS, single voxel magnetic resonance spectroscopy.

Lipids

Increased levels of lipids are believed to be caused by necrosis and membrane breakdown and are observed in metastasis (see **Fig. 4**),[25–28] aggressive high-grade primary brain tumors such as glioblastoma multiforme (GBM) (see **Figs. 1, 2**, and **5**) and lymphoma (**Fig. 6**), and in nonneoplastic

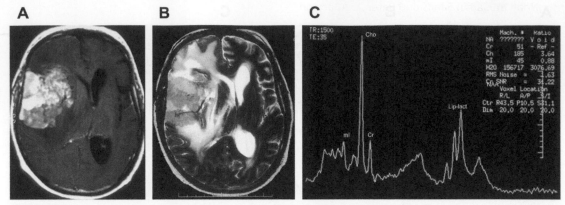

Fig. 2. GBM. There is a right frontal mass presenting with strong enhancement (*A*) and heterogeneous signal intensity on T2 (*B*). H-MRS (*C*) demonstrates significant reduction of NAA, Cr, and Myo. The Myo/Cr ratio is less than 1.0, which is typical for high-grade glioma. Note a significant increase in Cho and the presence of lipids and lactate. Cho, choline; Cr, creatine; H-MRS, proton magnetic resonance spectroscopy; mI, myo-inositol; Myo, myo-inositol; Myo/Cr, myo-inositol/creatine; NAA, N-acetyl-aspartate.

lesions such as inflammatory processes and abscesses. A prominent lipid peak is also characteristic for radiation necrosis.

Alanine

Alanine is an amino acid that has a doublet centered at 1.48 ppm. This peak is located above the baseline in spectra obtained with short or long TE and inverts below the baseline on acquisition using TE of 135 to 144 milliseconds.[5] In tumors, an increased level of alanine is considered specific for meningioma (**Fig. 7**).

Glutamine and Glutamate

Glutamine and glutamate (Glx) and Myo are metabolites better assessed with a TE of 30 milliseconds.[29] Except for meningiomas, in which an increased Glx peak may be seen (see **Fig. 7**), a significant increase in Glx levels should suggest nonneoplastic lesions.[19]

MAIN CLINICAL APPLICATIONS
Suggest Histology

Although conventional MR imaging is a sensitive modality available for detection of brain tumors,

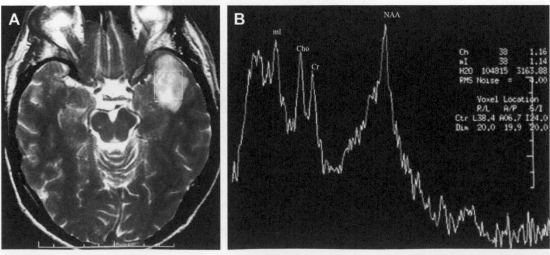

Fig. 3. Low-grade glioma (WHO grade II). A 51-year-old patient presenting with a circumscribed solid lesion in the left temporal lobe (*A*). The spectral pattern (*B*) is nearly normal: there is a discrete reduction in NAA as well a discrete increase in Cho with a Cho/Cr ratio of 1.16. The main abnormality in the curve is an increase in Myo (Myo/Cr 1.14), suggesting a low-grade tumor. Cho, choline; Cho/Cr, choline/creatine; mI, myo-inositol; Myo, myo-inositol; Myo/Cr, myo-inositol/creatine; NAA, N-acetyl-aspartate.

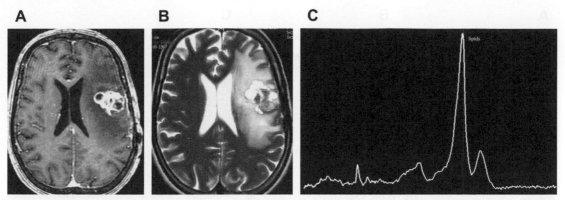

Fig. 4. Metastasis. There is a left frontal metastasis from breast cancer presenting with heterogeneous enhancement (A). A prominent lipid peak in the spectra (B, C) is related to extensive necrosis. No other metabolites are identified.

its specificity is low, and several tumor types may share a similar MR imaging appearance.[11] On the other hand, some tumors may present with a typical spectral pattern that may help to suggest the histology.

GBM

The spectral pattern of GBM is typical. There is a significant increase in Cho along with reduction of NAA, Cr, and Myo peaks. Increase of lipids and lactate is also common (see **Figs. 1** and **2**). When there is extensive necrosis, no increase in the Cho peak is seen. In this situation, prominent lipid and lactate peaks may be the only spectral abnormality (see **Fig. 5**). An overlap may be seen between the spectral pattern of GBM and metastasis. Although the absence of NAA in an intraaxial tumor generally implies an origin outside the central nervous system (metastasis) (see **Fig. 4**), a highly malignant tumor that has destroyed all neurons in that location may also demonstrate absence of NAA (see **Fig. 5**).[5] On the other hand,

NAA may be present in the spectra of a metastatic lesion if there is a partial volume effect with the adjacent parenchyma. For discriminating solitary metastases from primary high-grade tumors, it has been suggested that investigation of peri-enhancing tumor regions is useful. Metastases are encapsulated and do not show high Cho levels outside the region of enhancement, whereas gliomas are often invasive and show increased Cho in surrounding tissues.[7,30–35] However, if tumor infiltration is not significant, no increase in Cho is seen in the peritumoral area surrounding a GBM (**Fig. 8**).

Meningioma

Meningiomas are readily diagnosed based on conventional imaging features, but the diagnosis may be confirmed by the presence of alanine, which has been reported in many meningiomas.[36,37] A significant increase in Cho along with some increase in the Glx peak and the presence of alanine are common spectral findings (see **Fig. 7**).

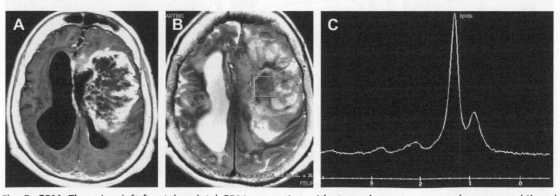

Fig. 5. GBM. There is a left frontal-parietal GBM presenting with strong heterogeneous enhancement (A) and heterogeneous signal intensity on T2 (B). Spectroscopy (C) demonstrates a prominent lipid peak. No other metabolites are identified.

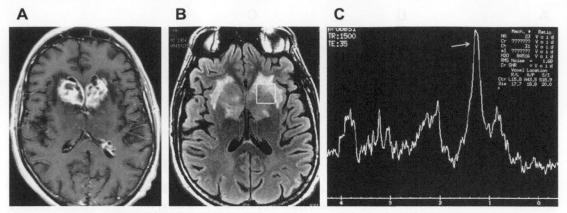

Fig. 6. Lymphoma. A 37-year-old man, human immunodeficiency virus (HIV) positive, diagnosed with brain lymphoma. There is a heterogeneously enhancing mass in the basal ganglia and adjacent to the frontal horns of the lateral ventricles (*A*). The spectra (*B, C*) demonstrate significant increase in the lipid peak (*arrow*).

Increase in Cho is characteristic and should not suggest malignancy. Meningiomas induced by radiation therapy tend to occur in younger patients, with equal frequency in males and females (sometimes more common in males), and present more atypia and higher nuclear/cytoplasm ratios.[38,39] In these cases, a large lipid peak along with reduction of all other metabolites including Cho may be seen. Their spectral pattern is similar to that of dural-based metastasis.

Lymphoma
Lymphomas may present as a solitary or multifocal solid lesion with no macroscopic evidence of necrosis in immunocompetent patients. On DW imaging, lymphoma shows hyperintensity with low ADC reflecting a higher nuclear/cytoplasm ratio.[40] The relative cerebral blood volume (rCBV) of lymphomas may be normal to slightly increased compared

with the rCBV of high-grade gliomas.[41,42] The spectral pattern of lymphomas is similar to that of other malignant tumors[6] and is characterized by increase in Cho, reduction in Myo, and prominent lipids. When lipids and lactate are found in a solid lesion, lymphoma should be suggested.[18,43,44] The spectral pattern described for solitary and multifocal (Fig. 9) lymphomas is similar to that seen in lymphomatosis cerebri (Fig. 10).

Gliomatosis cerebri
Gliomatosis cerebri is a distinct entity of glial tumors characterized by diffuse infiltration of the glial cell neoplasm throughout the brain. The WHO classification denotes grades II, III and IV gliomatosis cerebri.[45] Therefore, patients with this tumor have a variable prognosis. The most common finding in spectroscopy is reduction of NAA. Increase in Myo is characteristic of gliomatosis

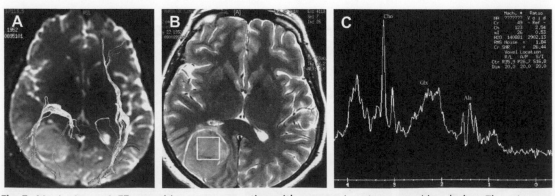

Fig. 7. Meningioma. A 57-year-old woman presenting with memory impairment and headaches. There is a meningioma in the right occipital region, displacing the optic radiations as seen on the diffusion tensor imaging (DTI) tractogram (*A*). Spectra (*B, C*) demonstrates elevation of Cho, some elevation of glutamine and glutamate (Glx), and presence of alanine. Ala, alanine; Cho, choline.

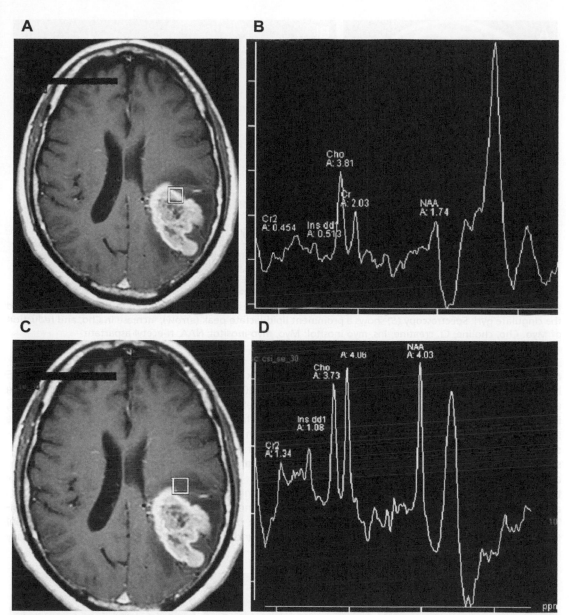

Fig. 8. *GBM.* 50-year-old man diagnosed with GBM. There is a heterogeneously enhancing lesion in the left parietal lobe (*A*). Spectrum from the margins of the lesion (*A, B*) demonstrates a significant increase in the lipid peak along with increases in Cho, Cho/Cr ratio, and Cho/NAA ratio as expected for a GBM. When the voxel is placed within the area of abnormal signal intensity surrounding the area of enhancement (*C*), no increase in the Cho peak, Cho/Cr ratio, or Cho/NAA ratio is demonstrated (*D*). Cho, choline; Cho/Cr, choline/creatine; Cho/NAA, choline/N-acetyl-aspartate; Cr, creatine; GBM, glioblastoma multiforme; Ins, Myo-inositol; NAA, N-acetyl-aspartate.

grade II, especially if there is no increase in Cho (**Fig. 11**).[46–49] Marked increases in Myo and Cr have been found in gliomatosis cerebri and may be attributed to glial activation rather than to glial proliferation because the Cho level is only moderately increased suggesting low glial cell density.[48] Sometimes Cho is reduced (see **Fig. 11**). A prominent lipid peak is seen in lymphomatosis cerebri (see **Fig. 10**), whereas a significant increase in Myo is characteristic of gliomatosis cerebri (see **Fig. 11**). In patients diagnosed with gliomatosis grade III, the Myo peak will be reduced and elevation of the Cho peak will be demonstrated (**Fig. 12**).

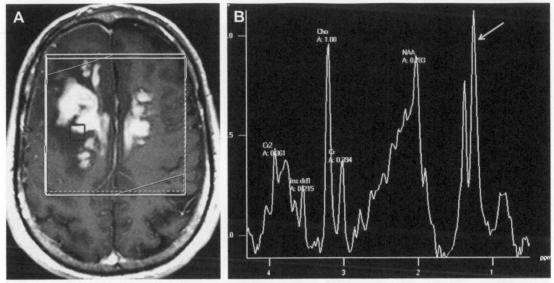

Fig. 9. Multifocal lymphoma. Multifocal solid enhancing nodules (A) are demonstrated in the frontal lobes and the cingulate gyri. Spectroscopy (B) shows a prominent lipid-lactate peak (arrow), increase in Cho, and reduction of Myo. Cho, choline; Cr, creatine; Ins, myo-inositol; Myo, myo-inositol; NAA, N-acetyl-aspartate.

Medulloblastoma

Medulloblastomas are more common in the pediatric population, although they may also present in adults aged 30 to 35 years. They are aggressive tumors (WHO grade IV) with a high propensity to disseminate throughout the cerebral fluid space. Their spectral pattern is characterized by a significant increase in Cho along with a reduction in the NAA and Myo peaks. Some lipids and lactate may be seen. Spectra with short TE show increased taurine at 3.3 ppm in patients.[50–55] Altering the TE can confirm that a peak at 3.3 ppm corresponds to taurine. At a TE of 30 milliseconds, taurine projects above the baseline, whereas at a TE of 144 milliseconds, the taurine peak is below the baseline.[50] It has been speculated that increased taurine is associated with increased cellular proliferation and tumoral aggressiveness.[50–52,55,56]

Ependymoma

Ependymomas are more common in the pediatric population, although they may also present around the age of 30 to 35 years. They typically

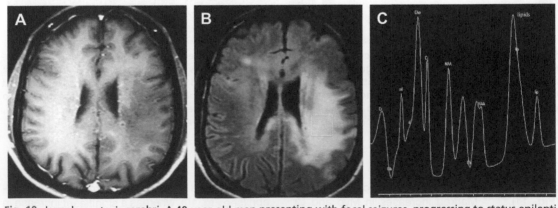

Fig. 10. Lymphomatosis cerebri. A 40-year-old man presenting with focal seizures, progressing to status epilepticus. There is a nonenhancing lesion compromising most of the left hemisphere (A), crossing the midline, and presenting with high signal intensity on the fluid attenuated inversion recovery (FLAIR) sequence (B). Spectroscopy (B, C) demonstrates a prominent lipid peak, increase in the Cho peak, and reduction of Myo. Cho, choline; Cr, creatine; mI, myo-inositol; Myo, myo-inositol; NAA, N-acetyl-aspartate. (Courtesy of Dr Leonardo Avanza, Espírito Santo, Brazil.)

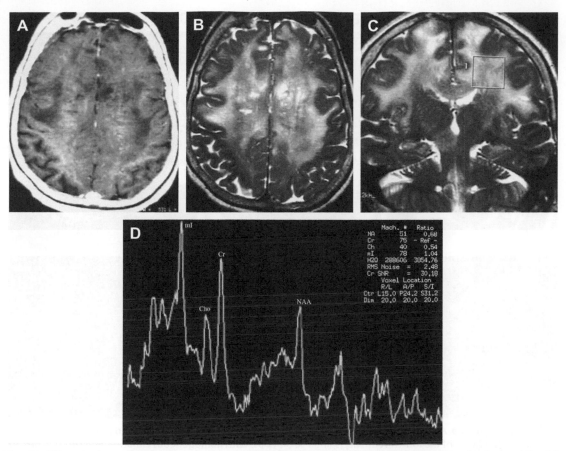

Fig. 11. Gliomatosis cerebri. A 49-year-old woman presenting with a nonenhancing infiltrative lesion (*A*) with high signal intensity on T2 (*B, C*) compromising the frontal and parietal lobes bilaterally. Spectroscopy (*C, D*) demonstrates increased Myo along with a reduction in the Cho and NAA peaks. Cr is also increased. Cho, choline; Cr, creatine; Myo, myo-inositol; NAA, N-acetyl-aspartate.

occur within the fourth ventricle. A most important imaging finding to identify ependymomas is extension of the tumor through the fourth ventricular outflow foramina (**Fig. 13**).[57–59] On computed tomography, the tumor reveals mixed density with punctate calcification in 50% of cases, with variable enhancement.[57] These tumors are heterogeneous on MR imaging, reflecting a combination of

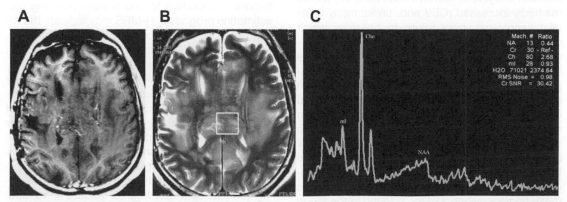

Fig. 12. Gliomatosis cerebri. There is an extensive infiltrating lesion compromising the frontal and parietal lobes, presenting with some tiny areas of discrete irregular enhancement (*A*) and high signal intensity on T2 (*B*). Spectroscopy (*B, C*) demonstrates prominent Cho and reduction in the Myo, Cr, and NAA peaks; a spectral pattern different from that shown in **Fig. 11**. Cho, choline; Cr, creatine; ml, myo-inositol; Myo, myo-inositol; NAA, N-acetyl-aspartate.

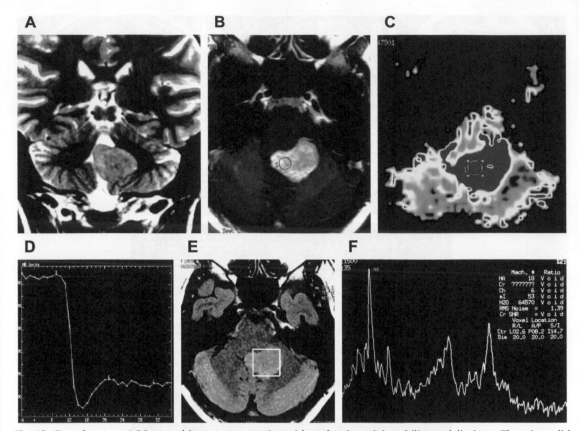

Fig. 13. Ependymoma. A 36-year-old woman presenting with neck pain, gait instability, and dizziness. There is a solid mass within the cavity of the fourth ventricle, isointense on T2 (*A*) with homogeneous enhancement (*B*). The mass extends through the fourth ventricular outflow foramina of Luschka into the left cerebello-pontine angle. A perfusion study (*C, D*) demonstrates a significant increase in rCBV with poor return to baseline indicating leaky tumoral blood vessels (*D*). The main finding on spectroscopy (*E, F*) is increased Myo. No increase in the Cho peak is demonstrated. Cho, choline; ml, myo-inositol; Myo, myo-inositol; rCBV, relative cerebral blood volume.

solid component, cyst, calcification, necrosis, edema, or hemorrhage.[60] When performed, perfusion MR imaging of ependymoma generally shows markedly increased rCBV and, unlike many other glial neoplasms, poor return to baseline, which may be attributable to fenestrated blood vessels and an incomplete blood-brain barrier (see **Fig. 13**C, D).[61,62] MRS shows considerable heterogeneity.[57] In general, ependymomas have low NAA and moderately increased Cho and Cr.[57] Harris and colleagues[63] stated that the presence of high Myo strongly suggests a diagnosis of ependymoma when short TE (30 milliseconds) is used at 1.5 T (see **Fig. 13**E–F). Another study also demonstrated that high Myo and glycine are found in ependymomas, more significant at short TE.[51] According to these findings, when a mass is found in the fourth ventricle, high Myo and glycine suggest ependymoma, whereas high Cho supports primitive neuroendocrine tumor.[64] Sometimes, no increase in Cho is seen in ependymomas (see **Fig. 13**F).

Suggest Tumor Grade

Differentiation between high-grade and low-grade tumors is important for therapeutic planning and estimating prognosis. H-MRS may indicate the tumor grade with more accuracy than a blind biopsy, because it assesses a larger amount of tissue than what is usually excised at biopsy.[43]

Tumors are commonly heterogeneous, and their spectra may vary depending on the region sampled by MRS.[65,66] Hence, the region of interest chosen for analysis has a large influence on the results, and, as stated earlier, MRS imaging is generally considered preferable because it allows metabolic heterogeneity to be evaluated. One recent MRS imaging study used MR perfusion imaging (arterial spin labeling) to guide the spectral measurement location; in regions with increased flow, Cho was found to be higher in high-grade gliomas compared with low-grade gliomas.[67] No metabolic differences between high-grade and low-grade gliomas were found in normal or hypo-perfused tumor regions.

H-MRS is considered 96% accurate in differentiating low-grade versus high-grade gliomas.[68] H-MRS may be readily integrated into a multimodality MR imaging examination for presurgical evaluation of patients with gliomas.[69-72]

Useful metabolites for suggesting tumor grade

Cho Increased Cho correlates with cellular proliferation and density. There is a high correlation between the in vivo concentration of Cho in brain tumors and in vitro tumor proliferation markers. Statistically significant higher Cho/Cr, Cho/NAA, and rCBV values in high-grade gliomas than in low-grade gliomas have been reported,[42] although threshold values of metabolite ratios for grading of gliomas are not well established. Cho/Cr is the most frequently used ratio. Some institutions use

a threshold value of 2.0 for Cho/Cr to differentiate low-grade from high-grade gliomas; others use a cutoff value of 2.5. Although increased Cho is related to tumor grade (higher Cho is found in higher-grade tumors than in lower-grade tumors), some studies have found grade IV GBM to have lower levels of Cho (see **Fig. 1C**) than grade II or grade III (**Fig. 14**) gliomas.[26] This may be due to the presence of necrosis in high-grade tumors, because necrosis is associated with a prominent lipid peak along with reduction of all other metabolites (see **Fig. 5**).[73]

Lipids and lactate The presence of lipids and lactate correlates with necrosis in high-grade gliomas (see **Figs. 1, 2**, and **5**). Di Constanzo and colleagues[69] evaluated 31 patients with either high-grade or low-grade tumors through multimodality 3-T MR imaging (including long TE MRS

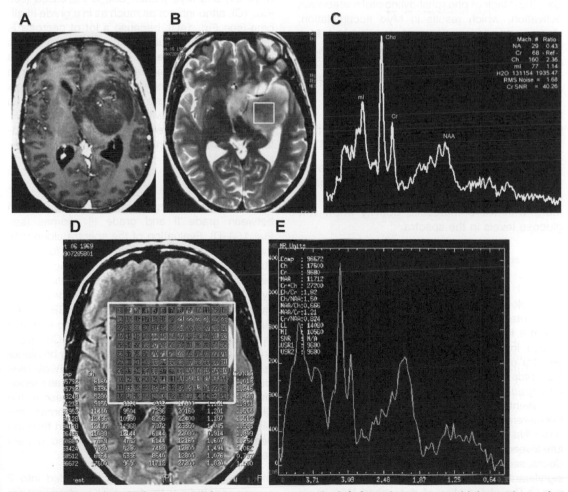

Fig. 14. Grade III glioma. There is a solid mass compromising the left frontal and temporal lobes with tiny foci of enhancement (*A*), isointense on T2 (*B*) suggesting high cell density. SV-MRS (*B, C*) demonstrates a significant increase in Cho along with a reduction in NAA and Cr. MV MRS (*D, E*) demonstrates the same findings. Cho, choline; Cr, creatine; mI, myo-inositol; NAA, N-acetyl-aspartate.

imaging). They concluded that high-grade and low-grade tumors and their margins could be differentiated based on the lactate/lipid signal and rCBV. Lipids are also the main spectral finding in metastasis (see **Fig. 4**). When lipids are demonstrated in solid lesions, lymphoma should also be considered (see **Fig. 9**).

Increase in the lipid peak is inversely correlated to survival.[74]

Lipids and lactate, although usually related to high-grade primary brain tumors and metastasis, may also be demonstrated in pilocytic astrocytomas.

Myo Useful information on tumor grade may be acquired by using a short TE (30–35 milliseconds) to assess Myo.[22] In low-grade tumors, the Myo/Cr ratio is typically higher (see **Fig. 3**) than in high-grade tumors (see **Figs. 1** and **2**).[24,26] This may be due to a low mitotic index in low-grade gliomas and, thus, lack of phosphatidylinositol metabolism activation, which results in Myo accumulation. Howe and colleagues[26] concluded that high Myo was characteristic of grade II astrocytomas. Increased levels of Myo have been reported to be useful for identifying low-grade astrocytomas in which the Cho/Cr ratio was not altered.[75,76]

NAA and Cr The greatest reductions in NAA and Cr levels occur in higher-grade tumors (compare **Figs. 1** and **2** with **Fig. 3**).

Glucose Short TE spectra may allow the evaluation of a peak around 3.67 ppm (probably glucose), which is directly related to survival. Tumors with more metabolic activity show low glucose levels in the spectra.[74]

Typical spectral findings in grade II, III, and IV gliomas

Grade II gliomas H-MRS in low-grade gliomas may look similar to normal spectra, demonstrating a discrete reduction in the NAA peak, along with a discrete increase in the Cho peak.[26,50,77] An increase in Myo can be the only finding in the spectra of a grade II astrocytoma (see **Fig. 3**).[13] No lipids or lactate are usually demonstrated. Low-grade glioma was studied in vivo at 4 T in 11 patients using H-MRS (incorporating the direct measurement of macromolecules in the spectrum) and [23]Na imaging. The results showed that absolute levels of glutamate and NAA were significantly decreased, whereas levels of Myo and [23]Na were significantly increased in low-grade glioma tissue.[78] The observation of decreased NAA levels is consistent with previous studies.[26,50,77–79] The observed decrease in glutamate contradicts a previous study[79] performed at 1.5 T that suggested

that increased Glx maybe characteristic of low-grade gliomas. The discrepancy may be due to the removal of the macromolecule baseline signal intensity in the current study before quantification. The observed increase in Myo is consistent with previous studies.[24,26]

Grade III gliomas In grade III gliomas, there is a significant increase in the Cho peak, which correlates well with high cell density in these tumors.[80] The NAA, Cr, and Myo peaks are reduced (see **Fig. 14**). Metastases and glioblastomas nearly always show increased lipid peaks; thus, if the lesion does not exhibit mobile lipid signals, anaplastic glioma is more likely.[81] In the authors' experience, however, some increase in lipids and lactate may be seen in grade III gliomas (**Fig. 15A, B**).

Grade IV gliomas The spectral pattern of grade IV gliomas is characterized by severe reduction of the NAA, Cr, and Myo peaks. Cho is increased (see **Fig. 1C**), although not as much as in a grade III glioma (see **Fig. 14C**), because a lot of necrosis is usually present in grade IV gliomas, which results in a significant increase in the lipid peak (see **Fig. 1C**). Typically, higher levels of Cho occur in grade III gliomas, whereas, in GBM, the Cho levels may be much lower as a result of necrosis.[82] When the voxel is placed within the necrotic area of a GBM, no Cho is detected and a prominent lipid-lactate peak is the only spectral abnormality (see **Fig. 5**).[82]

Special things to remember

Some overlap in the spectral pattern may be seen between grade II and grade III gliomas (see **Fig. 15A–D**). Evaluation of the spectra along with the information obtained from the other functional studies such as DW imaging, PW imaging, and permeability maps enhance the diagnostic capacity of brain tumors (see **Fig. 15E–J**). Some aggressive tumors, such as metastases, GBM, and gliomatosis cerebri may present with no increase in Cho (see **Figs. 4, 5**, and **11**). The Cho peak and the Cho/Cr and Cho/NAA ratios may be higher in grade III (see **Fig. 14C**) than in grade IV gliomas (see **Fig. 1C**). Some benign tumors such as meningiomas present with a significant increase in the Cho peak (see **Fig. 7**). Pilocytic astrocytomas usually present with a significant increase in the Cho peak. Some lipids and lactate are also usually seen in these tumors.

Oligodendroglioma This tumor is divided into 2 groups according to the WHO classification: grades II and III.[83] It originates from oligodendrocytes but often contains a mixed population of cells, particularly astrocytes. On dynamic

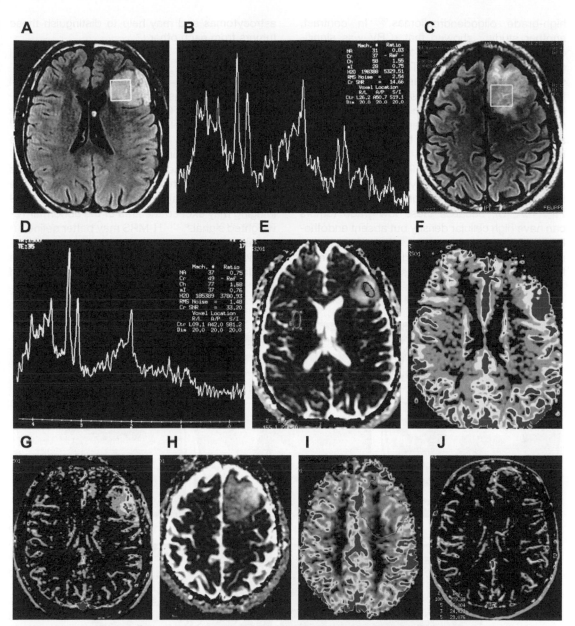

Fig. 15. Grade II versus grade III: a multimodality approach. (A, B) Conventional MR imaging and spectra obtained from a grade III glioma and from a grade II oligodendroglial tumor (C, D). In both cases there is an increase in the Cho peak. The Cho/Cr ratio is 1.55 in patient 1 (A, B) and 1.58 in patient 2 (C, D). There is a reduction in Myo in both cases, and the Myo/Cr ratio is 0.75 in patient 1 and 0.76 in patient 2. Despite similarities, some lipids and lactate are seen in the spectrum from patient 1 (B), suggesting a higher-grade lesion. In patient 1 (grade III glioma), an area of restricted diffusion is demonstrated within the lesion (E, ADC map) indicating high cell density. There is a significant increase in blood volume (F, rCBV map) and very high permeability (G), once again suggesting a high-grade tumor. In patient 2 (grade II glioma), no areas of restricted diffusion are seen (H, ADC map). There is a small area of discrete increased blood volume (I, rCBV) and no significant increase in permeability (J). ADC map, apparent diffusion coefficient map; Cho, choline; Myo, myo-inositol; rCBV map, relative cerebral blood volume map.

contrast-enhanced MR perfusion, low-grade oligodendrogliomas may demonstrate high rCBV because they contain a dense network of branching capillaries.[84,85] Thus, many oligodendrogliomas can be misinterpreted as high-grade tumors because of their high rCBV.

One study showed that rCBV was not significantly different between low-grade and high-grade oligodendrogliomas.[66] In contrast, another study[86] showed that rCBV was significantly different between low-grade and high-grade oligodendrogliomas. The results of H-MRS studies in oligodendrogliomas are more consistent than those of MR perfusion studies. Similar to astrocytomas, H-MRS of oligodendrogliomas demonstrates significantly higher Cho, Cho/Cr ratio, and a higher incidence of lactate and lipids in high-grade tumors than in low-grade tumors.[79,86,87] Nevertheless, low-grade oligodendrogliomas may show highly increased Cho (see Fig. 15C, D), mimicking high-grade tumors (see Fig. 15A, B), because these low-grade tumors can have high cellular density but absent endothelial proliferation and necrosis.[86] Apart from higher rCBV, the level of Glx is significantly higher in low-grade oligodendrogliomas than in low-grade

astrocytomas and may help to distinguish these tumors from each other.[79]

Assess Tumor Extension

In infiltrative lesions, tumor activity can be demonstrated by H-MRS beyond the enhanced area identified on gadolinium-enhanced conventional MR imaging (Figs. 16 and 17). Comparison of the extent (and location) of active tumor as defined by MR imaging and MRS imaging demonstrates the differences between the 2 techniques.[87] The area of metabolic abnormality as defined by MRS imaging may exceed the area of the abnormal T2-weighted signal.[87–90] H-MRS may better define tumor extension than conventional MR imaging.[91]

Cho has been found to correlate well with the cellular density of the tumor[80] and the degree of

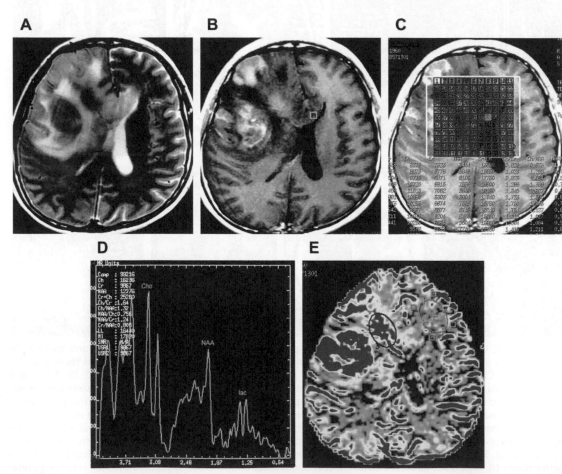

Fig. 16. Tumor extension. A 48-year-old woman diagnosed with GBM. There is a large infiltrative lesion in the right frontal lobe crossing the midline with heterogeneous signal intensity on T2 (A) and areas of contrast enhancement (B). MV MRS (C, D) demonstrates significant increase in Cho and the Cho/Cr and Cho/NAA ratios in the corpus callosum along with the presence of lactate compatible with tumor infiltration beyond the areas of enhancement. There is also an increase in blood volume in the same area (E, rCBV map). Cho, choline; lac, lactate; MV MRS, multivoxel magnetic resonance spectroscopy; NAA, N-acetyl-aspartate; rCBV map, relative cerebral blood volume map.

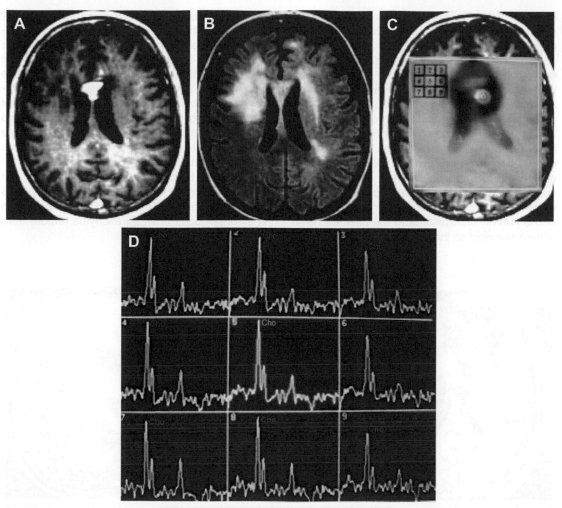

Fig. 17. Tumor extension. A 71-year-old man diagnosed with lymphoma. There is a solid enhancing nodule compromising the corpus callosum (*A*). FLAIR demonstrates an ill-defined high signal intensity abnormality in the frontal lobes surrounding the solid nodule, which could represent vasogenic edema and/or tumor infiltration (*B*). MV MRS (*C, D*) better defines tumor extension, demonstrating a significant increase in Cho, and the Cho/NAA and Cho/Cr ratios in all voxels. Cho, choline; Cho/Cr, choline/creatine; Cho/NAA, choline/N-acetyl-aspartate; MV MRS, multivoxel magnetic resonance spectroscopy.

tumor infiltration into brain tissue.[92] The use of MRS imaging to map Cho levels has been suggested as a method for defining tumor boundaries. To assess the degree of tumor infiltration, MRS imaging data obtained from 7 patients with untreated supratentorial gliomas (WHO grades II and III) were fused with three-dimensional MR imaging data sets and integrated into a frameless stereotactic system for image-guided surgery in an interactive manner.[89] Tissue samples were obtained from 3 regions, defined individually in each patient based on the Cho/NAA ratio: (1) a spectroscopically normal region, (2) a transitional region, and (3) a region with maximum spectroscopic abnormality. In all cases, the highest Cho/NAA ratios were obtained in the tumor center, and

intermediate values in the regions of low tumor invasion. In 4 patients, however, biopsies sampled in regions with normal Cho/NAA ratio showed tumor infiltration. One of the reasons may be the low resolution of MRS imaging with respect to glioma borders.[89] Based on this observation, it can be concluded that if the Cho/NAA ratio is increased outside the area of enhancement, tumor infiltration can be diagnosed. On the other hand, if no increase in the Cho/NAA ratio is demonstrated, tumor infiltration cannot be ruled out. The reason for this is probably the fact that increases in the Cho/Cr and Cho/NAA ratios are related to the number of neoplastic cells that have infiltrated outside the enhancing lesion. A retrospective study performed on 10 gliomas examined the relationship between metabolite levels and histopathologic parameters in the border zone of gliomas.[93] A strong negative correlation was detected between NAA concentration and both absolute and relative measures of tumor infiltration; no correlation for Cho was detected. The study concluded that NAA concentration is the most significant parameter for the detection of low levels of tumor cell infiltration.[93] MRS may demonstrate tumor infiltration not only in the area of vasogenic edema but also in the normal-appearing white matter (NAWM) contralateral to the affected hemisphere. Kallenberg and colleagues[94] have shown that, in patients with histopathologically confirmed primary GBM, H-MRS of the NAWM contralateral to the affected hemisphere revealed an increase in the concentrations of Myo and glutamine but otherwise normal metabolite levels. These results indicate increased density of cells of astrocytic origin in the NAWM of patients with GBM in the presence of still normal neuroaxonal tissue, as indicated by the absence of changes in the major metabolites. This observation may, in turn, be taken as a potential indicator of the presence of tumor cells in NAWM, representing an early sign of neoplastic infiltration, suggesting a new role for H-MRS in the treatment of patients with brain tumors.[94]

The results from this study are in agreement with findings observed in previous reports on H-MRS and conventional MR imaging of glioma infiltration in inconspicuous brain parenchyma remote from the tumor.[95–98]

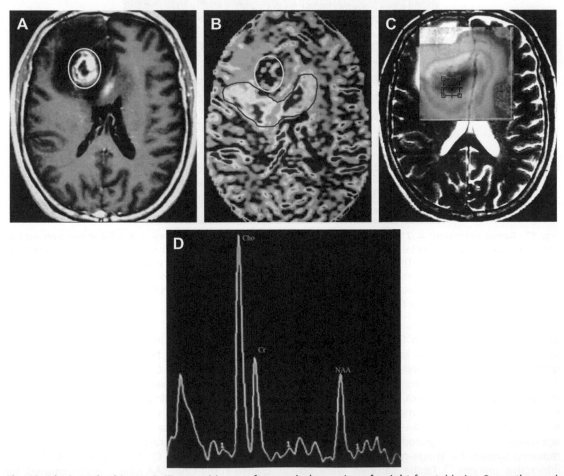

Fig. 18. Ideal site for biopsy. A 47-year-old man after surgical resection of a right frontal lesion 3 months previously; pathology was negative. The area that enhances (*circle A*) presents with low capillary density seen as low perfusion (*B, rCBV map*) and thus is not the ideal site for biopsy. Surrounding the area of enhancement posteriorly, there is an area of high capillary density (*B, red circle*) seen as high perfusion and high cell density (*C, D*) presenting with high Cho and high Cho/Cr and Cho/NAA ratios. This area is the best site for biopsy. Cho, choline; Cho/Cr, choline/creatine; Cho/NAA, choline/N-acetyl-aspartate; Cr, creatine; NAA, N-acetyl-aspartate; rCBV map, relative cerebral blood volume map.

Indicate the Ideal Site for Biopsy

Biopsy is not always performed in the area of the tumor with greatest cellularity so it may underestimate the pathology of the lesion.[43] By evaluating metabolic abnormalities, H-MRS may better define the ideal site for biopsy than conventional MR imaging.[42] Stereotactic brain biopsy is usually performed based on the anatomic appearance of the lesion or enhancement characteristics.[99] The area of enhancement does not necessarily represent the area of greater tumor activity. In high-grade heterogeneous tumors, there is a possibility that unspecific or lower-grade tumor tissue is sampled or that important functional tracts are damaged. Ideally, regions of increased angiogenesis, vascular permeability, and high metabolic activity should be sampled.[100] The role of H-MRS in biopsy guidance is to recognize regions of high metabolic activity: regions of increased Cho levels (and low NAA levels) indicating tumor tissue are a good target for biopsy (Fig. 18).[99,101–104] Regions with low Cho and NAA levels may indicate

radiation necrosis, astrogliosis, macrophage infiltration, or mixed tissue.

Follow Tumor Progression

Serial H-MRS examinations may be used to follow the progression of gliomas.[105,106] Anaplastic degeneration can be demonstrated early with H-MRS and perfusion mapping compared with conventional MR imaging. Tumor progression is characterized by increased Cho levels in serial examinations (Fig. 19).[105] Tedeschi and colleagues[105] demonstrated that interval percentage changes in Cho intensity in stable gliomas and progressive gliomas (malignant degeneration or recurrent disease) is less than 35 and more than 45, respectively. Interval increased Cho/Cr or Cho/NAA is suggestive of malignant progression.

Predict Prognosis and Survival

Histopathology remains the gold standard for prognostic assessment, providing insights into

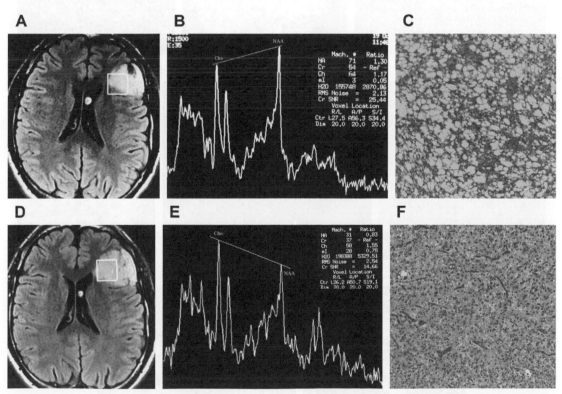

Fig. 19. Tumor progression. A 27-year-old man presenting with seizures. First examination demonstrates a left frontal lesion with high signal intensity on the FLAIR sequence (A). Spectroscopy demonstrates that the NAA peak is higher than the Cho peak (B). Biopsy results were compatible with a grade II glioma (C). Nine months later, (D, E) Cho is higher than NAA indicating higher cell density and suggesting anaplastic transformation. The lesion was resected and pathology demonstrated a high cell density and highly vascular lesion, compatible with grade III glioma (F), as suggested by the MRS study. Cho, choline; MRS, magnetic resonance spectroscopy; NAA, N-acetyl-aspartate. ([C, E] Courtesy of Dr Leila Chimelli, Rio de Janeiro, Brazil.)

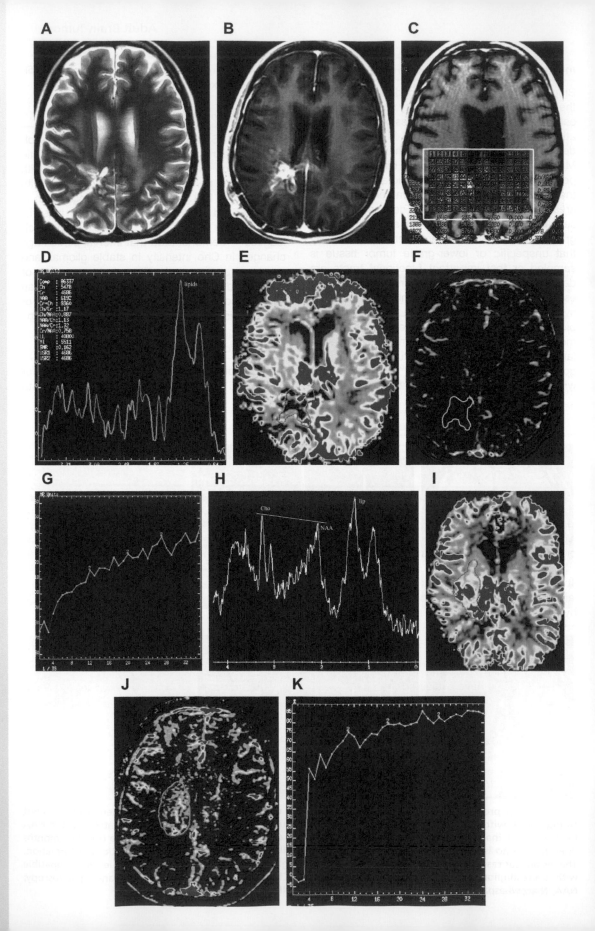

the morphologic cytostructure of the tumor. However, histopathology has limitations in providing prognostic value.[74] DW imaging, PW imaging, and H-MRS yield structural and metabolic information that may provide better insight into tumor functionality and improve the prognostic stratification of brain tumors.[74]

A pretreatment H-MRS study of 187 patients with high-grade astrocytomas produced 180 spectra at short TE (30 milliseconds) and 182 at long TE (136 milliseconds).[74] The study demonstrated that a high-intensity value of the peaks at 0.98 and 1.25 ppm, attributed to lipids, correlated with tumoral necrosis and with low survival. More interesting was the finding that another region of the short TE spectrum, around 3.67 ppm, showed a direct correlation with patient survival. This peak probably represents glucose. High metabolic activity and consequently poor prognosis correlate with depletion of glucose in the extracellular compartment and, accordingly, with low intensity of the resonances that represent this compound in the spectra, centered at 3.67 ppm. The investigators found that H-MRS could be used to stratify prognostic groups in high-grade gliomas and that this prognostic assessment could be made by evaluating the intensity values of 2 points on the spectrum at short TE (0.98 and 3.67 ppm) and another 2 at long TE (0.98 and 1.25 ppm). Short TE H-MRS may be considered somewhat superior to long TE H-MRS for prognostic assessment of high-grade gliomas. Nevertheless, spectra at both TEs may provide relevant information.[74]

Oh and colleagues[107] found a significantly shorter median survival time for patients with a large volume of metabolic abnormality, measured by H-MRS. Additional studies have evaluated some particular resonances of the spectrum such as Cho-containing compounds, NAA, Cr, lipids, and lactate, and have found them to be useful for predicting patient outcome in gliomas.[108,109] A series of articles have evaluated the role of MRS imaging in predicting survival of patients with GBM.[108,110–113] In a recent study, conventional MR imaging, MRS imaging, DW imaging, and perfusion MR imaging were used in a group of grade IV gliomas (examined before surgery and treatment). Survival was relatively poor in patients with lesions exhibiting large areas of contrast enhancement, abnormal metabolism, or restricted diffusion. Specifically, of the H-MRS parameters, high relative volumes of regions with increased Cho/NAA index were negatively associated with survival. Survival time was also negatively associated with high lactate and lipid levels (see **Fig. 1**) and the ADC within the enhancing volume.

Not all studies have found associations between metabolic indices and prognosis; for instance, in 16 patients with a B-cell lymphoma, the presence of lactate and lipids in the spectra collected before treatment was not associated with overall survival.[114] In another prospective H-MRS study, 50 patients with newly diagnosed low-grade gliomas (WHO grade II) evaluated before surgery showed no relationship between Cho and Cr levels in the tumor and survival.[115] Despite the few studies mentioned here,[114,115] most of the studies published in the literature agree that H-MRS is helpful for predicting the prognosis of brain tumors.

Assess Therapeutic Response

An important issue about postradiation therapy in patients with brain tumors is differentiation between recurrent brain tumor and radiation injury/change, particularly when new contrast-enhancing lesions are seen in previously operated and/or irradiated regions.[116–120] Typical conventional MR imaging appearance of radiation necrosis is a T2 hyperintense signal and enhancement after contrast administration, which is difficult to distinguish from tumor progression or pseudoprogression (a transient increase in edema, mass effect, and contrast enhancement that resolves over time).[115] Differentiating residual or recurrent tumors from treatment-related changes is limited on conventional MR imaging as well as on histologic examination; areas

Fig. 20. Radiation necrosis versus tumor recurrence. A 24-year-old woman diagnosed with GBM after surgical resection, radiation therapy, chemotherapy, and steroids. A surgical cavity is seen in the right parietal lobe (A) with some irregular enhancement in the surrounding parenchyma (B). MV MRS (C, D) demonstrates a significant reduction in the NAA, Cho, and Cr peaks along with a prominent lipid peak consistent with radiation necrosis. Perfusion is reduced in the surgical bed (E, rCBV map) and there is no increase in permeability (F, G) also indicating therapeutic response rather than tumor. Four months later, H-MRS shows an increase in Cho and the Cho/NAA ratio indicating tumor cell proliferation (H). A perfusion study (I) demonstrates high capillary density and there is increased permeability (J, K) in the same area. Results from H-MRS, perfusion, and permeability studies are compatible with tumor recurrence. Cho, choline; Cho/NAA, choline/N-acetyl-aspartate; Cr, creatine; H-MRS, proton magnetic resonance spectroscopy; lip, lipids; MV MRS, multivoxel magnetic resonance spectroscopy; NAA, N-acetyl-aspartate; rCBV map, relative cerebral blood volume map.

of T1 contrast enhancement after radiation treatment often contain both residual and recurrent tumor and tissue affected by therapy-related changes. In addition, the heterogeneity of gliomas before and after therapy and the inaccuracy of biopsy sampling pose another challenge in the histologic differentiation of tumors from necrosis.[121] On conventional MR imaging, the evaluation of treatment response and categorization as stable disease, responder (partial remission), and nonresponder (progression) are based predominantly on changes in tumor volumes.[122] MRS imaging may distinguish metabolic changes in the tumor before any change in volume. H-MRS has been applied to differentiate between radiation-induced tissue injury and tumor recurrence in adult and pediatric patients with brain tumors after radiation, gamma knife radiosurgery, and brachytherapy.[123] Significantly reduced Cho and Cr levels suggest radiation necrosis.[73,75,124–129] Necrotic regions may also show increased lipid and lactate signals (**Fig. 20A–G**).[75,130,131] On the other hand, increased Cho (evaluated as Cho levels relative to the Cho signal in normal-appearing tissue, Cho/Cr, or Cho/NAA ratios) suggests recurrence (see **Fig. 20H–K**).[112,125,128,129] Many studies have found that Cho/Cr and/or Cho/NAA ratios are significantly higher in recurrent tumor (or predominantly tumor) than in radiation injury.[117–120] In a retrospective MRS imaging study of 33 tumors using an intermediate TE of 144 milliseconds, Smith and colleagues[118] demonstrated that higher Cho/Cr and Cho/NAA ratios and a lower NAA/Cr ratio suggest recurrence compared with radiation change. According to this study, the Cho/NAA ratio demonstrated the best confidence interval to distinguish between tumor recurrence and radiation change. The distinction between recurrent tumor and radiation necrosis using the Cho/NAA ratio could be made with 85% sensitivity and 69% specificity.[118] According to Elias and colleagues,[132] the Cho/NAA and NAA/Cr ratios best differentiated recurrent brain tumor from radiation injury using H-MRS in previously treated patients diagnosed with primary intracranial neoplasm. Comparison with biopsy specimens revealed that MRS imaging cannot reliably differentiate between tissue containing mixed tumor/radiation necrosis and either tumor or radiation necrosis, although it did achieve good separation between pure necrosis and pure tumor.[75]

H-MRS is a promising, noninvasive tool for predicting and monitoring the clinical response to temozolamide in patients with low-grade gliomas.[133] In these patients, the H-MRS profile changes more widely and rapidly than tumor volume during relapse and represents an early predictive factor of outcome over 14 months of follow-up.

Tumor recurrence may be detected by H-MRS in a site remote from the irradiated area. In some cases, the development of a spectral abnormality may precede a coincident increase in contrast enhancement by 1 to 2 months.[126,134]

Some overlap may be seen in the H-MRS of tumors and radiation change. An increase in Cho-containing compounds after radiation therapy as a result of cell damage and astrogliosis may be seen in radiation necrosis misclassified as tumors.[135] In addition, both tumors and necrotic tissue have low levels of NAA, consistent with neuronal damage. Also, residual tumor may be present along with some radiation changes in the same patient. If the spectrum is indeterminate (ie, indicating the presence of both residual tumor and radiation change), repeated examination is suggested after an interval of 6 to 8 weeks.[130] If the increase in Cho is related to radiation change, it will normalize with time. Additional information from the perfusion and permeability studies may also help to correctly differentiate between tumors and radiation necrosis. Recurrent tumors have a higher rCBV (see **Fig. 20I**) and higher permeability (see **Fig. 20J, K**) compared with radiation necrosis (see **Fig. 20E–G**).[10,94]

A discrete and isolated increase in Cho in serial examinations should not be considered evidence of tumor recurrence. Interval increased Cho/Cr or Cho/NAA is suggestive of malignant progression/tumor recurrence if the percentage change in Cho is more than 45% and/or is associated with increased blood volume and permeability indicating vascular proliferation and significant compromise of the blood-brain barrier, respectively.

H-MRS is able to detect the effects of radiation on normal brain. The most commonly reported changes after radiation are decreases in NAA,[136] which can be detected 1 to 4 months after radiation in nontumoral regions receiving between 20 and 50 Gy[137] and decreases in Cho levels.[123] Radiation therapies may result in a decrease in whole-brain NAA with no corresponding changes in the mental status.

DIFFERENTIAL DIAGNOSIS BETWEEN LESIONS THAT LOOK ALIKE

In many cases, reliable differentiation of neoplastic from nonneoplastic brain masses is difficult or even impossible with conventional MR imaging.[137–147] Use of contrast agent may also not increase diagnostic specificity because various nonneoplastic processes are often associated with disruption of the blood-brain barrier and not all tumors enhance.[135] Studies have shown that the use of

H-MRS in specific cases improves the accuracy and level of confidence in differentiating neoplastic from nonneoplastic masses.[13,15,135,138,148–150] The differential diagnosis of a brain mass varies depending on its solid or necrotic aspect.[13] When a necrotic mass is encountered in the brain, the main diagnoses include aggressive brain tumors, abscess, tuberculous granuloma, parasitic infection, or radiation necrosis. On the other hand, when the lesion is solid, the main diagnoses include tumors without necrosis, lymphoma, and pseudotumoral demyelinating disease. Hourani and colleagues,[135] using cutoff points of NAA/Cho equal to or less than 0.61 and rCBV equal to or greater than 1.50 (corresponding to diagnosis of the tumors), achieved a sensitivity of 72.2% and specificity of 91.7% in differentiating tumors from nonneoplastic lesions. Although studies have shown that perfusion MR imaging and the combination of H-MRS imaging and perfusion MR imaging had were comparable with MRS imaging alone in differentiating tumors from nonneoplastic lesions, in the authors' experience, a multifunctional approach with DW imaging, PW imaging, permeability mapping, and H-MRS is the most accurate way to make a precise diagnosis.

Tumor Versus Stroke

Differentiation between a glioma and a vascular lesion may be difficult or impossible using conventional MR imaging. In these cases, increased Cho makes the diagnosis of neoplasm more likely, whereas no increase in Cho makes the diagnosis of tumor less likely. Increased lipids along with reduction of all other metabolites is characteristic of infarcts but these findings may also be present in tumors with extensive necrosis (see **Fig. 5**). On the other hand, increased Cho may be seen in infarction especially in the subacute stage, mimicking tumor (**Fig. 21**). In this situation, the clinical history and a multifunctional approach with DW imaging and perfusion mapping help in making the correct diagnosis.

Tumor Versus Demyelination

Differentiation between high-grade gliomas and some acute demyelinating lesions based on H-MRS alone may be difficult because of histopathologic similarities, which include hypercellularity, reactive astrocytes, mitotic figures, and areas of necrosis.[121,125,138,149] Both entities typically present with increased Cho and decreased NAA, and lactate and lipids are often increased (**Fig. 22**).[148–153]

In the acute stage of a demyelinating disease, increased lactate reflects the metabolism of inflammatory cells.[148–150]

Majós and colleagues[13] found that the increase in Cho and decrease in NAA at long TE are even higher in tumors and that these metabolites can discriminate between tumors and pseudotumoral lesions. However, in the authors' experience, a significant increase in Cho along with significant reduction of NAA may be demonstrated in acute demyelinating plaques (see **Fig. 22**). According to Cianfoni and colleagues,[150] increase in Glx helps differentiate demyelinating tumefactive lesions from neoplastic masses, avoiding unnecessary biopsy and potentially harmful surgery, as well as providing a more specific diagnosis during the initial MR examination, allowing the earlier institution of appropriate therapy.

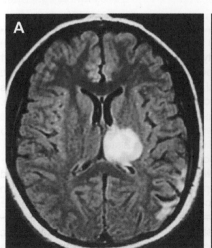
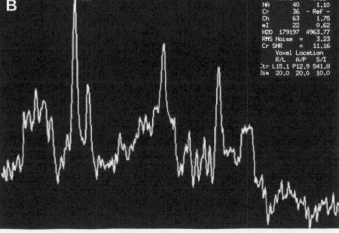

Fig. 21. Infarct with high Cho in the spectrum. A significant increase in the Cho peak is demonstrated in the spectrum from a left thalamic infarct. The spectral pattern resembles that of a brain tumor. Cho, choline.

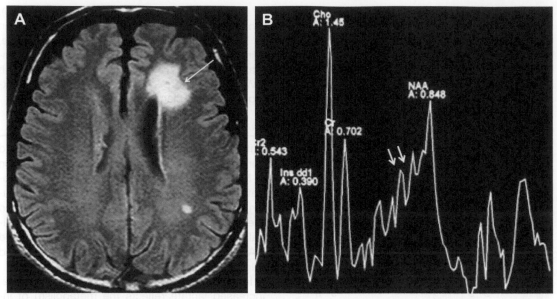

Fig. 22. Tumor versus demyelination. A 61-year-old man presenting with blurred vision. There is a left frontal lesion hyperintense on FLAIR (*A*) that shows a significant increase in Cho and the Cho/NAA and Cho/Cr ratios along with a reduction in NAA (*B*). A diagnosis of tumor was suggested and a stereotactic biopsy showed findings consistent with demyelination. A close inspection of the spectrum shows a high Glx peak (*B, arrows*), more consistent with demyelination than high-grade glioma. Cho, choline; Cho/Cr, choline/creatine; Cho/NAA, choline/N-acetyl-aspartate; Cr, creatine; Glx, glutamine and glutamate; Ins, myo-inositol; NAA, N-acetyl-aspartate.

Tumor Versus Focal Cortical Dysplasia

In some cases of focal cortical dysplasia, Cho may be moderately increased probably as a result of intrinsic epileptic ictal activity.[154]

Tumor Versus Abscess

The differential diagnosis between brain abscess and neoplasms (primary and secondary) is a challenge. Both appear as cystic lesions with rim enhancement on conventional MR imaging. Pyogenic abscesses have high signal intensity on DW imaging, which is usually not seen in tumors. Nevertheless, some neoplasms may occasionally have restricted diffusion and biopsy is inevitable. H-MRS may help to establish a diagnosis. In the case of a rim-enhancing lesion, to differentiate between a necrotic tumor and an abscess, the voxel should be placed within the cystic-necrotic area.[155] Abscesses and tumors both demonstrate high lactate peaks. Nonetheless, the presence of acetate, succinate, and amino acids such as valine, alanine, and leucine in the core of the lesion has high sensitivity for pyogenic abscess (**Fig. 23**).[82,155,156] To demonstrate the typical spectral abnormalities in the abscess cavity, an intermediate (144 milliseconds) or high (270 milliseconds) TE should be used.[155]

Typical spectra of anaerobic bacterial abscesses (acetate, succinate, and amino acids) do not exist in abscesses caused by *Staphylococcal aureus*, which are aerobic bacterial abscesses.[156] In this situation, lipids and lactate may be the only spectral findings and the spectrum is similar to that of a necrotic brain lesion.[155] Also, the resonances of acetate, succinate, and amino acids may disappear with effective antibiotic therapy. A high Cho peak and high Cho/NAA and Cho/Cr ratios may be seen in infection and should not be considered as evidence of tumor.

Tumor Versus Encephalitis

Among the encephalitis, herpes simplex encephalitis has a typical distribution of brain involvement at the hippocampus and cortex of the temporal, frontobasal, and insular lobes.[157] H-MRS shows marked reduction of NAA and the NAA/Cr ratio, and increase in Cho and the Cho/Cr ratio at the involved region, which reflect neuronal loss and gliosis and correlate with histopathologic findings. H-MRS findings may resemble those of brain tumors. However, increase in the Glx peak should favor encephalitis over tumor.

A practical MRI-based algorithm, including the results from postcontrast MR imaging, DW imaging, perfusion MR imaging, and MRS imaging, allowed the classification of tumors and nonneoplastic lesions with accuracy, sensitivity, and specificity of 90%, 97%, and 67%, respectively.[7,8]

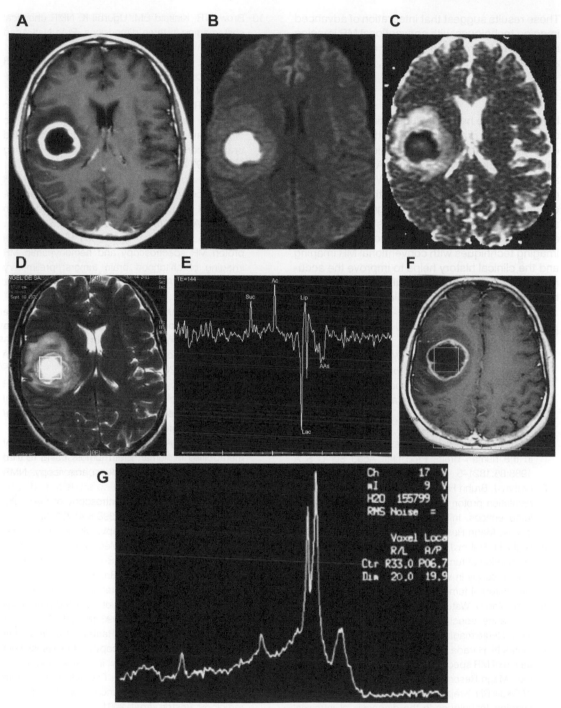

Fig. 23. Tumor versus abscess. A 39-year-old man, HIV positive, presenting with a ring-enhancing lesion in the right frontal lobe (A). There is restricted diffusion (high signal intensity on DW imaging (B) and low signal intensity on the ADC map (C)), compatible with the diagnosis of pyogenic abscess. Spectra from the abscess cavity performed with intermediate TE (144 milliseconds) (D, E) demonstrates lipids and lactate, which can also be seen in the necrotic core of a GBM (F, G) in the study obtained with low TE (30 milliseconds). However, amino acids (0.9 ppm), acetate (1.9 ppm), and succinate (2.4 ppm) are also seen in the abscess cavity (E). These findings have high sensitivity for the diagnosis of pyogenic abscesses and are not demonstrated within the necrotic core of a GBM. AAS, aminoacids; Ac, acetate; ADC, apparent diffusion coefficient; DW, diffusion weighted; GBM, glioblastoma multiforme; lac, lactate; lip, lipids; Suc, succinate; TE, echo time.

These results suggest that integration of advanced imaging techniques with conventional MR imaging may help to improve the reliability of the diagnosis and classification of brain lesions.[158]

SUMMARY

H-MRS may be helpful in suggesting tumor histology and tumor grade and may better define tumor extension and the ideal site for biopsy compared with conventional MR imaging. A multifunctional approach with DW imaging, PW imaging and permeability mapping, along with H-MRS, may enhance the accuracy of the diagnosis and characterization of brain tumors and estimation of therapeutic response. Also, integration of advanced imaging techniques with conventional MR imaging and the clinical history helps to improve the accuracy, sensitivity, and specificity in differentiating between tumors and nonneoplastic lesions.

REFERENCES

1. Bottomley PA, Edelstein WA, Foster TH, et al. In vivo solvent suppressed localized hydrogen nuclear magnetic resonance spectroscopy: a window to metabolism? Proc Natl Acad Sci U S A 1985;82: 2148–52.

2. Hanstock CC, Rothman DL, Prichard JW, et al. Spatially localized ^{1}H NMR spectra of metabolites in the human brain. Proc Natl Acad Sci U S A 1988;85:1821–5.

3. Frahm J, Bruhn H, Gynell ML, et al. Localized high resolution proton NMR spectroscopy using stimulated echoes: initial applications to human brain in vivo. Magn Reson Med 1989;9:79–93.

4. Bruhn H, Frahm J, Gynell ML, et al. Noninvasive differentiation of tumors with use of localized H-1 MR spectroscopy in vivo: initial experience in patients with cerebral tumors. Radiology 1989;172:541–8.

5. Bertholdo D, Watcharakorn A, Castillo M. Magnetic resonance spectroscopy: introduction and overview. Neuroimaging Clin North Am, in press.

6. Morita N, Harada M, Otsuka H, et al. Clinical application of MR spectroscopy and imaging of brain tumor. Magn Reson Med Sci 2010;9(4):167–75.

7. Al-Okaili RN, Krejza J, Wang S, et al. Advanced MR imaging techniques in the diagnosis of intraaxial brain tumors in adults. Radiographics 2006;26: 173–89.

8. Al-Okaili RN, Krejza J, Woo JH, et al. Intraaxial brain masses: MR-imaging-based diagnostic strategy–initial experience. Radiology 2007;243:539–50.

9. Majós C, Julià-Sapé M, Alonso J, et al. Brain tumor classification by proton MR spectroscopy: comparison of diagnostic accuracy at short and long TE. AJNR Am J Neuroradiol 2004;25:1696–704.

10. Brown TR, Kinkaid BM, Ugurbil K. NMR chemical shift imaging in three dimensions. Proc Natl Acad Sci U S A 1982;79:3523–6.

11. Horska A, Baker PB. Imaging of brain tumors: MR spectroscopy and metabolic imaging. Neuroimaging Clin N Am 2010;20:293–310.

12. Hourani R, Horska A, Albayram S, et al. Proton magnetic resonance spectroscopic imaging to differentiate between non neoplatic lesions and brain tumors in children. J Magn Reson Imaging 2006;23:99–107.

13. Majós C, Aguilera C, Alonso J, et al. Proton MR spectroscopy improves discrimination between tumor and pseudotumoral lesion in solid brain masses. AJNR Am J Neuroradiol 2009;30:544–51.

14. Tzika AA, Vajapeyam S, Barnes PD. Multivoxel proton MR spectroscopy and hemodynamic MR imaging of childhood brain tumors: preliminary observations. AJNR Am J Neuroradiol 1997;18: 203–18.

15. Butzen J, Prost R, Chetty V, et al. Discrimination between neoplastic and non neoplastic brain lesions by use of proton MR spectroscopy. The limits of accuracy with a logistic regression model. AJNR Am J Neuroradiol 2000;21:1213–9.

16. Voge TJ, Jassoy A, Söllner O, et al. The proton MR spectroscopy of intracranial tumors. The differential diagnostic aspects for gliomas, metastases and meningeomas. Rofo 1992;157:371–7 [in German].

17. Kinoshita Y, Yokota A. Absolute concentrations of metabolites in human brain tumors using in vitro proton magnetic resonance spectroscopy. NMR Biomed 1997;10:2–12.

18. Castillo M. Proton MR spectroscopy of the brain. Neuroimaging Clin N Am 1998;8(4):733–52.

19. Rand SD. MR spectroscopy: single voxel. Presented at the 39th Annual Meeting of the American Society of Neuroradiology. Boston, April, 2001.

20. Michaelis T, Merboldt KD, Bruhn H, et al. Absolute concentrations of metabolites in the adult human brain in vivo: quantification of localized proton MR spectra. Neuroradiology 1993;187:219–27.

21. Herminghaus S, Pilatus U, Raab P, et al. Impact of in vivo proton MR spectroscopy for the assessment of the proliferative activity in viable and partly necrotic brain tumor tissue. Presented at the 39th Annual Meeting of the American Society of Neuroradiology. Boston, April, 2001.

22. Palasis S. Utility of short TE MR spectroscopy in determination of histology, grade and behavior of pediatric brain tumors. Presented at the 39th Annual Meeting of the American Society of Neuroradiology. Boston, April, 2001.

23. Herholz K, Heindel W, Luyten PR, et al. In vivo imaging of glucose consumption and lactate concentration in human gliomas. Ann Neurol 1992;31: 319–27.

24. Castillo M, Smith JK, Kwock L. Correlation of myo-inositol levels and grading of cerebral astrocytomas. AJNR Am J Neuroradiol 2000;21: 1645–9.

25. Pilatus U, Reichel C, Raab P, et al. ERM detectable lipid signal in low- and high-grade glioma, recurrent gliomas, metastases, lymphomas and abscesses. Presented at the 39th Annual Meeting of the American Society of Neuroradiology. Boston, April, 2001.

26. Howe FA, Barton SJ, Cudlip SA, et al. Metabolic profiles of human brain tumors using quantitative in vivo ^{1}H magnetic resonance spectroscopy. Magn Reson Med 2003;49:223–32.

27. Kuesel AC, Sutherland GR, Halliday W, et al. ^{1}H MRS of high-grade astrocytomas: mobile lipid accumulation in necrotic tissue. NMR Biomed 1994;7:149–55.

28. Di Costanzo A, Scarabino T, Trojsi F, et al. Proton MR spectroscopy of cerebral gliomas at 3 T: spatial heterogeneity, and tumour grade and extent. Eur Radiol 2008;18:1727–35.

29. Hawley J, Pennizi A, Paul C, et al. Clinical evaluation of ultrashort TE proton spectroscopy imaging of the brain. Presented at the 39th Annual Meeting of the American Society of Neuroradiology. Boston, April, 2001.

30. Fan G, Sun B, Wu Z, et al. In vivo single-voxel proton MR spectroscopy in the differentiation of high-grade gliomas and solitary metastases. Clin Radiol 2004;59:77–85.

31. Law M, Cha S, Knopp EA, et al. High-grade gliomas and solitary metastases: differentiation by using perfusion and proton spectroscopic MR imaging. Radiology 2002;222:715–21.

32. Chiang IC, Kuo YT, Lu CY, et al. Distinction between high-grade gliomas and solitary metastases using peritumoral 3-T magnetic resonance spectroscopy, diffusion, and perfusion imagings. Neuroradiology 2004;46:619–27.

33. Ricci R, Bacci A, Tugnoli V, et al. Metabolic findings on 3T H-MR spectroscopy in peritumoral brain edema. AJNR Am J Neuroradiol 2007;28: 1287–91.

34. Burtscher IM, Skagerberg G, Geijer B, et al. Proton MR spectroscopy and preoperative diagnostic accuracy: an evaluation of intracranial mass lesions characterized by stereotactic biopsy findings. AJNR Am J Neuroradiol 2000;21:84–93.

35. Weber MA, Zoubaa S, Schlieter M, et al. Diagnostic performance of spectroscopic and perfusion MR for distinction of brain tumors. Neurology 2006;66: 1899–906.

36. Demir MK, Iplikcioglu AC, Dincer A, et al. Single voxel proton MR spectroscopy findings of typical and atypical intracranial meningiomas. Eur J Radiol 2006;60:48–55.

37. Bulakbasi N, Kocaoglu M, Örs F, et al. Combination of single-voxel proton MR spectroscopy and apparent diffusion coefficient calculation in the evaluation of common brain tumors. AJNR Am J Neuroradiol 2003;24:225–33.

38. Rabin BM, Meyer JR, Berlin JW, et al. Radiation-induced changes in the central nervous system and head and neck. Radiographics 1996;16: 1055–72.

39. Kado H, Ogawa T, Hatazawa J, et al. Radiation-induced meningioma evaluated with positron emission tomography with fludeoxyglucose F 18. AJNR Am J Neuroradiol 1996;17:937–8.

40. Zacharia TT, Law M, Naidich TP, et al. Central nervous system lymphoma characterization by diffusion-weighted imaging and MR spectroscopy. J Neuroimaging 2008;18:411–7.

41. Hakyemez B, Erdogan C, Bolca N, et al. Evaluation of different cerebral mass lesions by perfusion-weighted MR imaging. J Magn Reson Imaging 2006;24:817–24.

42. Law M, Yang S, Wang H, et al. Glioma grading: sensitivity, specificity, and predictive values of perfusion MR imaging and proton MR spectroscopic imaging compared with conventional MR imaging. AJNR Am J Neuroradiol 2003;24: 1989–98.

43. Brandão L, Domingues R. Intracranial neoplasms. In: McAllister L, Lazar T, Cook RE, editors. MR spectroscopy of the brain. Philadelphia: Lippincott Williams & Wilkins; 2002. p. 130–67.

44. Knopp EA. Advanced MR imaging of tumors: using spectroscopy and perfusion. Presented at the 39th Annual Meeting of the American Society of Neuroradiology. Boston, April, 2001.

45. Taillibert S, Chodkiewicz C, Laigle-Donadey F, et al. Gliomatosis cerebri: a review of 296 cases from the ANOCEF database and the literature. J Neurooncol 2006;76:201–5.

46. Mohana-Borges AV, Imbesi SG, Dietrich R, et al. Role of proton magnetic resonance spectroscopy in the diagnosis of gliomatosis cerebri. J Comput Assist Tomogr 2004;28(1):103–5.

47. Sarafi-Lavi E, Bowen BC, Pattany PM, et al. Proton MR spectroscopy of gliomatosis cerebri: case report of elevated myoinositol with normal choline levels. AJNR Am J Neuroradiol 2003;24:946–51.

48. Guzmán-de-Villoria JA, Sánchez-González J, Muñoz L, et al. ^{1}H MR spectroscopy in the assessment of gliomatosis cerebri. AJR Am J Roentgenol 2007;188:710–4.

49. Galanaud D, Chinot O, Nicoli F, et al. Use of proton magnetic resonance spectroscopy of the brain to differentiate gliomatosis cerebri from low-grade glioma. J Neurosurg 2003;98:269–76.

50. Tong Z, Yamaki T, Harada K, et al. In vivo quantification of the metabolites in normal brain and brain

tumors by proton MR spectroscopy using water as an internal standard. Magn Reson Imaging 2004; 22:1017–24.

51. Panigrahy A, Krieger MD, Gonzalez-Gomes I, et al. Quantitative short echo time [1]H-MR spectroscopy of untreated pediatric brain tumors: preoperative diagnosis and characterization. AJNR Am J Neuroradiol 2006;27:560–72.

52. Schneider JF, Gouny C, Viola A, et al. Multiparametric differentiation of posterior fossa tumors in children using diffusion-weighted imaging and short echo-time [1]H-MR spectroscopy. J Magn Reson Imaging 2007;26:1390–8.

53. Majós C, Aguilera C, Cós M, et al. In vivo proton magnetic resonance spectroscopy of intraventricular tumors of the brain. Eur Radiol 2009;19: 2049–59.

54. Jouanneau E, Tovar RA, Desuzinges C. Very late frontal relapse of medulloblastoma mimicking a meningioma in an adult. Usefulness of ^{1}H magnetic resonance spectroscopy and diffusion-perfusion magnetic resonance imaging for preoperative diagnosis: case report. Neurosurgery 2006;58(4): E789.

55. Yamasaki F, Kurisu K, Satoh K, et al. Apparent diffusion coefficient of human brain tumors at MR imaging. Radiology 2005;235:985–91.

56. Peeling J, Sutherland G. High-resolution ^{1}H NMR spectroscopy studies of extracts of human cerebral neoplasms. Magn Reson Med 1992;24:123–6.

57. Raybaud C, Barkovich AJ. Intracranial, orbital and neck masses of childhood. In: Barkovich AJ, Raybaud C, editors. Pediatric neuroimaging. 5th edition. Philadelphia: Lippincott Williams & Wilkins; 2012. p. 637–711.

58. Barkovich A. Intracranial, orbital and neck masses of childhood. In: Barkovich AJ, Raybaud C, editors. Pediatric neuroimaging. 5th edition. Philadelphia: Lippincott Williams & Wilkins; 2005. p. 637–750.

59. Blaser SI, Harwood-Nash DC. Neuroradiology of pediatric posterior fossa medulloblastoma. J Neurooncol 1996;29:23–34.

60. Kleihues P, Cavenee WK. World Health Organization classification of tumors: pathology and genetics of tumors of the central nervous system. Lyon (France): IARC Press; 2000.

61. Yuh EL, Barkovich AJ, Gupta N. Imaging of ependymomas: MRI and CT. Childs Nerv Syst 2009; 25:1203–13.

62. Uematsu Y, Hirano A, Llena JF. Electron microscopic observations of blood vessels in ependymoma. No Shinkei Geka 1988;16:1235–42 [in Japanese].

63. Harris L, Davies N, MacPherson L, et al. The use of short-echo time ^{1}H MRS for childhood cerebellar tumors prior to histopathological diagnosis. Pediatr Radiol 2007;37:1101–9.

64. Bourgouin PM, Tampieri D, Grahovac SZ, et al. CT and MR imaging findings in adults with cerebellar medulloblastoma: comparison with findings in children. AJR Am J Roentgenol 1992; 159:609–12.

65. Movsas B, Li BS, Babb JS. Quantifying radiation therapy–induced brain injury with whole-brain proton MR spectroscopy: initial observations. Radiology 2001;221:327–31.

66. Ricci PE, Pitt A, Keller PJ, et al. Effect of voxel position on single-voxel MR spectroscopy findings. AJNR Am J Neuroradiol 2000;21:367–74.

67. Chawla S, Wang S, Wolf RL, et al. Arterial spin labeling and MR spectroscopy in the differentiation of gliomas. AJNR Am J Neuroradiol 2007;28: 1683–9.

68. Hollingworth W, Medina LS, Lenkinski RE, et al. A systematic literature review of magnetic resonance spectroscopy for the characterization of brain tumors. AJNR Am J Neuroradiol 2006;27: 1404–11.

69. Di Costanzo A, Scarabino T, Trojsi F, et al. Multiparametric 3T MR approach to the assessment of cerebral gliomas: tumor extent and malignancy. Neuroradiology 2006;48:622–31.

70. Chang SM, Nelson S, Vandenberg S, et al. Integration of preoperative anatomic and metabolic physiologic imaging of newly diagnosed glioma. J Neurooncol 2009;92:401–15.

71. Arnold DL, Shoubridge EA, Villemure JG, et al. Proton and phosphorus magnetic resonance spectroscopy of human astrocytomas in vivo. Preliminary observations on tumor grading. NMR Biomed 1990;3:184–9.

72. Gill SS, Thomas DG, Van Bruggen N, et al. Proton MR spectroscopy of intracranial tumours: in vivo and in vitro studies. J Comput Assist Tomogr 1990;14:497–504.

73. Preul MC, Leblanc R, Caramanos Z, et al. Magnetic resonance spectroscopy guided brain tumor resection: differentiation between recurrent glioma and radiation change in two diagnostically difficult cases. Can J Neurol Sci 1998;25:13–22.

74. Majós C, Bruna J, Julià-Sapé M, et al. Proton MR spectroscopy provides relevant prognostic information in high-grade astrocytomas. AJNR Am J Neuroradiol 2011;32:74–80.

75. Rock JP, Hearshen D, Scarpace L, et al. Correlations between magnetic resonance spectroscopy and image-guided histopathology, with special attention to radiation necrosis. Neurosurgery 2002;51:912–9.

76. Covarrubias DJ, Rosen BR, Lev MH. Dynamic magnetic resonance perfusion imaging of brain tumors. Oncologist 2004;9:528–37.

77. Isobe T, Matsumura A, Anno I, et al. Quantification of cerebral metabolites in glioma patients with

proton MR spectroscopy using T2 relaxation time correction. Magn Reson Imaging 2002;20:343–9.

78. Bartha R, Megyesi JF, Watling CJ, et al. Low-grade glioma: correlation of short echo time ^{1}H-MR spectroscopy with ^{23}Na MR imaging. AJNR Am J Neuroradiol 2008;29:464–70.

79. Rijpkema M, Schuuring J, van der Meulen Y, et al. Characterization of oligo-dendrogliomas using short echo time ^{1}H MR spectroscopic imaging. NMR Biomed 2003;16:12–8.

80. Gupta RK, Cloughesy TF, Sinha U, et al. Relationships between choline magnetic resonance spectroscopy, apparent diffusion coefficient and quantitative histopathology in human glioma. J Neurooncol 2000;50: 215–26.

81. Ishimaru H, Morikawa M, Iwanaga S, et al. Differentiation between high-grade glioma and metastatic brain tumor using single-voxel proton MR spectroscopy. Eur Radiol 2001;11:1784–91.

82. Grand S, Passaro C, Ziegler A, et al. Necrotic tumor versus brain abscess: importance of aminoacids detected at ^{1}H MR spectroscopy–initial results. Radiology 1999;213:785–93.

83. Louis DN, Ohgaki H, Wiestler OD, editors. WHO classification of tumours of the central nervous system. Lyon (France): IARC; 2007. 978-92-832-2430-2.

84. Lev MH, Ozsunar Y, Henson JW, et al. Glial tumor grading and outcome prediction using dynamic spin-echo MR susceptibility mapping compared with conventional contrast-enhanced MR: confounding effect of elevated rCBV of oligodendrogliomas [corrected]. AJNR Am J Neuroradiol 2004;25:214–21.

85. Cha S, Tihan T, Crawford F, et al. Differentiation of low-grade oligodendrogliomas from low-grade astrocytomas by using quantitative blood-volume measurements derived from dynamic susceptibility contrast-enhanced MR imaging. AJNR Am J Neuroradiol 2005;26:266–73.

86. Spampinato MV, Smith JK, Kwock L, et al. Cerebral blood volume measurements and proton MR spectroscopy in grading of oligodendroglial tumors. AJR Am J Roentgenol 2007;188:204–12.

87. Xu M, See SJ, Ng WH, et al. Comparison of magnetic resonance spectroscopy and perfusion-weighted imaging in presurgical grading of oligodendroglial tumors. Neurosurgery 2005;56:919–26.

88. Pirzkall A, McKnight TR, Graves EE, et al. MR-spectroscopy guided target delineation for high-grade gliomas. Int J Radiat Oncol Biol Phys 2001; 50:915–28.

89. Ganslandt O, Stadlbauer A, Fahlbusch R, et al. Proton magnetic resonance spectroscopic imaging integrated into image-guided surgery: correlation to standard magnetic resonance imaging and tumor cell density. Neurosurgery 2005;56:291–8.

90. McKnight TR, Von Dem Bussche MH, Vigneron DB, et al. Histopathological validation of a three-dimensional magnetic resonance spectroscopy index as a predictor of tumor presence. J Neurosurg 2002;97:794–802.

91. Poussaint TY. Pediatric brain tumors. In: Newton HB, Jolesz FA, editors. Handbook of neuro-oncology neuroimaging. New York: Academic Press; 2008. p. 469–84.

92. Croteau D, Scarpace L, Hearshen D, et al. Correlation between magnetic resonance spectroscopy imaging and image-guided biopsies: semiquantitative and qualitative histopathological analyses of patients with untreated glioma. Neurosurgery 2001;49:823–9.

93. Stadlbauer A, Nimsky C, Buslei R, et al. Proton magnetic resonance spectroscopic imaging in the border zone of gliomas: correlation of metabolic and histological changes at low tumor infiltration initial results. Invest Radiol 2007;42:218–23.

94. Kallenberg K, Bock HC, Helms G. Untreated glioblastoma multiforme: increased myo-inositol and glutamine levels in the contralateral cerebral hemisphere at proton MR spectroscopy. Radiology 2009;253(3):805–12.

95. Luyten PR, Marien AJ, Heindel W, et al. Metabolic imaging of patients with intracranial tumors: H-1 MR spectroscopic imaging and PET. Radiology 1990;176:791–9.

96. McBride DQ, Miller BL, Nikas DL, et al. Analysis of brain tumors using ^{1}H magnetic resonance spectroscopy. Surg Neurol 1995;44:137–44.

97. Nelson SJ, Huhn S, Vigneron DB, et al. Volume MRI and MRSI techniques for the quantitation of treatment response in brain tumors: presentation of a detailed case study. J Magn Reson Imaging 1997;7:1146–52.

98. Kelly PJ, Daumas-Duport C, Scheithauer BW, et al. Stereotactic histologic correlations of computed tomography- and magnetic resonance imaging-defined abnormalities in patients with glial neoplasms. Mayo Clin Proc 1987;62:450–9.

99. Martin AJ, Liu H, Hall WA, et al. Preliminary assessment of turbo spectroscopic imaging for targeting in brain biopsy. AJNR Am J Neuroradiol 2001;22: 959–68.

100. Klingebiel R, Bohner G. Neuroimaging. Recent Results Cancer Res 2009;171:175–90.

101. Dowling C, Bollen AW, Noworolski SM, et al. Preoperative proton MR spectroscopic imaging of brain tumors: correlation with histopathologic analysis of resection specimens. AJNR Am J Neuroradiol 2001;22:604–12.

102. Hall WA, Martin A, Liu H, et al. Improving diagnostic yield in brain biopsy: coupling spectroscopic targeting with real-time needle placement. J Magn Reson Imaging 2001;13:12–5.

103. Hall WA, Galicich W, Bergman T, et al. 3-Tesla intraoperative MR imaging for neurosurgery. J Neurooncol 2006;77:297–303.

104. Hermann EJ, Hattingen E, Krauss JK, et al. Stereotactic biopsy in gliomas guided by 3-Tesla [1]H-chemical-shift imaging of choline. Stereotact Funct Neurosurg 2008;86:300–7.

105. Tedeschi G, Lundbom N, Ramon R, et al. Increased choline signal coinciding with malignant degeneration of cerebral gliomas: a serial proton magnetic resonance spectroscopy imaging study. J Neurosurg 1997;87:516–24.

106. Castillo M, Kwock L. Proton MR spectroscopy of common brain tumors. Neuroimaging Clin N Am 1998;8:733–52.

107. Oh J, Henry RG, Pirzkall A, et al. Survival analysis in patients with glioblastoma multiforme: predictive value of choline-to-N-acetylaspartate index, apparent diffusion coefficient, and relative cerebral blood volume. J Magn Reson Imaging 2004;19:546–54.

108. Kuznetsov YE, Caramanos Z, Antel SB, et al. Proton magnetic resonance spectroscopic imaging can predict length of survival in patients with supratentorial gliomas. Neurosurgery 2003;53: 565–74 [discussion: 574–76].

109. Li X, Jin H, Lu Y, et al. Identification of MRI and ^{1}H MRSI parameters that may predict survival for patients with malignant gliomas. NMR Biomed 2004; 17:10–20.

110. Saraswathy S, Crawford FW, Lamborn KR, et al. Evaluation of MR markers that predict survival in patients with newly diagnosed GBM prior to adjuvant therapy. J Neurooncol 2009;91:69–81.

111. Crawford FW, Khayal IS, McGue C, et al. Relationship of pre-surgery metabolic and physiological MR imaging parameters to survival for patients with untreated GBM. J Neurooncol 2009;91:337–51.

112. Arslanoglu A, Bonekamp D, Barker PB, et al. Quantitative proton MR spectroscopic imaging of the mesial temporal lobe. J Magn Reson Imaging 2004;20:772–8.

113. Chan AA, Lau A, Pirzkall A, et al. Proton magnetic resonance spectroscopy imaging in the evaluation of patients undergoing gamma knife surgery for Grade IV glioma. J Neurosurg 2004;101:467–75.

114. Raizer JJ, Koutcher JA, Abrey LE, et al. Proton magnetic resonance spectroscopy in immunocompetent patients with primary central nervous system lymphoma. J Neurooncol 2005;71:173–80.

115. Hattingen E, Raab P, Franz K, et al. Prognostic value of choline and creatine in WHO grade II gliomas. Neuroradiology 2008;50:759–67.

116. Yang I, Aghi MK. New advances that enable identification of glioblastoma recurrence. Nat Rev Clin Oncol 2009;6:648–57.

117. Rabinov JD, Lee PL, Barker FG, et al. In vivo 3-T MR spectroscopy in the distinction of recurrent glioma versus radiation effects: initial experience. Radiology 2002;225:871–9.

118. Smith EA, Carlos RC, Junck LR, et al. Developing a clinical decision model: MR spectroscopy to differentiate between recurrent tumor and radiation change in patients with new contrast-enhancing lesions. AJR Am J Roentgenol 2009; 192:W45–52.

119. Weybright P, Sundgren PC, Maly P, et al. Differentiation between brain tumor recurrence and radiation injury using MR spectroscopy. AJR Am J Roentgenol 2005;185:1471–6.

120. Zeng QS, Li CF, Liu H, et al. Distinction between recurrent glioma and radiation injury using magnetic resonance spectroscopy in combination with diffusion-weighted imaging. Int J Radiat Oncol Biol Phys 2007;68:151–8.

121. Cha S. Update on brain tumor imaging: from anatomy to physiology. AJNR Am J Neuroradiol 2006; 27:475–87.

122. Weber MA, Giesel FL, Stieltjes B. MRI for identification of progression in brain tumors: from morphology to function. Expert Rev Neurother 2008;8: 1507–25.

123. Sundgren PC. MR spectroscopy in radiation injury. AJNR Am J Neuroradiol 2009;30:1469–76.

124. Nelson SJ, Graves E, Pirzkall A, et al. In vivo molecular imaging for planning radiation therapy of gliomas: an application of ^{1}H MRSI. J Magn Reson Imaging 2002;16:464–76.

125. Taylor JS, Langston JW, Reddick WE, et al. Clinical value of proton magnetic resonance spectroscopy for differentiating recurrent or residual brain tumor from delayed cerebral necrosis. Int J Radiat Oncol Biol Phys 1996;36:1251–61.

126. Graves EE, Nelson SJ, Vigneron DB, et al. Serial proton MR spectroscopic imaging of recurrent malignant gliomas after gamma knife radiosurgery. AJNR Am J Neuroradiol 2001;22: 613–24.

127. Lichy MP, Plathow C, Schulz-Ertner D, et al. Follow-up gliomas after radiotherapy: [1]H MR spectroscopic imaging for increasing diagnostic accuracy. Neuroradiology 2005;47:826–34.

128. Wald LL, Nelson SJ, Day MR, et al. Serial proton magnetic resonance spectroscopy imaging of glioblastoma multiforme after brachytherapy. J Neurosurg 1997;87:525–34.

129. Chernov MF, Hayashi M, Izawa M, et al. Multivoxel proton MRS for differentiation of radiation-induced necrosis and tumor recurrence after gamma knife radiosurgery for brain metastases. Brain Tumor Pathol 2006;23:19–27.

130. Law M. MR spectroscopy of brain tumors. Top Magn Reson Imaging 2004;15:291–313.

131. Li X, Vigneron DB, Cha S, et al. Relationship of MR-derived lactate, mobile lipids, and relative blood

volume for gliomas in vivo. AJNR Am J Neuroradiol 2005;26:760–9.

132. Elias AE, Carlos RC, Smith EA, et al. MR spectroscopy using normalized and non-normalized metabolite ratios for differentiating recurrent brain tumor from radiation injury. Acad Radiol 2011;18: 1101–8.

133. Murphy PS, Viviers L, Abson C, et al. Monitoring temozolomide treatment of low-grade glioma with proton magnetic resonance spectroscopy. Br J Cancer 2004;90:781–6.

134. Lewin JS. Percutaneous MR image-guided procedures in neuroradiology. Presented at the 39th Annual Meeting of the American Society of Neuroradiology. Boston, April, 2001.

135. Hourani R, Brant LS, Rizk T, et al. Can proton MR spectroscopic and Perfusion Imaging Differentiate Between Neoplastic and Nonneoplastic Brain Lesions in Adults? AJNR Am J Neuroradiol 2008;29: 366–72.

136. Sundgren PC, Nagesh V, Elias A, et al. Metabolic alterations: a biomarker for radiation-induced normal brain injury–an MR spectroscopy study. J Magn Reson Imaging 2009;29:291–7.

137. Esteve F, Rubin C, Grand S, et al. Transient metabolic changes observed with proton MR spectroscopy in normal human brain after radiation therapy. Int J Radiat Oncol Biol Phys 1998;40:279–86.

138. Rand SD, Prost R, Haughton V, et al. Accuracy of single-voxel proton MR spectroscopy in distinguishing neoplastic from non neoplastic brain lesions. AJNR Am J Neuroradiol 1997;18:1695–704.

139. Paley RJ, Persing JA, Doctor A, et al. Multiple sclerosis and brain tumor: a diagnostic challenge. J Emerg Med 1989;7:241–4.

140. Giang DW, Poduri KR, Eskin TA, et al. Multiple sclerosis masquerading as a mass lesion. Neuroradiology 1992;34:150–4.

141. Hunter SB, Ballinger WE Jr, Rubin JJ. Multiple sclerosis mimicking primary brain tumor. Arch Pathol Lab Med 1987;111:464–8.

142. Kurihara N, Takahashi S, Furuta A, et al. MR imaging of multiple sclerosis simulating brain tumor. Clin Imaging 1996;20:171–7.

143. Mastrostefano R, Occhipinti E, Bigotti G, et al. Multiple sclerosis plaque simulating cerebral tumor: case report and review of the literature. Neurosurgery 1987;21:244–6.

144. Silva HC, Callegaro D, Marchiori PE, et al. Magnetic resonance imaging in five patients with a tumefactive demyelinating lesion in the central nervous system. Arq Neuropsiquiatr 1999;57:921–6.

145. Tate AR, Underwood J, Acosta D, et al. Development of a decision support system for diagnosis and grading of brain tumours using in vivo magnetic resonance single voxel spectra. NMR Biomed 2006;19:411–34.

146. Preul MC, Caramanos Z, Collins DL, et al. Accurate, noninvasive diagnosis of human brain tumors by using proton magnetic resonance spectroscopy. Nat Med 1996;2:323–5.

147. Majós C, Alonso J, Aguilera C, et al. Proton magnetic resonance spectroscopy (^{1}H MRS) of human brain tumors: assessment of differences between tumour types and its applicability in brain tumour categorization. Eur Radiol 2003;13:582–91.

148. De Stefano N, Caramanos Z, Preul MC, et al. In vivo differentiation of astrocytic brain tumors and isolated demyelinating lesions of the type seen in multiple sclerosis using ^{1}H magnetic resonance spectroscopic imaging. Ann Neurol 1998;44: 273–8.

149. Saindane AM, Cha S, Law M, et al. Proton MR spectroscopy of tumefactive demyelinating lesions. AJNR Am J Neuroradiol 2002;23:1378–86.

150. Cianfoni A, Niku S, Imbesi SG, et al. Metabolite findings in tumefactive demyelinating lesions utilizing short echo time proton magnetic resonance spectroscopy. AJNR Am J Neuroradiol 2007;28: 272–7.

151. Srinivasan R, Sailasuta N, Hurd R, et al. Evidence of elevated glutamate in multiple sclerosis using magnetic resonance spectroscopy at 3 T. Brain 2005;128:1016–25.

152. Bitsch A, Bruhn H, Vougioukas V, et al. Inflammatory CNS demyelination: histopathologic correlation with in vivo quantitative proton MR spectroscopy. AJNR Am J Neuroradiol 1999;20: 1619–27.

153. Fernando KT, McLean MA, Chard DT, et al. Elevated white matter myo-inositol in clinically isolated syndromes suggestive of multiple sclerosis. Brain 2004;127:1361–9.

154. Vuori K, Kankaanranta L, Häkkinen AM, et al. Low-grade gliomas and focal cortical developmental malformations: differentiation with proton MR spectroscopy. Radiology 2004;230(3):703–8.

155. Pal D, Bhattacharyya A, Husain M, et al. In vivo proton MR spectroscopy evaluation of pyogenic brain abscesses: a report of 194 cases. AJNR Am J Neuroradiol 2010;31:360–6.

156. Lai PH, Ho JT, Chen WL, et al. Brain abscess and necrotic brain tumor: discrimination with proton MR spectroscopy and diffusion-weighted imaging. AJNR Am J Neuroradiol 2002;23(8):1369–77.

157. Samann PG, Schlegel J, Muller G, et al. Serial proton MR spectroscopy and diffusion imaging findings in HIV-related herpes simplex encephalitis. AJNR Am J Neuroradiol 2003;24:2015–9.

158. Law M, Hamburger M, Johnson G, et al. Differentiating surgical from non-surgical lesions using perfusion MR imaging and proton MR spectroscopic imaging. Technol Cancer Res Treat 2004; 3:557–65.

Index

Note: Page numbers of article titles are in **boldface** type.

Neuroimag Clin N Am 23 (2013) 557–561
http://dx.doi.org/10.1016/S1052-5149(13)00069-5
1052-5149/13/$ – see front matter © 2013 Elsevier Inc. All rights reserved.

Moving?

Make sure your subscription moves with you!

To notify us of your new address, find your **Clinics Account Number** (located on your mailing label above your name), and contact customer service at:

Email: journalscustomerservice-usa@elsevier.com

800-654-2452 (subscribers in the U.S. & Canada)
314-447-8871 (subscribers outside of the U.S. & Canada)

Fax number: 314-447-8029

Elsevier Health Sciences Division
Subscription Customer Service
3251 Riverport Lane
Maryland Heights, MO 63043

*To ensure uninterrupted delivery of your subscription, please notify us at least 4 weeks in advance of move.

Printed and bound by CPI Group (UK) Ltd, Croydon, CR0 4YY

03/10/2024

01040378-0002